Human–Computer Interaction Series

Editors-in-chief
Desney Tan, Microsoft Research, USA
Jean Vanderdonckt, Université catholique de Louvain, Belgium

More information about this series at http://www.springer.com/series/6033

Boris Galitsky

Computational Autism

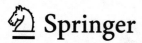

Springer

Boris Galitsky
Knowledge-Trail Inc.
San Jose, CA, USA

Additional material to this book can be downloaded from http://extras.springer.com.

ISSN 1571-5035
Human–Computer Interaction Series
ISBN 978-3-319-82005-7   ISBN 978-3-319-39972-0   (eBook)
DOI 10.1007/978-3-319-39972-0

Printed on acid-free paper

This Springer imprint is published by Springer Nature
The registered company is Springer International Publishing AG Switzerland

To teach a child with autism, one might first consider learning how to program a robot

Contents

Chapter 1
Introduction: Phenomena of Autistic Reasoning

List of Abbreviations

CwA child (children) with autism. In most cases we assume high-functioning verbal individuals, unless specified otherwise
CC   control child (children), normal, typically developing children
AwA adult(s) with autism
PwA people (person) with autism (CwA ∪ AwA)
ASD autistic spectrum disorder
ACS autistic spectrum condition
AC   autistic condition
AS   Asperger's syndrome
NL   natural language
AI   Artificial Intelligence
ML   Machine Learning

In this book we evaluate the accounts and models of autistic reasoning and cognition from the computational standpoint. Autism is a development disorder characterized by restrictive, stereotyped and repetitive behavior as well as limited social interaction and communication, and narrow interest (DSM-IV, 1994). Although autism is being researched intensively, little is known about how people with autism reason. Most scientists have focused on the intuitive Theory-of-Mind reasoning (Baron-Cohen 1995), which attributes beliefs and intentions to other people to understand, predict and control behavior. A small number of studies including (Leevers and Harris 2000; Scott and Baron-Cohen 1996; Peterson and Bowler 2000; Stenning and van Lambalgen 2008; Pijnacker et al. 2008) investigated broader aspects of logical reasoning and so far the finding are not very consistent.

Let us formalize some decision-making problems from the real world and consider how humans and machines can solve them. Control humans, people with autism and intelligent machines each have characteristic limitations in solving these

© Springer International Publishing Switzerland 2016
B. Galitsky, *Computational Autism*, Human–Computer Interaction Series,
DOI 10.1007/978-3-319-39972-0_1

problems. One of the key question of this book is how can these limitations be characterized in terms of specific features of algorithms. That would make the current science of autism much more formal, more systematic, more concise and hopefully more efficient in terms of rehabilitation strategies.

Today, computational and psychological studies of autism are very sparse and disconnected, and in this book we try to describe their results in the unified framework. We select the studies with experimental results with models that are computationally plausible in our view. Then we describe a model of autistic reasoning that is consistent with these studies on one hand and also generalizes our own experiments with exploration and training of autistic reasoning on the other hand. The main feature of our model is that it is axiom level – based and describes the autistic syndrome from the standpoint of axioms that have not been properly acquired and therefore should be trained. These axioms are backed up by our computational frameworks for reasoning about mental states and autistic active learning. We then investigate how these trained axioms improve reasoning as a first step and the overall behavior of children with autism as a second step.

Recent psychological studies have revealed that autistic children can neither reason properly about mental states nor understand emotions (Perner 1991; Leslie 1987; Pilowsky et al. 2000). There is a strong need for efficient educational support for such children with special needs. Autism is a developmental disorder which is currently defined in terms of its symptoms (Eigsti and Shapiro 2003). The three main accounts of the psychology of autism can be outlined as follows:

Theory of mind account, which refers to the ability to infer and understand what oneself and others are thinking (knowing, believing, desiring) in order to plan one's own behavior and predict the behavior of others. This ability to reason about mental attitudes is impaired in patients with autism (Baron-Cohen 2000). This reasoning disability leads to difficulties with such mental reasoning-based forms of behavior as pretend play, problems in understanding false beliefs, and the ability to tell lies.

Weak central coherence account, which refers to the inability of individuals with autism to process information in context, even having a remarkable ability to remember details (Frith 1989, 2001). For example, autistic individuals seem to have more difficulty than controls in recalling sentences or a main plot of a story, being as good as controls at recalling unconnected word strings (Hermelin and O'Connor 1967).

Executive dysfunction account, which refers to the inability of autistic individuals to maintain appropriate problem-solving behavior (Pennington and Ozonoff 1996; Russell 1997). This is often manifested in the form of behavior that perseveres inappropriately despite changing goals (Ozonoff 1997).

In this book we mainly focus on formalization and computational implementation of the first account and develop a tool that assists the learning process of reasoning about mental attitudes. To do that, we subject the Theory of Mind (ToM) and its impairment under autism to a formal analysis, propose a formal model of reasoning about mental attitudes (adequate for such learning), and build a training tool in accordance to this model. This tool is based on a simulation of reasoning about mental states and actions by conflicting software agents. We present the deployment of the natural language multiagent mental simulator NL_MAMS for mental and emotional development of autistic children.

In this book we treat the ToM from the perspective of logical artificial intelligence, providing a more systematic way to characterize mental states, mental actions and how their representation is corrupted under autism. Building the adequate model of the mental world and emotions is important for teaching the individuals, whose understanding of mental world is impaired.

In our previous studies we have analyzed each of the above three accounts in terms of models of underlying reasoning. The theory of mind account has been a subject of the systematic exploration of the reasoning about mental states by individuals with mental disorders (Galitsky 2000, 2001). The ToM account has been extended to reflect the computational experience of "teaching" computers to reason about mental attitudes: an adequate formalization of the mental world has been built to represent a number of autism phenomena. These studies addressed the peculiarities of autistic reasoning about knowledge, beliefs, intentions, and about other mental states and actions. Involving the formalisms of logical artificial intelligence, and the BDI (Belief-Desire-Intention) model in particular (Bratman 1987), the system for representation of reasoning about mental states and actions has been built. Our system is capable of simulating the verbal behavior of autistic as well as control patients (Galitsky 2002b). We have also analyzed various forms of autistic reasoning about action, time, space and probabilities, and have found that their deductive reasoning skills are stronger than their inductive, abductive, and analogical forms of reasoning (Galitsky and Goldberg 2003). We developed a set of exercises and built the software implementations focusing on selected reasoning patterns, teaching autistic trainees to reason properly about mental states in accordance to the traditions of axiomatic method, since the natural ways of teaching (by example) usually do not help (Galitsky 2003). Also, it has been shown that the training of reasoning about beliefs, desires and intentions assists the emotional development (Galitsky 2001). A series of interactive rehabilitation software tools have been developed which stimulate various forms of commonsense reasoning, conversation and decision-making in autistic trainees (Peterson et al. 2004).

The second and third accounts of autism above have been characterized in terms of default reasoning (Peterson et al. 2004; Galitsky and Peterson 2005), where typical and atypical situations are treated differently, in contrast to classical reasoning.

In this book, we propose a new conceptual reasoning model for autism in which the core deficits, and other related symptoms, emerge as a result of a basic problem with symbolic reasoning. Our model attempts to provide the developmental mechanism required to explain why primary deficits related to social orientation may be the cause for autism and its broader features, and why intensive early intervention by means of stimulating reasoning about mental attitudes frequently helps to improve autistic reasoning.

Beyond the Introduction, the book is organized as follows. We firstly discuss computational models and generally accepted accounts of autism (Chap. 2) and then proceed to intuitive Theory of Mind (Chap. 3) and its formalization (Chap. 4). The reader who prefers to avoid technical details may want to skip Chaps. 4, 5, 6, and 7 and proceed to Chaps. 8 and 9.

In Chap. 5 the mental simulator NL_MAMS is presented, the system that is capable of automated reasoning within our framework of the mental world. User interface and implementation of the simulator is followed by evaluation of its reasoning capabilities and the description of its deployment for the rehabilitation of reasoning. Chapter 8 presents the NL_MAMS-assisted rehabilitation strategy and describes its evaluation. Towards the end of the book we analyze educational value of the proposed rehabilitation strategy and describe a case study. In describing the theory of mind, we will be relying on the language of logic programming, this being a convenient way to introduce the mental world both to computers and autistic children.

1.1   How Computer Scientists Can Help Individuals with Autism

The main behavioral problem of children with autism (CwA) lays in the area of reasoning, decision making, control, and cognition as reflected in their behavior and motion. These are the areas of expertise of engineers, building the reasoning, search, recommend, recognition and control systems. Today, in the second decade of the twenty-first century, these specialists and these systems are very common, and plenty of experience is accumulated on how these systems malfunctions and how they can be repaired.

At the same time, a high number of models for the malfunction of autistic reasoning, control and cognition has been proposed by psychologists, neurobiologists, geneticists and specialists in neural networks, specialists without a hands-on experience with respective engineering systems. The mystery of autism still has a long way to be solved, and there is a tremendous amount of inconsistencies between today accounts and models of autism. Some of these inconsistencies are, in our opinion, due to computational implausibility of some proposed models. These models can be realistic in terms of how a correct sensory or reasoning system might work, according to their authors, but indeed they look faulty to an engineer who might have tried respective architecture, failed and now knows a reason for it.

In this book we take a number of models of autism and apply a computational plausibility test to them. We attempt at combining the best of two words: computer scientists are inspired by psychological experiments on how intelligence works, and autism specialists learn from the experience of computer scientists and engineers building systems and solving problems similar to those where children with autism have deficiencies. Applying the computational plausibility criteria, we reduce the number of models of autistic dysfunctions and attempt to convert them to a form acceptable by members of computer science community.

Traditionally, strict (formalized, mathematical) thinking is considered as an opposite entity to the emotional (fuzzy, approximate) thinking and behavior. However, for autistic patients the strict rule-based learning is much easier than the direct introduction of the various forms of emotional behavior, hence the latter is achieved via the former. Therefore, we are teaching autistic kids the "mechanic" forms of mental and especially emotional behavior. Regretfully, the attempts to directly introduce the emotional interaction with the others in a natural manner (teaching by examples, imitating) frequently fail.

In this book, we want to characterize autistic reasoning patterns from the perspective of axiomatic logic, similar to how a behavior of an automatic agent is expressed. Our interest is how various forms of autistic reasoning are connected with each other and determine the observable decision-making and behavior. We will also address the issue of how can our experience with reasoning of automatic agents, accumulated in artificial intelligence, help with understanding and treatment of reasoning of autistic individuals.

In the current body of research on autism there is no accurate model for how the correct reasoning in various reasoning domains should work. There is a lack of formal interconnection between the reasoning patterns in different domains (mental, physical, spatial/temporal, probabilistic, etc.). To overcome this, we need a systematic approach to reasoning that is based on practical experience building software agents with decision-making capabilities, acting in the above domains.

Frequently, CwA are good at some analytical tasks, including reasoning and calculations. At the same time, they lack communicative and cognitive skills, and their orientation in the mental world is limited. Such children are the primary target of the methodology developed in this book, they can learn axioms directly from multiple sources including their teachers. The best teachers for them are computer scientists because they literally use a similar language of rigidity and attention to details. High-functioning CwA with advances analytical skills can then infer theorems from acquired axioms and apply these theorems to their decision-making and behavior, being guided by rehabilitation professionals. Such CwA are the part of the broader audience of computer scientists who would be happy to learn reasoning patterns from this book skipping the psychological and general humanitarian wrapper of reasoning (the latter is required by the rest of CwA for whom the boundary between reasoning and behavior is not that crisp).

1.2 Developing Deductive Reasoning Skills of Machines and Children with Autism

The issue of training to overcome various deficiencies of autistic reasoning has been addressed in a number of studies (Green 1996; Baron-Cohen 2000). There is a series of peculiar techniques developed to teach children with autism certain forms of reasoning, mainly reasoning about mental states and actions, reasoning about generic actions, default and defeasible reasoning, deductive, inductive, abductive and analogical reasoning patterns, probabilistic decision-making etc. Skills of reasoning in some of these domains are lacking in every child with autism (Howlin 1998).

Teaching by analogy is the standard technique for both junior students and adults in a majority of subject domains. However, autistic trainees experience significant difficulties learning from examples, they can imitate some forms of behavior and actions of other people but do it without understanding. Also, visual programming tools is an efficient way to introduce abstract and general programming concept, they are quite efficient for both education of programming and efficient software development (Grandin 2006). In spite of the appeal to use visual programming tools, autistic children do not learn abstract reasoning patterns from them most of times.

Hence in terms of reasoning patterns, controls learn by induction and analogy, and reinforce learning results by deduction (explicit rules) in most of real-world domain (excluding e.g. math). At the same time, autistic trainees learn by deductive rules most of the time, and other reasoning patterns play auxiliary roles only (Galitsky 2005).

Therefore, teaching autistic trainees in any domain must be preceded by formulating exact and explicit rules. Otherwise, the teaching approach that might be adequate for a control trainee would be unacceptable for an autistic trainee, as our experience shows (Galitsky and Goldberg 2003). Teaching a new entity to a child with autism, one needs to make sure that all entities the current one refers to are fully conceptually understood. On the contrary, a child from a control group is ready to acquire a new entity in the environment where some features are uncertain, assuming she can learn them later (Fig. 1.1).

The idea of this book is to explore the similarity between formulating domain knowledge in a way acceptable by a computer and formulation of this knowledge to be acquired by an autistic trainee. We enumerate the commonalities in cognitive demands of computers and autistic trainees with respect to teaching them knowledge representation and reasoning in real-world domains:

1. All concepts have to be *clearly* and *explicitly* defined. A basis of indefinable concepts may be selected, but a programmer/teacher should be aware that a computer or trainee will not be able to freely operate and provide explanations with these concepts from the basis. For example, when taught the rules for basic mental states of the mental world (knowledge and intention), followed

Learn to reason (*formally, symbolically*) about mental states ⇒

Capable of applying rules to subjects of real world ⇒

Can understand others and behave properly in real world

Fig. 1.1 Main steps of our proposal

by the rules by derived mental/communicative actions derived from this basis, the autistic trainees are capable of explaining what is *pretending* and *deceiving* (derived) but not what is *knowledge* and *intention* (basic).

2. Definitions for concepts can be either *procedural* or *declarative*. A trainee can be taught a sequence of actions to achieve a goal, or a clause for a sequence of conditions an environment should satisfy to achieve this goal. To be capable of training in a declarative way, respective trainees' skills have to be developed. For example, if a child with autism is requested to be at the top of a rock in the middle of a puddle with a fishing pole, the child needs some skills to determine the order of operations: put on rubber boots, take a fishing pole, cross the puddle and climb the rock. In contrast to a control child who would acquire this skill independently on the basis of trial-and-error, a child with autism needs a substantial guidance to learn how to search for a proper sequence of actions independently.

3. All special cases should be addressed. For example, for an arbitrary predicate like *want* we would expect a smart trainee to operate with *want(Who, What)* with arbitrary *Who* and *What*. It is not the case for a child with autism who does not understand that other people may *want* something,

When we refer to an autistic or computer software trainee, we assume a medium-to-high-functioning individuals with autism and a standard software environment without sophisticated machine learning systems like explanation-based generalization (Mitchell et al. 1986) or inductive logic programming (Muggleton and De Raedt 1994).

In this book we will demonstrate that experimental cognitive science is relevant to a number of important AI problems in reasoning and machine learning. We focus on the domain of autistic reasoning that is a curious mixture of topics in AI and cognitive sciences. We will outline the commonalities of teaching autistic children and teaching computers (programming) to solve real-world problems, and provide a simplified illustration on how the experience of the former can be applied to the latter. Our claim is that it is significantly easier to teach control children to solve these problems than to teach children with autism, and, obviously, it is even more so for programming, where much more details have to be provided for robust functioning.

We will also demonstrate that lessons learned in teaching reasoning about mental world, adjusting one's action to an environment and can be naturally applied to improve the performance of machine reasoning in the respective domains. The conclusion will be that theoretical and experimental cognitive science of autistic reasoning might contribute to such traditionally "technical" areas as machine learning and reasoning.

1.3   Prior Work in Intelligent Systems for Autistic Education

Learning behavior in mental space based on rules, as described in this study, can be viewed as a special way of learning programming, in particular, object–oriented programming. Galvez et al. (2009) present a blended e-learning experience consisting of supplying an undergraduate student population with a problem-solving environment in which students can resolve programming exercises. The system applies an assessment for learning strategy where students are formatively assessed and also generates feedback and hints to help students to understand and overcome their misconceptions and to reinforce correctly learned concepts.

The synergies, functional effectiveness and integration of behavior simulation within an e-learning environment have attracted little interest for serious research so far, despite the overarching importance of knowledge acquisition by students for fostering their innovation and creativity. Learners often fail to reach their desired learning objects due to the failure of methods to provide them with a ubiquitous learning grid. Lau and Tsui (2009) discuss how knowledge management can be used effectively in e-learning, and how it can provide a learning grid to enable the learner to identify the right learning objects in an environment which is based on the learner's context and personal preferences.

The use of ontologies to model the knowledge of specific domains such as mental attitudes represents a key aspect for the integration of information coming from different sources, for supporting collaboration within virtual communities, and for reasoning on available knowledge. In the e-learning field, ontologies can be used to model educational domains and to build, organize and update specific learning resources (i.e. learning objects, learner profiles, learning paths, etc.). One of the main problems of educational domains modeling is the lacking of expertise in the knowledge engineering field by the e-learning actors. Gaeta et al. (2009) present an integrated approach to manage the life-cycle of ontologies, used to define personalized e-learning experiences supporting blended learning activities, without any specific expertise in knowledge engineering. Also, collaborative learning serves as an important part of e-learning. It increases interactivity and accessibility to various learning resources either synchronously or asynchronously among users. Distributed interactivity through Web services thus forms the focus of (Fang and Sing 2009) who review service-oriented architecture, distributed infrastructure and highlight the need to integrate service-oriented technologies for meaningful and interactive collaborative learning processes.

The need for providing learners with web-based learning content that match their accessibility needs and preferences, as well as providing ways to match learning content to user's devices has been identified as an important issue in accessible educational environment. For a web-based open and dynamic learning environment, personalized support for learners becomes more important. In order to achieve optimal efficiency in a learning process, individual learner's cognitive learning style should be taken into account. Due to different types of learners using these systems, it is necessary to provide them with an individualized learning support system. However, the design and development of web-based learning environments for people with special abilities has been addressed so far by the development of hypermedia and multimedia based on educational content. Guo and Zhang (2009) presented a framework of individual web-based learning system by focusing on learner's cognitive learning process, learning pattern and activities, as well as the technology support needed. Based on the learner-focused mode and cognitive learning theory, the authors demonstrate an online course design and development that supports the students with the learning flexibility and adaptation.

Multiple technologies have been suggested for mental rehabilitation, including playing LEGO (Resnick 1987), video-clips together with a set of dolls (Blocher and Picard 2002), autonomous mobile robots and the interactive tool for browsing and recognizing emotional expressions. Recent advances in mobile and ubiquitous technologies provide an opportunity to efficiently and accurately capture important information preceding and associated with problematic behaviors of children with autism. The ability to obtain this type of data will help with both intervention and behavioral rehabilitation efforts. Through collaboration with behavioral scientists and therapists, Sano et al. (2012) identified relevant design requirements and created an easy-to-use mobile application for collecting, labeling, and sharing in-situ behavior data in individuals diagnosed with autism.

These computer-based tools assist the development of a wide spectrum of behavioral and cognitive skills. However, our focus is teaching reasoning about the mental world, which then naturally leads to communication and other skills (Galitsky 2002a). The goal of this book is to describe an intelligent education system that is at least capable of reasoning on its own, in contrast to the approaches mentioned above which are the infrastructures for providing access to various media.

To differentiate the proposed educational environment from existing software packages for children with autism, we address the following issues:

- The software needs to stimulate *reasoning* with an accent on rule-base reasoning. In particular, reasoning about *intention, knowledge* and *beliefs* of others should be developed after the basic entities are introduces via rules.
- The software has to be *intelligent*. This requirement is due to the fact that in contrast to conventional learning process, such software has to be capable of substituting interaction with humans in a certain degree. Frequently, autistic trainees prefer to deal with software agents rather than with humans. These software agents need to demonstrate the reasoning skills, which are expected to be developed by the learners, rather than just to introduce a domain for reasoning.
- While identifying three core deficits outlined above certainly helps in the study and diagnosis of autism, it does not provide a causal explanation of the disorder, nor does it provide a rehabilitation mechanism. It is worth mentioning a number of neural network-based models of autistic phenomena (see e.g. Cohen 1994); however there is no explicit connection between these models and reasoning or possible rehabilitation strategies.

1.4   Teaching Theory of Mind to Autistic Patients

Teaching children with autism can be overwhelming, but it also can be a triumph at the same time. The possibility to teach autistic children theory of mind has been assessed in multiple studies because of potentially important clinical implications.

If it is true that a deficit in reasoning about mental attitudes leads to impairment in social interaction and understanding of oneself and others, then an efficient method for teaching theory of mind may assist in overall autism rehabilitation. Autism training studies, including the current one, are valuable sources of knowledge regarding how improved reasoning patterns affect trainees' behavior including social interaction.

The theory of mind training studies conducted so far have shown that some individuals with autism can be taught to pass the particular tasks of reasoning about mental states (Swettenham 1996; Baron-Cohen and Swettenham 1997; Sutton et al. 1999; Scott et al. 2002). In most cases, it is natural to assume that trainees indeed apply one or another reasoning pattern rather than memorizing exact answers. Regrettably, in most cases, the studies of how individuals with autism acquire mental reasoning patterns are lacking an accurate formulation of these patterns, backed up by computational experiments. We believe the latter is essential to differentiate between mental and non-mental components of reasoning process.

Another problem with teaching particular patterns of reasoning about mental states is a verification of how children can generalize from acquired mental reasoning patterns. Because the majority of ToM training studies have not considered deductive links between the mental reasoning patterns *involved in a given thought*, it is unclear how the acquisition of one pattern should have affected others. We believe that the question of mutual dependence of reasoning patterns should be addressed from a computational perspective. Indeed, applying axioms about intention, knowledge and beliefs to be introduced, we subject their generalizations to a formal treatment and observe how they can be taught (Chaps. 4 and 8).

A number of earlier studies have focused on theory of mind tasks, demonstrating that members of high-functioning group of individuals with autism are able to pass first-order (Baron-Cohen 1989; Swettenham et al. 1996), second order and even third-order tasks (Happe 1994). Also, the tasks include interaction and conversational skills concerning maintaining the topic of conversation and adjustment of conversation topics for others, interpretation and expression of non-verbal signals, listening and expressing interest in others have been investigated.

The results of these ToM training studies are that the performance of the group which has undergone training has improved (at least with the second order tasks) with respect to controls. However, frequently children were able to apply non-mental state rules, and were not able to show the results of their training in their behavior. Only a smaller proportion of high-functioning autistic children are believed by these authors to improve their social skills as a result of training. In terms of generalization, children were able to apply acquired mental rules to other subjects and objects. However, it is still unclear what was being generalized – new knowledge about inferring mental states or a non-mental-state rule that allowed participants to pass tests. Disappointingly, children with autism can hardly transfer their reasoning skills from one mental domain to another (e.g. recognition of emotion, pretense, false belief; Hadwin et al. 1997, Fig. 1.2).

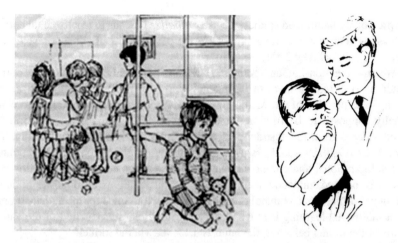

Fig. 1.2 On the *left*: a typical posture, position and avoidance of the other children. On the *right*: an autistic child is subject to repeated attempts of adult to make eye-to-eye contact (Both reproduced from Hutt and Hutt 1970)

We believe that the reasons for the rather low efficiency of the above training, in addition to autism-specific reasoning impairments, concern the consistency and persistency of the training and the thoroughness of coverage of the domain of mental reasoning. Here we discuss how to develop the experimental studies, verifying whether treatment of autistic theory of mind reasoning is efficient or not, into long-term rehabilitation strategies which are viable for a wide audience of individuals with autism.

Firstly, the training has to be consistent. A totality of the first-order mental entities should be introduced first, followed by the totality of second-order entities, if acquired properly. The third-order rules should be introduced only after the trainees can consistently demonstrate not only passing the simpler exercises, but respective behavior and understanding second-order entities of others.

Secondly, in terms of persistence, the training should be attempted from the earliest possible age and as long as a trainee is interested in practicing the exercises. If no success is observed at a given age, the training should be attempted again in a few months assuming a trainee has acquired some necessary background knowledge and/or reasoning skills to adopt certain mental-state reasoning patterns failed earlier.

Thirdly, trainees would benefit from the complete coverage of mental domain, which is rather compact in comparison with other domains. The totality of basic mental entities (intention, knowledge and belief) should be introduced together with derived mental entities (including pretending, deceiving, explaining, forgiving etc.). Such coverage is assured by the formal model specifying how to derive mental entities from the basic ones; this formal model will be introduced in Chap. 4.

Similar to the theory of mind training settings introduced above, we teach individuals with autism mental entities and their combinations. However, unlike the previously mentioned studies, we use *formalized* means to teach mental entities, suggesting that they are more suitable to the peculiarities of autistic development (Peterson and Galitsky 2004).

We use the non-human (computer) resources, readily acceptable by autistic children, to introduce them to the mental world (of humans) via formalized reasoning. The paradox of our methodology is that reasoning about the mental world, usually supposed to be irrational and displayed as an emotion, can nevertheless be considered from the abstract perspective, formalized and used in training. This hypothesis (Galitsky 2002b) is used as a framework of our rehabilitation strategy to develop rational and emotional behavior in the real mental world. Traditionally, strict (formalized, mathematical) thinking is considered as an opposite notion to emotional (fuzzy, approximate) thinking and behavior. Since for the autistic trainees strict rule-based learning is much easier than the direct introduction of the various forms of emotional behavior, the latter is achieved via the former.

Our model of the human agent is based on the supposition that there are a number of standard axioms for mental entities, including emotions; these axioms are genetically set for normal children and are corrupted in the autistic brain (Galitsky 2013). The patterns of corruption vary from trainee to trainee and are correlated with the specifically outlined groups of individuals with autism. They have to acquire these axioms explicitly, by means of direct training, using the specific scenarios. Frequently, autism is not accompanied by learning disabilities, so the patents willingly participate in training programs. Our practical experience shows that using a software-based training allows us to hold the attention of autistic trainees for much longer periods than traditional means of one-to-one treatment by a human trainer.

1.5 How to Read This Book

The main targets of this book are software engineers, computer scientists and mathematicians interested in theory and practice of autism. This category of readers is expected to learn about autism and remediation strategies in their native language. Describing the problems children with autism experience in various circumstances, we describe similar problems in engineering artificial intelligence systems and try to find common solutions. Specialists in logical Artificial Intelligence should focus on Chaps. 4, 5, and 6, and machine learning and cognitive system professionals – on Chap. 7. Software engineers might find Sections 4–7 equally appealing. Computer engineers and natural scientists who are parents of children with autism can briefly familiarize themselves with Chaps. 2, 3, 4, 5, 6, and 7 and read in depth Chaps. 8 and 9.

For those who prefer to avoid the language of logic and computation, we recommend Chaps. 3, 6, 7, 8, and 9. Rehabilitation professionals can briefly look at Chaps. 2 and 3 and proceed to Chaps. 8 and 9.

References

American Psychiatric Association (1994) Quick reference to the diagnostic criteria from DSM-IV. American Psychiatric Association, Washington, DC

Baron-Cohen S (1989) Perceptual role-taking and proto-declarative pointing in autism. Br J Dev Psychol 7:113–127

Baron-Cohen S (1995) Mindblindness: an essay on autism and theory of mind. MIT Press/Bradford Books, Boston

Baron-Cohen S (2000) Theory of mind and autism: a fifteen year review. In: Baron-Cohen S, Tagar- Flusberg H, Cohen DJ (eds) Understanding other minds, vol. A. Oxford University Press, Oxford, pp 3–20

Baron-Cohen S, Swettenham J (1997) Theory of mind in autism: its relationship to executive function and central coherence. In: Cohen DJ, Volkmar FR (eds) Handbook for autism and pervasive developmental disorders. Wiley, New York, pp 880–893

Blocher K, Picard R (2002) Affective social quest: emotion recognition therapy for autistic children. Socially intelligent agents: creating relationships with computers and robots, p 133

Bratman ME (1987) Intention, plans and practical reason. Harvard University Press, Cambridge, MA

Cohen IL (1994) An artificial neural network analogue of learning in autism. Biol Psychiatry 36: 5–20

Eigsti IM, Shapiro T (2003) A systems neuroscience approach to autism: biological, cognitive, and clinical perspectives. Ment Retard Dev Disabil Res Rev 9:205–215

Fang CF, Sing LC (2009) Collaborative learning using service-oriented architecture: a framework design. Knowl-Based Syst 22(4):271–274

Frith U (1989) Autism and "theory of mind". In: Gillberg C (ed) Diagnosis and treatment of autism. Plenum Press, New York, pp 33–52

Frith U (2001) Mind blindness and brain in autism. Neuron 32:969–979

Gaeta M, Orciuoli F, Ritrovato P (2009) Advanced ontology management system for personalised e-learning. Knowl-Based Syst 22(4):292–301

Galitsky B (2000) Simulating autistic patients as agents with corrupted reasoning about mental states. AAAI FSS-2000 symposium on human simulation, Cape Cod, MA

Galitsky B (2001) Learning the axiomatic reasoning about mental states assists the emotional development of the autistic patients. AAAI FSS-2001 symposium on emotional and intelligent II, Cape Cod, MA

Galitsky B (2002a) On the training of mental reasoning: searching the works of literature. FLAIRS – 02, Pensacola Beach, FL

Galitsky B (2002b) Extending the BDI model to accelerate the mental development of autistic patients. Second international conference on development & learning. Cambridge, MA

Galitsky B (2003) Natural language question answering system: technique of semantic headers. Advanced Knowledge Intl, Adelaide

Galitsky B (2005) On a distance learning rehabilitation of autistic reasoning. Encyclopedia of online learning and technologies, vol 4. Idea Publishing Group

Galitsky B (2013) A computational simulation tool for training autistic reasoning about mental attitudes. Knowl-Based Syst 50:25–43

Galitsky B, Goldberg S (2003) On the non-classical reasoning of autistic patients. International conference on neural and cognitive systems Boston University, MA

Galitsky B, Peterson D (2005) On the peculiarities of default reasoning of children with Autism. FLAIRS-05

Galvez J, Guzmἴn E, Conejo R (2009) A blended E-learning experience in a course of object oriented programming fundamentals. Knowl-Based Syst 22(4):279–286

Grandin T (2006) Thinking in pictures, expanded edition. Vintage Press, New York

Green G (1996) Early behavioral interventions for autism: what does the research tell us? In: Maurice C (ed) Behavioral intervention for young children with autism. Pro-Ed, Austin

Guo Q, Zhang M (2009) Implement web learning environment based on data mining. Knowl-Based Syst 22(6):439–442

Happe FG (1994) Autism: an introduction to psychological theory. UCL Press, London

Hermelin B, O'Connor N (1967) Remembering of words by psychotic and subnormal children. Br J Psychol 58(3/4):213–218

Howlin P (1998) Children with autism and Asperger syndrome: a guide for practitioners and carers. Wiley, New York

Hutt SJ, Hutt C (1970) Direct observation and measurement of behaviour. Charles C. Thomas, Springfield

Lau A, Tsui E (2009) Knowledge management perspective on e-learning effectiveness. Knowl-Based Syst 22(4):324–325

Leevers HJ, Harris PL (2000) Counterfactual syllogistic reasoning in normal 4-year-olds, children with learning disabilities, and children with autism. J Exp Child Psychol 76:64–87

Leslie AM (1987) Pretence and representation: the origins of "theory of mind". Psychol Rev 94:412–426

Mitchell TM, Keller RM, Kedar-Cabelli ST (1986) Explanation-based generalization: a unifying view. Mach Learn 1(1):47–80

Muggleton S, De Raedt L (1994) Inductive logic programming: theory and methods. J Log Program 19–20:629–679

Ozonoff S (1997) Components of executive function in autism and other disorders. In: Russell J (ed) Autism as an executive disorder. Oxford University Press, Oxford, pp 179–211

Pennington BF, Ozonoff S (1996) Executive function and developmental psycopathology. J Child Psychol Psychiatry 37(1):51–87

Perner J (1991) Understanding the representational mind. MIT Press, Cambridge, MA

Peterson DM, Bowler DM (2000) Counterfactual reasoning and false belief understanding in children with autism. Autism: Int J Res Pract 4(4):391–405

Peterson D, Galitsky B (2004) Handling default rules by autistic reasoning. KES 3215:314–320

Peterson D, Galitsky B, Goldberg S (2004) Literal handling of conflicting default rules leads to inadequate reactions of autistic patients. In: Seventh international conference of cognitive and neural systems, Boston, MA

Pijnacker J, Hagoort P, Buitelaar J, Teunisse J-P, Geurts B (2008) Pragmatic inferences in high-functioning adults with autism and Asperger syndrome. J Autism Dev Disord 39(4):607–618

Pilowsky T, Yirmiya N, Arbelle S, Mozes T (2000) Theory of mind abilities of children with schizophrenia, children with autism, and normally developing children. Schizophr Res 42(2):145–155

Resnick M (1987) LEGO, LOGO, and life. In: Langton CG (ed) Proceedings on interdisciplinary workshop on the synthesis and simulation of living systems, Sept 87, Los Alamos, NM, pp 397–406

Russell J (1997) Autism as an executive disorder. Oxford University Press, Oxford

Sano A, Hernandez J, Deprey J, Eckhardt M, Picard RW, Goodwin MS (2012) Multimodal annotation tool for challenging behaviors in people with autism spectrum disorders, Workshop on ubiquitous mobile instrumentation at the international conference on ubiquitous computing, Pittsburgh, PA, 5–8 September 2012

Scott F, Baron-Cohen S (1996) Imagining real and unreal things: evidence of a dissociation in autism. J Cogn Neurosci 8:400–411

Scott F, Baron-Cohen S, Bolton P, Brayne C (2002) Brief report: prevalence of autism spectrum conditions in children aged 5–11 years in Cambridgeshire, UK. Autism 6:231–237

Stenning K, Van Lambalgen M (2008) Human reasoning and cognitive science. MIT Press, Cambridge, MA

Sutton J, Smith PK, Swettenham J (1999) Social cognition and bullying: social inadequacy or skilled manipulation? Br J Dev Psychol 17(3):435–450(16)

Swettenham J (1996) Can children with autism be taught to understand false belief using computers? J Child Psychol Psychiatry 37:157–165

Swettenham J, Baron-Cohen S, Gomez J-C, Walsh S (1996) "What is inside someone's head? Conceiving of the mind as a camera helps children with autism acquire an alternative to a "theory of mind. Cogn Meuropsychiatry 1:73–88

Chapter 2
Computational Models of Autism

2.1 Autistic Deficits

Speaking about the deficits, we describe observable features of CwA irrespectively of how these features can be connected. For example, deficits of a car with a flat tire would be making an unpleasant noise, not following directions, having a rim of the wheel riding on the tire tread, irreparable damage to the tire, loud noise, and flat tire itself. Although all these symptoms are due to the same cause, we enumerate them as car deficits at the same level, as a list.

Our second example will be a set of search engine deficits. Anything in which a given search engine deviates from an ideal one where we can quickly find everything we want is its deficit:

1. There are documents I know exist but the search engine does not give them to me when I search for the corresponding topic. This is called a search recall deficit.
2. It gives me some documents that are misleading, and it should not have given them to me. This is called a search precision deficit.
3. I have to wait for more than a second for search results to show. This is a slowness deficit.
4. When I search with in given topic or context, it gives me documents with the search query keywords but belonging to a different topic. This is called a user intent recognition deficit.

There are multiple reasons for a search engine to display deficits, including its implementation, structure of a search index, relevance model, how keywords are treated and ontologies are employed. A baseline search system such as Lucene/SOLR/Elastic Search without use of learning from users, linguistic processing or domain ontology would possess deficits 1, 2 and 4, but not 3. Any engineering system has some advantages and some deficits (Fig. 2.1).

© Springer International Publishing Switzerland 2016
B. Galitsky, *Computational Autism*, Human–Computer Interaction Series,
DOI 10.1007/978-3-319-39972-0_2

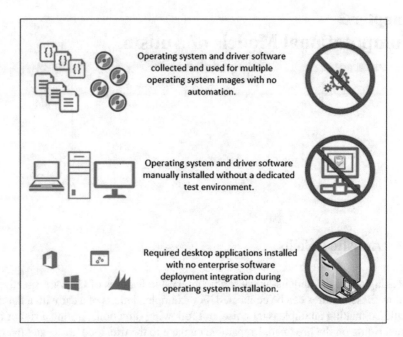

Fig. 2.1 Some symptoms for a problematic operating system (technet.microsoft.com)

Having considered the deficits of an engineering system, we are now ready to enumerate a broad range of deficit of CwA (Fig. 2.2):

1. Higher-level *abstract thinking*, including making inferences (Minshew 1996; Minshew and Goldstein 1998). This has long been known to be an area of deficit in autism. The notable finding of this study is the dissociation between intact performance on rule-learning tasks and deficits on concept formation tasks. Rule-learning tasks are ones in which there is a rule to solve the problem and the task is to discover the rule. Although the individuals in this study typically identified the rule correctly, they had difficulty changing rules when the context changed. Changing the rule to fit changing contexts adds to the information processing demands of the task, and is the basis of generalization. Concept formation tasks have no set solutions but require the individual to create one. Concept formation tasks are essentially problem solving in novel situations. This pattern is consistent with the behavior typical of autism, which is typically rule-dependent, lacking in flexibility, failing to consider the implications of context, and inability to cope with novel situations.
2. *Shared attention*, including social referencing and problem-solving (Mundy et al. 1990).
3. *Joint Attention* deficit. By 15 months of age, children are eager to share their interests with others. They show things to others, they try to share their

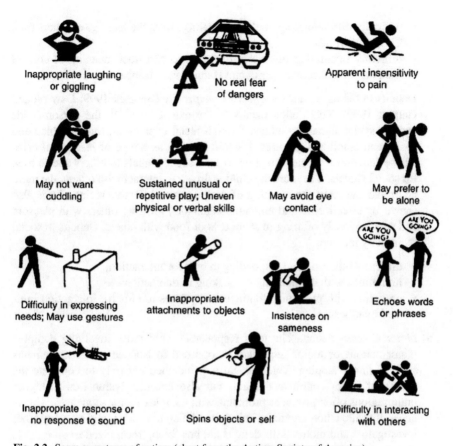

Fig. 2.2 Some symptoms of autism (chart from the Autism Society of America)

enjoyment, they babble reciprocally and they direct others' attention to objects which interest them. Later, when they have language, they ask about others' interests and ideas, and they share others' enjoyment.

4. *Social cognition* refers to the mental processes involved in perceiving, attending to, remembering, thinking about, and making sense of the people in our social world (Moskowitz 2005). Deficits in social cognition include

   • deficits in social and emotional learning including difficulty

      – managing emotions,
      – appreciating the perspectives of others,
      – developing pro-social goals,
      – using interpersonal skills to handle developmentally appropriate tasks (Payton et al. 2000);

- difficulty differentiating one's own feelings from the feelings of others (i.e., Theory of Mind);
- difficulty integrating diverse information to construct meaning in context (i.e., central coherence) (Frith and Happe 1994; Happe et al. 1996).

5. Deficits in the capacities for *affective reciprocity* (Baranek 1999; Dawson and Galpert 1990). This deficit occurs to the extent to which the person sends various social signals to others, through facial expression, tone of voice and social and emotional gestures. It could be seen as a type of instinctual drive whose function is to cause a child to send social signals to others and to look for social signals. The more the child is driven to interact with others, the more he or she can learn the meaning of such signals. Affective reciprocity is also shown by affectionate and empathic behaviors, greeting others with pleasure and spontaneously offering to share toys or food with others. Deficits in social reciprocity include:

- difficulty initiating and responding to bids for interaction,
- limitations with maintaining turn-taking in interactions,
- problems with providing contingent responses to bids for interaction initiated by others.

6. *Motor domain* deficit. The tests responsible were those involving complex motor actions or motor sequences as opposed to isolated motor movements such as finger tapping. This domain was included not only to complete the survey of major cognitive domains but also because dysfunction in higher brain regions often produces problems with complex motor sequences. This is generally called motor apraxia. This motor deficit has been found by many other investigators and motor skills deficits are now being recognized as an integral part of autism and the other disorders in this category. In young children, motor apraxia causes the problems with operating mechanical devices such as door knobs and wind up toys, whereas button pressing is not a problem. Later, motor apraxia is responsible for difficulty holding pencils, cutting with scissors, and tying shoe laces. In school age children, it is responsible for the problems with handwriting, either slowness or sloppiness. In the gross motor area, it is responsible for the lack of coordination in sports and contributes to the inability of many to ride bicycles or rollerblades. It is likely also responsible for the stilted quality to facial expressions.

7. Deficits in language and related cognitive skills include:

- impaired acquisition of words, word combinations, and syntax
  (i) initial words are often nouns and attributes, while words representing social stimuli, such as people's names (i.e., subjects) and actions (i.e., verbs), are delayed;
  (ii) the child loses words previously acquired;

- use and understanding of nonverbal and verbal communication

    (i) facial expressions, body language, and gestures as forms of communication are delayed in the latter part of the first year of life and remain unconventional throughout development;

    (ii) unconventional gestures (e.g., pulling a caregiver's hand toward an item) emerge prior to more conventional gestures (e.g., giving, pointing, and head nods/headshakes);

    (iii) understanding of gaze shifting, distal gestures, facial expressions, and rules of proximity and body language is limited;

    (iv) receptive language appears more delayed than expressive;

    (v) use of immediate echolalia and/or delayed echolalia (scripted language) is observed;

- vocal development deficits, including

    (i) atypical response to caregiver's vocalizations,

    (ii) atypical vocal productions beyond the first year of life,

    (iii) abnormal prosody once speech emerges (speech may sound robotic);

- symbolic play deficits, including

    (i) delayed acquisition of functional and conventional use of objects,

    (ii) repetitive, inflexible play,

    (iii) limited cooperative play in interactive situations;

- conversation deficits, including

    (i) limitations in understanding and applying social norms of conversation (e.g., balancing turns, vocal volume, proximity, and conversational timing);

    (ii) provision of inappropriate and unnecessary information in conversational contexts;

    (iii) problems taking turns during conversation;

    (iv) difficulty initiating topics of shared interest;

    (v) preference for topics of special interest;

    (vi) difficulties in recognizing the need for clarification;

    (vii) challenges adequately repairing miscommunications;

    (viii) problems understanding figurative language, including idioms, multiple meanings, and sarcasm;

- literacy deficits, including difficulty

8. *Complex language* deficit, i.e., the interpretative aspects of language. These include reading comprehension, story comprehension, comprehension of idioms and metaphors, verbal inference making, and comprehension of complex sentence structure. The latter is particularly important because it is the language of everyday life. It typically involves sentences like: before

you do this, I want you to do that and then do this and so on. These sentences place particularly heavy demands on information processing because they require processing of each segment and then a second stage of processing to determine the meaning of each bit to the next bit. Understanding the meaning of such a sentence requires yet a third level of processing. A similar process occurs with the understanding of a story. The combination of superior formal language abilities and inferior comprehension produces a wide gap between the listener's estimate of the autistic individual's language comprehension and his or her actual comprehension. The failure to understand what the person with autism understands is a major contributor to their dysfunction in many settings.

9. *Memory for complex information* deficit. Complexity can result from increasing amounts of simple information or increasing inherent complexity of the information. In essence, individuals with autism have difficulty with recall of complex material, because they fail to make use of cognitive organizing strategies or to benefit from the meaning of the material. Secondly, this pertained to both visual and auditory information. CwA remember less from the material presented to them than age and IQ matched peers; this has also been shown to reduce the amount of information they remember from recently experienced events. Thus, this memory impairment is likely to contribute to the social, language, and problem solving deficits. Knowledge of this impairment can be used to improve learning. Memory and learning can be improved by reducing the amount of material presented (smaller chunks), preprocessing the information (give the bottom line rather than patterns that require deduction of the bottom line), and increasing the processing time. Visual presentation of information often accomplishes all of these, and likely explains why they benefit from such adaptations. Visual material is constantly present for reference and re-reading, to guide behavior.

10. Deficit in the ability to *selectively manipulate sensory representation*. A different, perhaps more fundamental deficit should be entertained as being present in many persons with autism, particularly if they are low-functioning: a deficit in the ability to selectively manipulate sensory representations, concepts, and thoughts themselves (although these may also be deficient). In basic terms, this is a problem with the ability to imagine. However, it is not a deficit in simple visual imagery; there is self- reported evidence that high-functioning persons with autism not only have visual imaginations but rely upon them (Grandin 2006). Instead, what is referred to here is the ability to select elements of mental states and manipulate them. Normally, humans are able to focus on different aspects of an object or experience, and even seem to break these aspects away from the original experience and manipulate them separately. A person can see a white ball and separate out its whiteness from its shape. PwA are however well known for not being able to do this. They are notorious for context dependence and for apparently focusing on the "wrong" features of everyday objects.

11. Deficit in *social referencing*. Social referencing is known as the seeking and use of information from another individual to help evaluate a situation

(Bruinsma et al. 2004). The reason this may be difficult for individuals with autism is that they may prefer not interact with others and may not find this behavior reinforcing, and would rather engage in self-stimulatory type behaviors instead. Lacking these skills in the classroom can present teaching challenges to the teacher during whole class instruction, choral responding and teaching in the natural environment.

A number of patterns of deficits have been proposed in autism over the years; some of these are still being debated. These include:

- a single primary cognitive-single neural system deficit versus multiple primary co-existing cognitive-multiple neural systems deficit;
- auditory and not visual information processing deficit;
- information acquisition deficit versus information processing deficit,
- and simple versus complex information processing deficit(s).

Instances of essential autistic deficits can be visualized (Fig. 2.3).

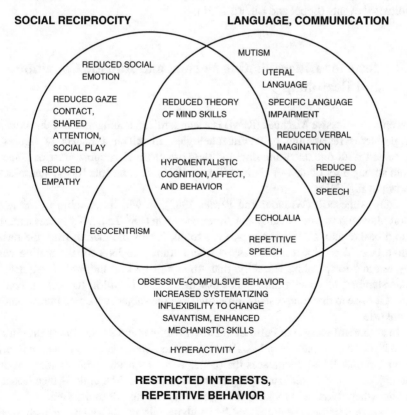

Fig. 2.3 Essential autistic deficits and their inter-relations

2.1.1   Hypotheses for the Origin of Autistic Reasoning

There are a number of other hypotheses concerning autistic reasoning, including (Gopnik et al. 2000) stating that children with autism are impaired in their ability to form theories about the world. Theories provide an understanding of causality to enable children to generate explanations about their environment. Not only mental domain but also reasoning about physical world is corrupted as well (not as strongly as about mental world (Leslie and Keeble 1987; Oakes and Cohen 1990)). Children with autism are less likely to generate "wh-" questions and are impaired on probe questions of causal explanations of emotions and thoughts (Tager-Flusberg 1989). Overall impairment in causal language across two narrative contexts (Losh and Capps 2006) is reported, as well as impairment on causal language relating to mental states and emotions (Capps et al. 2000). Also, a correlation between mental ability or false belief performance and an ability of these children to explain observed scenarios has been established. Relative to controls, CwA have a lower overall ability to provide explanations for voluntary actions and impossible physical and biological events (Sobel and Lillard 2001).

2.2   Tests for Differentiating Normal and Autistic Cognition and Reasoning

Raven's Progressive Matrices (RPM) is a standardized intelligence test that consists of problems resembling geometric analogies, in which a matrix of figures is presented with one entry missing and the correct missing entry must be selected from among a set of answer choices (Raven 1936). An example Raven's problem is shown in Fig. 2.4.

Sally-Anne task (Wimmer and Perner 1983), in which the subject is shown a short play with two dolls, Sally and Anne, shown in (Fig. 2.5). Sally places a marble into a basket and, after Anne leaves the room, moves the marble from the basket into a box. The subject is then asked where Anne will look for the marble when she returns. Responding correctly, that Anne will look in the basket, requires an understanding of Anne's false belief that the marble is still in the basket; Anne's belief is false in that it represents something that the subject watching the skit knows is not true.

In a standard version of False Belief task (Wimmer and Perner 1983), the child is introduced to two characters, Maxi and his mother. Maxi places an object of interest into a cupboard, and then leaves the scene. While he is away, his mother removes the object from the cupboard and places it in a drawer. The child is then asked to predict where Maxi will look for the object when he returns to the scene.

A box of Smarties is emptied, refilled with pencils and then shown to a child who is ignorant of the change. The child is asked: "What do you think is in the box?", and it answers: 'Smarties!' It is then shown the contents of the box. The pencils are

Fig. 2.4 An example
Raven's problem

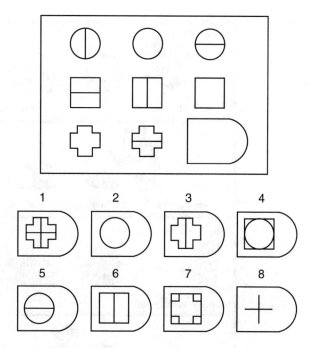

put back into the box, and the child is now asked: 'What do you think your [absent] mother will say is in the box?'

A famous experiment, the 'false belief' task investigates how autistic subjects reason about other people's belief. The standard design of the experiment is as follows. A child and a doll (Maxi) are in a room together with the experimenter. Maxi and child witness a bar of chocolate being placed in a box. Then Maxi is brought out of the room. The child sees the experimenter move the chocolate from the box to a drawer. Maxi is brought back in. The experimenter asks the child: 'Where does Maxi think the chocolate is?' The answers to this question reveal an interesting cut-off point, and a difference between CwA and CC.

Before the age of about 4 years, the normally developing child responds where the child knows the chocolate to be (i.e. the drawer); after that age, the child responds where Maxi must falsely believe the chocolate to be (i.e. the box). By contrast, CwA continue to answer 'in the drawer' for a long time. This experiment has been repeated many times, in many variations, with fairly robust results. There is for instance the 'Smarties' task, which goes as follows. Not shown to the child-subject, a box of Smarties is emptied and refilled with pencils. The child is asked: "What do you think is in the box?", and it happily answers: 'Smarties!' It is then shown the contents of the box. The pencils are put back into the box, and the child is now asked: 'What do you think your [absent] mother will say is in the box?'

We may then observe the same critical age: before age 4 the child answers: 'Pencils!', whereas after age 4 the child will say: 'Smarties!' Even more strikingly,

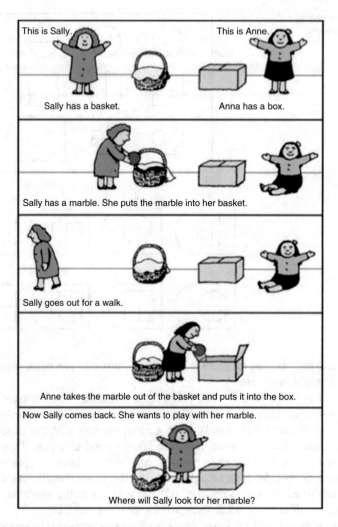

This is Sally.   This is Anne.

Sally has a basket.   Anna has a box.

Sally has a marble. She puts the marble into her basket.

Sally goes out for a walk.

Anne takes the marble out of the basket and puts it into the box.

Now Sally comes back. She wants to play with her marble.

Where will Sally look for her marble?

Fig. 2.5 Sally-Ann test (From visualsupportsandbeyond 2016)

when asked what it believed was in the box before seeing the actual contents, the younger child will say 'Pencils', even though it has just answered 'Smarties!'.

Feelings, Attitudes, and Behaviors Scale for Children (FAB-C) (Beitchman et al. 1996). The FAB-C is a self-report instrument designed to assess problems in children 6–13 years of age. It consists of 48 yes/no statements. Children are asked to indicate whether or not the statements describe them by circling yes or no. The questionnaire consists of five scales that measure conduct problems, self-image, worry, negative peer relations and antisocial attitudes.

Conners' Rating Scales-Revised (CRS-R) It provides a parental report of the behavioral, emotional and social functioning of the sibling. This questionnaire is composed of 80 items. Four response choices were available for each question, not true at all (never, seldom), just a little true (occasionally), pretty much true (often, quite a bit), very much true (very often, very frequent), and the score on each item ranged from 0 to 3.

N-back test is a continuous performance task that is commonly used as an assessment in cognitive neuroscience to measure a part of working memory. The n-back was introduced by Kirchner (1958). The subject is presented with a sequence of stimuli, and the task consists of indicating when the current stimulus matches the one from n steps earlier in the sequence. The load factor n can be adjusted to make the task more or less difficult. The visual n-back test is similar to the classic memory game of "Concentration". However, instead of different items that are in a fixed location on the game board, there is only one item, that appears in different positions on the game board during each turn. 1-N means that you have to remember the position of the item, ONE turn back. 2-N means that you have to remember the position of the item TWO turns back, and so on.

For example, an auditory three-back test could consist of the experimenter reading the following list of letters to the test subject:

T L H C H O C Q L C K L H C Q T R R K C H R

The subject is supposed to indicate when the letters marked in bold are read, because those correspond to the letters that were read three steps earlier.

Test for Pretend Play is designed to assess the three types of symbolic play, substituting one object for another object, or person attributing an imagined property to an object or person. Another type of symbolic play is a reference to an absent object, person or substance.

Test for Pretend Play can be used with a wide variety of children to assess a child's level of conceptual development and ability to use. This test also indicates a child's imaginative ability, creativity and emotional status. The test presents two versions of the test using structured conditions:on-verbal version – children up to 3 years and older children with insufficient comprehension to follow the language used in the verbal version, and verbal version – children of 3 years and above.

2.3   Neural Network Models

Advocates of neural network approaches believe that neural simulations act at the middle level, between molecular and behavioral levels. They give a chance for the understanding of the real reasons of causing behavior and linking network dynamics with molecular and genetic properties.

2.3.1   The Bridge Between Neural Models and Reasoning

If one considers an abstract reasoning system and looks at its input, output and interaction between black boxes as reasoning units, very little judgment can be obtained about its functioning. The information that can be extracted as a result of such observation is just a communication protocol between the reasoning units, but not the meaning of what each unit is reasoning about. A simulation of such system, based on this data, would be an attempt to reproduce a reasoning protocol and no information about the subjects of reasoning or reasoning domain would be obtained.

Hence neural network models targets the protocol of autistic reasoning, not the reasoning domain itself. Furthermore, numerical simulation of interaction between reasoning and cognitive units only gives a limited, one-sided view of such protocol. To better reproduce autistic reasoning and then all the way towards representing autistic behavior, a logical, not numerical model is required to match the model and its outcomes with experimental observations.

Neural network models are inspired by the fact that brain includes neurons. However, decoding of neuron signals into a semantic representation can be done very superficially, with almost complete loss of information. We believe that unlike reasoning models, neural network models help with neither prediction of health treatment nor some mechanism that can be potentially discovered experimentally.

Reasoning patterns, the subjects of this book, are the most insightful chunks of information that can be obtained, observing autistic phenomenology at different levels, from genetic to neural and to behavioral level. It is rather hard to build a bridge from neural circuitry to reasoning patterns directly. What can be done is establishing some features of existence. Building a neural model of some reasoning patterns, one can show that to implement certain reasoning patterns, there should exist a neural layer with certain patterns of firing. If a neural network can solve a particular AI problem, the conclusion is that *there exists* a way of a biological neural network to implement this functionality in the brain.

Let us imagine a search engine as a part of a brain, implemented as an inverse index searcher. There are certain patterns of activity for how the search engine reads this index from a disk, which can be observable from outside, without knowing semantics of search. Depending of search queries, different areas of index on the disk can be loaded. This pattern of activity becomes much more complicated when a search index is shared between multiple servers and some forms of shards are implemented (Fig. 2.6). Imagine that we have activity patterns data for disk access timing somewhat similar to neuron firing. How much can be said about search algorithms, given the observations of the patterns of activity of a search engine disk reading, having knowledge about Java implementation of memory management? Obviously not much. This example helps to explain our skepticism related to how the neural network models of the brain shed a light on how the brain implements reasoning.

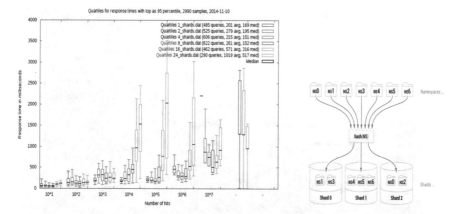

Fig. 2.6   The data on activity of distributed search system (on the *left*) and its architecture (on the *right*)

The idea that cognitive processes arise from the interaction of neurons through synaptic connections has been popular for a few decades. The knowledge in interactive and distributed neural systems is stored in the strengths of the connections and is acquired step-by-step in the course of accumulating experience. How can autistic reasoning and a degradation of semantic knowledge associated with this be explained via neural network models?

McClelland and Rogers (2003) hypothesize that degradation of semantic knowledge occurs through degradation of the patterns of neural activity that attempts to retrieve the knowledge stored in the connections. The authors demonstrate that through simulation models for development and disintegration of cognitive processes, with the focus on domain-specific patterns of generalization in young children and structure change of conceptual knowledge as a function of experience.

Rumelhart and Todd (1993) connectionist network is shown in Fig. 2.7. Inputs, consisting from concept-relation pair, are on the left and activation propagates to the right. Every unit in the pool on the sending side on the left projects to every unit on the receiving side on the right. The network is trained to turn on all these output units that represent the correct completions of the input patterns.

The connectionist neural model suggest there exists a representation unit such as temporal pole that ties together all objects properties with various types of information. Temporal pole is strongly affected by the semantic dementia disease. Temporal lobe can also be a region that stores addresses for conceptual representations. Patterns of activations in the temporal lobe capture semantic similarity between concepts and serve as means of semantic generalization on one hand. Also, damage in these areas disrupts the abilities to activate more specific properties of concepts elsewhere. The parallel distributed processing accounts of cognitive activity have

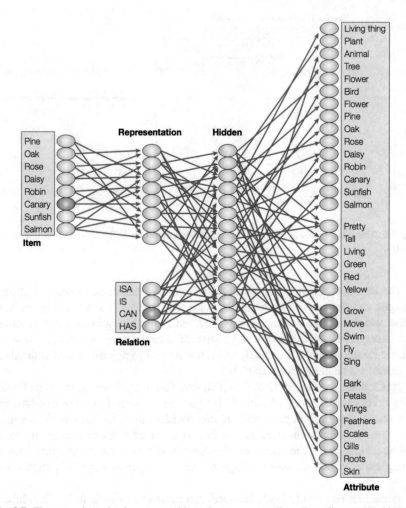

Fig. 2.7 The network used to learn propositions about concepts (From Rumelhart and Todd 1993)

posed a serious and pressing challenge to the view of the mind as a serial symbol manipulator (Clark 1989; Rumelhart and McClelland 1986).

Major brain structures implicated in autism are shown in Fig. 2.8.

2.3.2 Sensory Hyper-sensitivity

The combination of sensory hyperarousal and abnormal attentional selectivity suggests that autism may involve over-connected neural networks, in which signal is insufficiently differentiated from noise or irrelevant information and in which

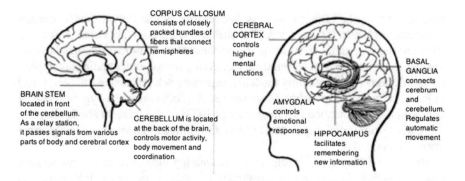

Fig. 2.8 The brain structures implicated in autism

information capacity is therefore reduced (Belmonte et al. 2004). This idea is consistent with genetic and neurochemical results, such as linkage to the 15q11–13 region, which contains a cluster of γ -amino-butyric acid (GABA) receptor genes (Buxbaum et al. 2002), low GABA receptor binding in hippocampus (Blatt et al. 2001), and low GABA levels in blood platelets (Rolf et al. 1993), and with the substantial comorbidity of epilepsy with autism. Also, substantial amount of noise in neural networks is associated with autistic psychophysical anomalies such as high visual motion coherence thresholds (Milne et al. 2002).

Low level visual, tactile and proprioceptive inputs are intact or even improved in CwA. At the same time, visual impairments occur at the level of image interpretation and integration of visual signals; it is still unclear if this is true for other modalities. Hyper-sensitivity and enhanced ability to detect details in input stimulus is augmented with difficulties in integrating sensory information into a coherent pattern. It is hypothesized that these difficulties contribute to motor deficits. The measures of motor coherence are correlated with motor skills of CwA. Gowen and Miall (2005) found out that CwA's performance is worse on motor tasks which require more sensory processing, such as pointing and timing, compared to repetitive tapping and hand turning. A miscalculated sensory input affects determination of the spatial state used to plan and modify movements. Babies who are visually hypersensitive or auditorily hypersensitive will need a more soothing type of enticement to take an interest in that outside world. Babies who are underreactive will require more animated interactions.

Baron-Cohen et al. (2008) argue that the excellent attention to detail in PwA is itself a consequence of sensory hyper-sensitivity. The authors review an experiment from our laboratory demonstrating sensory hyper-sensitivity detection thresholds in vision and conclude that the origins of the association between autism and talent begin at the sensory level, include excellent attention to detail and end with hyper-systemizing.

Mottron and Burack (2001) suggested an approach called 'enhanced perceptual functioning' of CwA associated with a stronger low-level perceptual processing.

Studies using questionnaires such as the sensory profile have revealed sensory abnormalities in over 90 % of CwA (Tomchek and Dunn 2007). In visual processing, PwA are more accurate at detecting the orientation of first-order gratings (simple, luminance-defined) but less accurate at identifying second-order gratings (complex, texture-defined). In the auditory modality, superior pitch processing has been found in PwA. In the tactile modality, Blakemore et al. (2006) showed a hyper-sensitivity to vibro-tactile stimulation to a frequency of 200 Hz but not for 30 Hz. In addition, the CwA group rated supra-threshold tactile stimulation as significantly more intense than CC did.

Hyper-sensitivity could result from a processing difference at various sensory levels including the density or sensitivity of sensory receptors, inhibitory and exhibitory neurotransmitter imbalance or speed of neural processing. Belmonte et al. (2004) suggested local range neural over-connectivity in posterior, sensory parts of the cerebral cortex is responsible for the sensory 'magnification' in CwA.

2.3.3   High or Low Connectivity?

The apparent contradiction between theories of over-connectivity and under- connectivity in autism may arise because of the multiple ways the term *connectivity* can be defined. One should differentiate local connectivity within neural assemblies from long-range connectivity between functional brain regions. On the other hand, one can separate physical connectivity (associated with synapses and tracts) from computational connectivity (associated with information transfer). Physically, in the autistic brain, high local connectivity may develop at the same time as low long-range connectivity develops (Just et al. 2004; Belmonte et al. 2004). It might be caused by frequent changes in synapse reduction and formation that breaks the computationally optimal balance between local and long-range connections. A decrease in network entropy due to indiscriminately high connectivity within local networks could yield abnormally low information capacity and may develop in tandem with abnormally low computational connectivity with other regions.

According to the under-connectivity theory there is an excess of low-level (sensory) processes, with under-functioning of high-level neural connections and synchronization (Gepner and Feron 2009). fMRI and EEG studies suggest local over-connectivity in the cortex and weak functional connections to/from frontal lobes. Under-connectivity is observed mainly within each hemisphere of the cortex. Autism may be in this view a disorder of the association cortex. The theory does not explain how and why this under -connectivity can arise, and how does it explain many specific autistic symptoms.

"Default brain network" (cingulate cortex, mPFC, lateral PC) shows low activity for goal-related actions; it is active in social and emotional processing, mind-wandering, daydreaming. Activity of the default network is negatively correlated with the "action network" (conscious goal-directed thinking), but this is not the case in autism. Perhaps this is a manifestation of under – connectivity, and shows disturbance of self-referential thought, necessary for development of the theory of mind.

There is an abnormal brain activation in a number of circuits under autism in a mirror neuron system (responsible for imitation) as well as other systems, and at the same time the performance of CwA on various imitation tasks may be normal. Another large neural subsystem related to the representation of the self-structures, the default mode network, has also been affected. The impairment of these two systems may be the result of general under-connectivity between spatially separated brain areas (Gepner and Feron 2009).

2.3.4 Deviation of Neural Network Functioning

The majority of studies in the area of computational autism focuses on autistic perception as most prominent autistic features and attempt to explain how the deviation of perception system architecture might explain what has been observed in experimental studies of autistic cognition. Peculiarities of visual, auditory and tactile autistic perceptions are analyzed.

Neural networks theories of cognitive processes state that many mental operations are carried out through successive sets (layers) of neuronal processing elements (Gordon 1997). With the proper input and training criteria, and the proper learning of rules, such networks have proven to be extremely efficient at extracting rules and patterns that are implicit in the data presented to them. However, the accuracy of this extraction is very dependent on the number of processing elements in the active learning layer (Baum and Hausler 1989). If there are too few elements then the network does not learn with very good accuracy: it, in fact, tends to over-generalize. If there are too many elements, then the network learns each specific situation presented to it and doesn't generalize enough. If some number of working elements leads to adequate performance, a somewhat greater number can result in truly superior performance in learning implicit rules and patterns, as long as it avoids becoming too specific.

This observation might be tied in to normal development, and to the abnormal development(s) that occur in autism, in the following way: the normal development of higher cerebral functions in a child's cortex appears to be driven by at least two major influences:

1. predetermined connections;
2. activity and use.

It has often been noted that the number of genes coding for the brain and neural tissue (about fifty thousand) are insufficient to specify all the connections of the mature brain. Thus, the development of these connections must be guided in part by experience. Edelman (1987) and (Edelman et al. 1997) have suggested that whether an uncommitted area develops connections with one region or another is based on the outcome of a competition for use. The developing child's brain normally has several primary sensory inputs which are hard-wired, including vision, audition, and touch. Such sensory inputs will attempt to stimulate upstream neuronal processing resources that are not yet employed.

Normally, the multiple influences on a child lead to a balance of forces, with the normal balance of lower and higher processing abilities (and neuroanatomic maps) as a result. The amount of neural tissue that is devoted to each higher function therefore represents a tradeoff between several forces: an attempt to optimize processing, the practical limits on optimization (because of lack of enough experience and training time), and competition with other functions for those same neuronal processing elements.

The hypothesis is that a developing brain of CwA has all those same forces at work, but for some reason some processing systems are impaired or delayed in their development. The systems in question are those involved in speech perception and speech production. Specific genetic deficits in speech generation have been tentatively identified, and it is plausible that there are combinations of deficits with more widespread effects on both speech generation and perception.

We continue to hypothesize that if the systems related to speech perception and speech production were developmentally impaired, then many higher abilities correlated with appropriate auditory input and output would never develop properly. Whatever cerebral tissue would have been devoted to those higher functions would then be free to be incorporated into other processes (assuming the tissue itself was not too badly affected by the same defects). If vision were intact, then visual-related abilities would be expected to rely on extra cerebral tissue. The result would be a child's brain that was not capable of *all* of the normal functions of a child, but that was capable of performing some functions satisfactorily. The brain would not be capable of those abilities that are related to speech and language capability, such as a long-term component of working memory (the part normally dependent upon an articulatory loop), and perhaps even such higher functions as the "inner voice" aspects of consciousness. It would, however, be extraordinarily good at wordless visual perception and analysis. Neuropathologically, such a brain might have only a few, apparently nonspecific, abnormalities. It would not have to have fewer neurons than normal.

In reality, the autistic brain is average or larger-than-average in size (Courchesne et al. 1999). It might be possible to detect additional areas responsible for visual-related functions, but perhaps not with current behavioral tasks and instrumentation. Autism may therefore represent disorders of activity-dependent plasticity during brain development that occur at several different levels: gene, synapse, neuron, network, and neuronal group.

In Fig. 2.9 solid arrows indicate direction of neural transmission, based on current information; large striped arrow depicts uncertain cerebellar effects. Large scissors depict cellular "lesions" in important structures that might contribute to network dysfunction or a "disconnection syndrome." Small scissors show potential sites for disconnection within networks and an example of "functional" (correct: globus

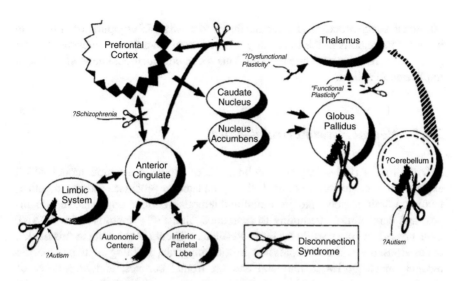

Fig. 2.9 Putative neural networks in autism

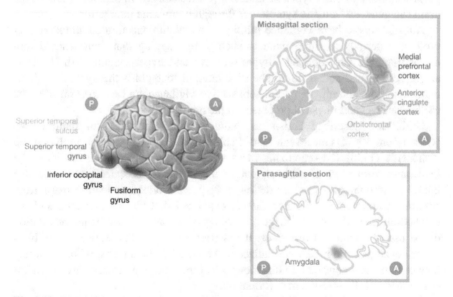

Fig. 2.10 The social brain (Adapted from Talairach and Tournoux 1988)

pallidus to thalamus) or "dysfunctional" (aberrant) repair that might occur from bypassing the globus pallidus. In schizophrenia, a disconnection is thought to occur between the dorsolateral prefrontal area and the anterior cingulate cortex (Benes et al. 1993).

Medial and inferior frontal and superior temporal cortices in Fig. 2.10, along with the amygdala, form a network of brain regions that implement computations relevant to social processes. Perceptual inputs to these social computations may arise in part from regions in the fusiform gyrus and from the adjacent inferior occipital gyrus that activate in response to faces. This social computational network has been implicated in autism.

2.3.5 Neural Network Architecture

iSTART model (Grossberg and Seidman 2006) proposes a neural model which explains how cognitive, emotional, timing and motor processes interact together, involving brain regions like prefrontal and temporal cortex, amygdala, hippocampus, and cerebellum, attempting to reproduce "autistic" symptoms. The iSTART model based on Grossberg's Adaptive Resonance Theory. According to this model, under-aroused emotional depression in the amygdala, learning of hyper-specific recognition categories in temporal and pre-frontal cortices, and breakdown of attention-based and motor circuits in hippocampus and cerebellum. The model proposes how particular types of imbalanced mechanisms in different parts of the brain can generate "autistic symptoms" through brain-wide interactions.

Autistic people have vigilance (ability to maintain concentrated attention over prolonged periods of time) fixed at such a high setting that their learned representations are very concrete, hyper-sensitive and hyper-specific. While this is an interesting and rather comprehensive attempt to build a theory that explains many symptoms of autism, parameters such as vigilance are hard to connect to the molecular level and physical processes in the brain.

Gustafsson described autism as deficient self-organization of feature map (Gustafsson 1997; Gustafsson and Paplinski 2003). His model is based on Kohonen's (1995) self-organizing maps where excessive inhibition results in the inadequate formation of cortical feature maps. He hypothesized that excessive lateral inhibition, as a primary deficit, may prevent adequate feature maps from forming. Courchesne and Allen (1997) explained that the parietal lobe and the cerebellum are both involved in the physiology of autism with cerebellar modulation of the use of attentional resources. It has been suggested that autism stems from under-developed and highly specialized and focused cortical maps, without overlap between different concepts. In this model, the initial amount of nerve-growth factor is assumed to influence the map formation.

Björne and Balkenius (2005) proposed a computational model with three interacting components for context sensitive reinforcement learning, context processing and automation to autonomously learn a focus attention and a shift attention task. The performance of the model is similar to that of normal children, and when a single parameter is changed, the performance on the two tasks approaches that of autistic children. To learn associations between stimuli and responses in a context dependent way, the authors use an extension of the Q-learning algorithm (Watkins and Dayan 1992). A ContextQ system learns associations between stimuli and responses based on the reinforcement. The CONTEXT system controls in what

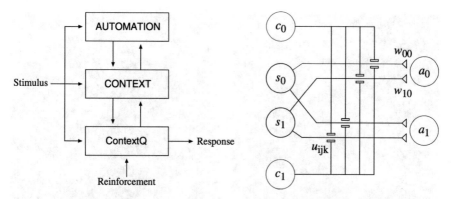

Fig. 2.11 Overview of the reinforcement learning model (on the *left*) and neural network-based implementation of the estimating function (on the *right*)

context each stimulus-response association should be used. The AUTOMATION system learns to produce stimulus-triggered contextual shifts (Fig. 2.11). The function of the context system is to integrate sensory input over time to create a code for the current context (Balkenius 2000). Here, it operates as a working memory for the last potential target that the system reacted to.

The function which assigns a value to each action in each states is approximated via an artificial neural network with shunting inhibition from the context nodes c_k to the association between a state node s_i and an action node a_j (Fig. 2.11 on the right).

Deuel (2002) proposed to represent autism as a common phenotype, characterized and explainable by an early onset of dysfunction in a circuit that involves cerebellar adaptive timing, the limbic and neocortical systems.

Overall, neural network models describe the features of meta-reasoning, and it is hard to correlate them with the feature of object-level reasoning. Majority of information is communicated in object-level, and only its specific parts is in meta-level.

2.3.6 Neural Simulation of Attention Deficit Disorder

To shift attention, neurons need to desynchronize and then synchronize again. In the language of dynamical systems this means that the trajectory of the system, describing neural activity has to leave one attractor basin and jump to another basin. However, neural dysfunctions may make this process difficult. One cause may be due to the damage of leak ion channels that slow down the process of spontaneous depolarization of neurons. Neurons stay in the same activity patterns for extended time, leading to hyper-specific memories, problems with disengagement of attention, and a general lack of flexibility of changing brain states. Lack of frequent changes of brain states in the developmental process will lead to under-connectivity.

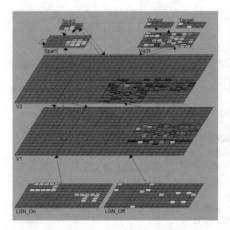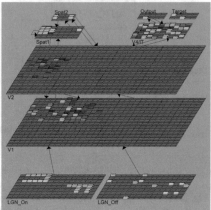

Fig. 2.12 Model of visual recognition (O'Reilly and Munakata 2000) based on Casanova (2007). Two steps of visual recognition simulation: on the *left* the first object was recognized, on the *right* after attention shifted to the second object

This is due to the fact that Hebbian learning mechanisms will not naturally increase the strength of distal connections. Attractor dynamics of two models implemented in the Emergent simulator has been studied to verify the attention hypothesis.

The first example is based on a model of visual recognition (Fig. 2.12), and it involves:

- recognition of two objects presented in the visual field;
- information is first processed by the on-off cells in the retina and passed to the thalamic lateral geniculate nuclei (LGN);
- from the LGN it is passed to the V1 and larger receptive fields of V2;
- the dorsal stream includes the V5/MT layers (Spat 1 and 2 in Fig. 2.12) that help to localize where the object is in the visual field and through the feedback connection helps to maintain the V2 and V1 activity focused on this object;
- the ventral stream includes V4/IT for object recognitions, and has connections with the V5/MT region.

Spat1 has recurrent activations and inhibition, focusing on a single object. In normal situations after a short time neurons desynchronize and synchronize on the second object, and as a result attention is shifted and the second object recognized. Damage to leak channels disables this process and the system cannot disengage attention from the first object for a long time. It is interesting that leak channels may also be damaged in the other direction letting large depolarizing current out, and thus ma- king the system unstable, jumping from one object to the other. This is characteristic of the attention deficit hyperactivity disorder (ADHD).

Thus, relatively simple low-level problem with properties of neurons may lead to autism and ADHD. Considering the influence of such problems on the development, a variety of symptoms may be explained.

2.4   Game-Theoretic Approach

The precise cognitive dysfunctions that determine the heterogeneity at the heart of this spectrum, however, remains unclear. Furthermore, it remains possible that impairment in social interaction is not a fundamental deficit but a reflection of deficits in distinct cognitive processes. To better understand heterogeneity within autistic spectrum, Yoshida et al. (2010) employed a game-theoretic approach to characterize unobservable computational processes implicit in social interactions.

Using a social hunting game with autistic adults, the authors found that a selective difficulty representing the level of strategic sophistication of others, namely inferring others' mindreading strategy, specifically predicts symptom severity.

In contrast, a reduced ability in iterative planning was predicted by overall intellectual level. Our findings provide the first quantitative approach that can reveal the underlying computational dysfunctions that generate the autistic "spectrum."

The game success score was significantly higher for the CwA group than for the control group, while there was no significant difference between the groups for both verbal and strategic intelligence scores. Both the control and the autistic group had a higher game score when they behaved more cooperatively, when the computer agent was more sophisticated. The participants in the autistic group showed a larger variety of behavior than the control participants.

To identify functional abnormalities in the computational processes involved in the task, Yoshida et al. (2010) used the Theory of Mind model and the fixed strategy model. The Theory of Mind model included two model parameters characterizing the cognitive processing: one is the upper bound of sophistication, which defines the capacity of strategic planning, and the other is a forgetting effect, which controls how quickly a player responds to changes in the other's sophistication, thereby representing a measure of cognitive flexibility. For the fixed strategy model, as it is assumed that players do not change their strategy, only the sophistication level is estimated.

Bayesian model selection based on the log likelihoods showed that the Theory of Mind model of CC with belief inference accounted for the behavior significantly better than the fixed strategy model without belief inference. At the same time the fixed strategy model explained individual behavior better for more than two-third of CwA. CwA were guided to a significantly lower degree of belief inference than that of the control participants. CwA also showed deficits in cognitive flexibility as they tend to be tied to their past strategies during the social game rather than a capability to flexibly change rules and strategies by paying attention the other's new actions (Sect. 6.4). Also the level of nested expressions of the mental world (*you think that I think that you think*, etc.) for PwA participants was related to IQ scores. A study using a "Beauty Contest" game has indicated an association between higher-level reasoning in CC and higher intelligence scores (Coricelli and Nagel 2009). Highly intelligent PwA behave cooperatively as if they make predictions over a longer time-horizon. This suggests that the level of sophistication, a key component of higher-level reasoning, can be inferred in more complex dynamic social exchanges.

Bermudez (2005) claims that a mechanism of emotional sensitivity including "social referencing" is a form of low-level mindreading that is required for proper social understanding and social coordination without involving the attribution of propositional attitudes. In game theory there are social interactions that are modeled without assuming that the agents involved are engaged in explaining or predicting each other's behavior. In social situations that have the structure of the iterated prisoner's dilemma: "start out cooperating and then mirror your partner's move for each successive move" (Axelrod 1984). Applying this heuristic rule relies on understanding the players' moves such as cooperation and defection, based on the information of what has happened in the last round. These are the patterns of social interaction that are conducted on the basis of a heuristic strategy that involves the results of previous interactions rather than their psychological flavor. To play these kinds of games successfully, one does not need to reason about other players' intents; one only have to coordinate our behavior with theirs.

2.5 Accounts of Autism

A number of psychological theories of autism have been proposed with varied relevance to autistic reasoning and computational interpretation. We will look at these theories from the computational perspective, analyzing which system architecture might be causing the respective algorithmic limitation. Each account is framed as a feature of information processing, which is explained to cause autistic behavior deficits (Sect. 2.1). The competition between the accounts of autism is grounded in how well the link

Reasoning, cognition & *information processing* → *behavior & skills*

is established, how many features of autistic behavior it can explain (Fig. 2.13), how mutually consistent is the explanation of the causal link, and how compatible is the given account with other popular accounts of autism.

Some of the most popular ones are:

- the Theory-of-Mind (ToM) deficit theory (Leslie 1987). We devote a separate chapter to it since it is mostly computationally feasible among other theories.
- the weak central coherence theory (Happe and Frith 2006)
- the executive function deficit theory (Russell 1997),
- joint attention, and
- the affective foundation theory (Hobson and Lee 1999).

One of the examples of autistic behavior caused by peculiar perception capabilities is stereotypy (Fig. 2.14).

Fig. 2.13 Causes of autistic behavior

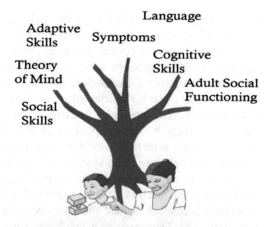

Fig. 2.14 Holding a palm near the mouth is not caused by social habits but stereotypy

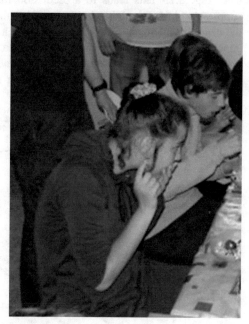

2.5.1 Weak Central Coherence Account

(Frith and Happe's 1994) weak central coherence theory of autism refers to an abnormally weak tendency to bind local details into global percepts. This theory is also built on the observation that CwA show certain supernormal abilities, including hyper-sensitivity. PwA are good at things which can be done by attention to detail while ignoring 'the big picture', particularly in some visual tasks. They show a lack of susceptibility to some visual illusions (e.g. Muller-Lyer 1889). Furthermore, they perform very well on the hidden figures task. The theoretical basis of weak central coherence is (Fodor 1983) theory of the modularity of mind.

Fodor postulated a central processing unit which processes the information supplied by the modules in a modality-free manner. Fodor viewed analogy and metaphor as the essential operations of the central processor. Weak central coherence states that under the distributed architecture in CwA the central processor does not fully perform its integrative function, resulting in the separate modules sharing their own specific information with other modules. As additional support for this account one may refer to the well-known inability of CwA to understand metaphor, and also their failure to exploit analogies in problem solving.

O'Loughlin and Thagard (2000) analyse several tasks on which autistic people are known to fail, such as the false belief task and the box task, and find that these tasks have a common logical structure that is identical to that of the suppression task (Fig. 2.15 This leads to a prediction for autistic people's behavior on the suppression task, which has been verified. This latter result is analyzed in terms of the neural implementation, which then gives a chance to make a connection to the genetics of autism. However, a structure of excitation and inhibition is fairly trivial and obviously not expressive enough to reproduce logical reasoning in its general form. Hence we believe that although such analysis is useful in understanding

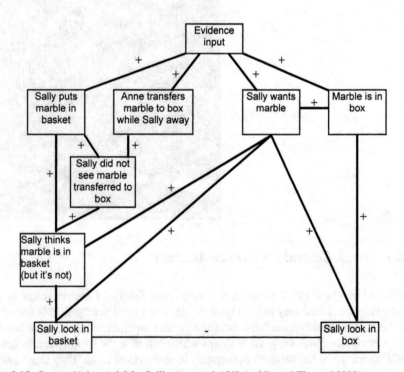

Fig. 2.15 Connectionist model for Sallie-Anne task (O'Loughlin and Thagard 2000)

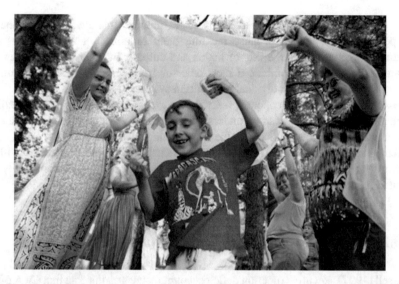

Fig. 2.16 Getting lost in a number of stimuli of various natures

a probable mechanism of integrative function, it cannot systematically advance our understanding of the reasoning capability of neither CwA nor neural-based intelligent machines.

Weak central coherence in autism has been demonstrated in the context of superior performance on visuo-motor tasks such as the Embedded Figures Test (Jolliffe and Baron-Cohen 1997), the Wechsler Block Design subtest (Shah and Frith 1983), tasks of visual discrimination and visual search (Plaisted et al. 1998), as well as impaired performance on more abstract tasks such as arranging sentences to form a coherent context (Jolliffe and Baron-Cohen 2000). The general pattern is one of superior segmentation of stimuli and attention to detail within these stimuli.

The week central coherence theory thus predicts that people with autism spectrum conditions will perform best on the tasks and occupations with focus on individual details (Fig. 2.16). At the same time, CwA are also mostly driven by the problems involving tons of details. Also, the Emphasizing-Systemizing theory predicts that people with autism spectrum conditions will be most driven by tasks and occupations that involve analysis of rule-based systems instead of generalization from data.

To a great extent, these predictions overlap: systemizing demands excellent attention to detail to isolate parameters that may then be tested individually for their effects on the system's output. From the ML point, CwA have decent skills to apply individual learning systems but are not capable of integrating them, applying, for example, a family of bagging and boosting algorithms (Zhi-Hua 2012).

However, differences in theoretical predictions arise in complex multimodal systems where a manipulation of inputs produces widespread effects on outputs, or when outputs vary with complex interactions among widely separated inputs.

The central coherence theory, taken by itself, predicts that PwA will be unable to perceive such stimuli because tackling them requires a global view of the interrelations between large sets of inputs and outputs. In other words, this is the engineering ability to combine a meta-detector from individual detectors, meta-recognizer from partial, individual recognition systems.

According to central coherence, CwA are expected to be capable of dealing with simple systems that can be understood in terms of relations between one or a few inputs and outputs. Conversely the Empathizing-Systemizing theory (Sect. 3.2), taken by itself, predicts that (relative to their mental age) people with autism will be able to learn how any sort of regular system works, regardless of its complexity, so long as it can be described by familiar and formalized rules.

2.5.2 Executive Function Deficit Account

Russell (1997) executive function deficit account focuses on the data that CwA often exhibit severe perseveration. They go on carrying out some routine when it is no longer appropriate. CwA show great difficulty in adjusting their action to a context (Fig. 2.17).

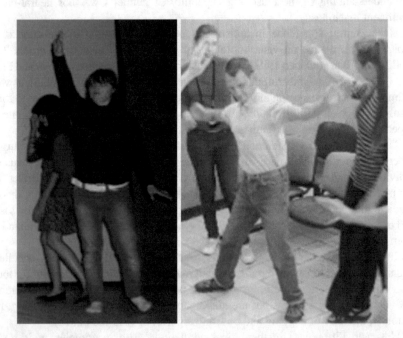

Fig. 2.17 CwA experience difficulties switching tasks with different movement and perception modes

They experience problems in switching tasks when the context calls for a switch, but it is not governed by any explicit rule. This perseveration gives rise to many of the symptoms of autism: obsessiveness, insensitivity to context, inappropriateness of behavior and literalness of carrying out instructions.

Task-switching is the brief of executive function, a process (or processes) responsible for high-level action control such as planning, initiation, co-ordination, inhibition and control of action sequences. Executive Function deficit also exists in the mental space, maintaining a goal, and pursuing it in the real world under possibly adverse circumstances. In this respect Executive Function deficit is correlated with extreme behavioral rigidity of CwA.

The origin of the concept of "Executive Function" deficit was heavily influenced by the analysis of neuropsychological patients. This has the important consequence that it is often most discussed in terms of its malfunctioning, and it is unclear how the proper executive function performs in humans and machines.

Situation calculus, AI theories of planning are expected to be relevant since they provide analyses of what is involved in planning action. On the contrary, the psychological study of normal planning of CC is mainly explored in the problem solving studies. Note that although CwA lack spontaneity, they may be able to carry out tasks involving fantasy play when instructed, as is indeed necessary if they are to engage with diagnostic tests such as the false belief task at all.

CwA's problem solving in turn has been most extensively studied in terms of the level of expertise, analyzing the difference between expert and novice problem solving. When discussing cognitive analyses of the malfunctioning of reasoning about mental states, it is natural that much clinical literature is oriented toward giving patients a unique categorization. A popular opinion of the contemporary psychiatry is that the existence of clusters of such categories is not always transparent. PwA are substantially more depressed, as measured by the relevant clinical diagnosis instruments, than the controls are.

It is unclear if executive dysfunction observed in autism is the same as the executive dysfunction observed in depression. The latter can be referred to as meta-executive dysfunction since depression affects reasoning about reasoning, not the object-level reasoning patterns like autism does. It is unclear if one could fractionate autistic problems, could the executive function subset be due to the accompanying depression. Studies (Ozonoff and Strayer 2001) challenge the view that PwA perform the Tower problems, WCST and similar complex problem solving tasks poorly because of a deficiency in working memory itself. Alternative theories have proposed that individuals with autism perform poorly on executive function tasks because of primary or inherent deficiencies in conceptual reasoning and planning abilities (Frith 1989; Frith and Happe 1994; Just et al. 2004). These models, the central coherence, complex information processing and underconnectivity models (Sect. 2.3) were proposed on the basis of the observation of a spectrum of deficits in higher order cognitive abilities and intact basic abilities in the same domains. In more detailed studies of individual cognitive domains, a relationship between increasing information processing demands and the emergence of deficits has been shown.

Following along these lines, we observe that successfully applying simple axioms for reasoning about mental states, CwA fail to apply more complex ones. At the same time one cannot say that ALL axioms in a given domain are absent. A reasoning system can possess an executive processing unit in the form of meta-reasoning, or reasoning about reasoning process that helps to control it. However, it is hard to imagine how a deep learning neural network system has a central coherence or executive function capability. Given a training set, it can be trained to solve a given problem, and it needs to be re-trained to solve another problem. An ensemble of deep learning systems would need an executive processor, but it has to have the same layered architecture so it is hard to imagine how it can implement the executive, meta-reasoning functionality that is totally different from multidimensional optimization functionality implemented by layered deep learning network.

Over last few decades, the popularity of neural networks was going up and down. After being a popular trend in the 1980s, they were dismissed as bunk by the AI establishment and the idea of "deep learning" was seen as scientific lunacy. At the time of writing of this book the neural network approach became popular again in the form of deep learning. Deep learning has become seen as technology's next big thing, sparking bidding wars among companies like Google to acquire companies researching ways to use deep learning. Deep learning applications are already working in major search engines including the image search. These algorithms allow users to image search terms like "handshake", get Smart Replies to their Gmail accounts and rely on machine translation. Deep learning is expected to be applied to other major problems like climate science, energy conservation, and in genomics.

Human brain has 1000-trillion synapses (10 to the power of 15). The largest computers have about a billion synapses, a million times less than brain. Deep learning scientist believe that expanding computer power and the size of training sets they can achieve the performance of the human brain. However, the observation of autistic brain does not support this belief: a huge sufficiently uniform neural network such as autistic brain is unable to learn from experience even simplest rules, such as that other people might have intent. It means that a uniform layered topology of a neural network, which includes fully functional neurons, cannot learn even very simple facts such as a basic binary relation between a subject and a mental object. Therefore, the claims about a connection between the deep neural network and the brain are premature.

Due to peculiar deviation in active learning process, as we will show in Sect. 7.3, people with autism spectrum conditions show unusually strong repetitive behaviors, a desire for routines, and a need for sameness.

The executive dysfunction theory also states that autism involves a form of frontal lobe pathology leading to perseveration or inability to shift focus. Although evidence for such executive deficits does exist (Pennington and Ozonoff 1996; Russell 1997), the high variance in measures of executive function in autism spectrum conditions, along with the lack of correlation between measures of executive function and measures of reciprocal social interaction and repetitive behaviors (Joseph and Tager-Flusberg 2004), suggests that executive dysfunction is unlikely to be a core feature of autism spectrum conditions.

The executive account has also traditionally ignored the content of repetitive behaviors. There are different ways repetitive behavior is explained. We demonstrate it by the deficiency in autistic active learning system, as a result of autistic cognitive development. On the contrary, Empathizing-Systemizing theory draws attention to the fact that much repetitive behavior involves the child's obsessional or strong interests, the foci of which cluster in the domain of strongly regular systems (Baron-Cohen and Wheelwright 1999). Rather than primary executive dysfunction, these behaviors may reflect an unusually strong interest in systems. Our explanation of this is that CwA have such strong interest in behavior patterns because they are unable to recognize less repetitive ones, not because of superior analytical skills.

Whilst some forms of repetitive behavior in autism, such as "stereotypies" (e.g., twiddling the fingers rapidly in peripheral vision) may be due to executive deficits, the executive account has traditionally ignored the content of "repetitive behavior".

The current account draws attention to the fact that much repetitive behavior involves the child's "obsessional" or strong interests with mechanical systems (such as light switches or water faucets) or other systems that can be understood in physical-causal terms. Rather than these behaviors being a sign of executive dysfunction, these may reflect the child's intact or even superior development of their folk physics. The child's obsession with machines and systems, and what is often described as their "need for sameness" in attempting to hold the environment constant, might be signs of the child as a superior folk-physicist: conducting mini-experiments in his or her surroundings, in an attempt to identify physical-causal principles underlying events.

A recent study of obsessions suggests that these are not random with respect to content (which would be predicted by the content-free executive dysfunction theory), but that these tests are clustered in the domain of folk physics (Baron-Cohen and Wheelwright 1999).

2.5.3 Autistic Memory

In the case of verbal linguistic tasks, increasing grammatical complexity of sentences leads to the emergence of deficits in high functioning autistic individuals, as did the transition from syntax to discourse (words to sentences to stories). In a study of memory using an extensive battery of tests, memory for simple information was demonstrated to be intact, documenting the preservation of basic associative memory processes (Minshew and Goldstein 2001). However, as the complexity of the task is getting higher, autistic deficits became more and more visible, as the use of contextual structure and organizational strategies to support memory diminishes (Fig. 2.18).

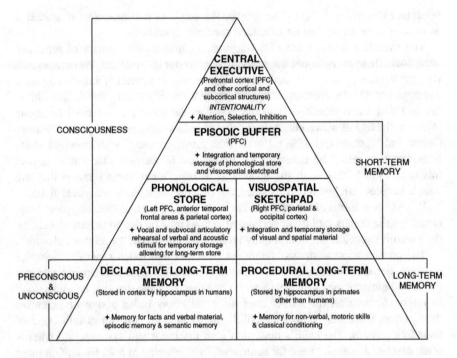

Fig. 2.18 The architecture of consciousness and working memory

An interesting discovery in autism research is that having verbal working memory intact, CwA' s spatial working memory may possibly be corrupted. Ozonoff and Strayer (2001) used a spatial memory-span task (recall of the location of three to five geometric shapes on a computer screen) and a box search task (participants had to search for objects hidden behind colored boxes using a method that required holding the color of the boxes in working memory during the search). Significant differences between CwA and CC were not found for either of these two tasks. Other measures of spatial working memory such as eye movement studies have also provided different results. The delayed oculomotor response task (memory-guided saccade) has been used as a measure of spatial working memory since the development of the technique with non-human primates by (Kojima and Goldman-Rakic 1982). In this procedure, the participant fixates on a central point, a peripheral target is presented and then extinguished, and the task is to make an eye movement to the remembered location of the target following a delay. Minshew et al. (1999) showed that CwA did significantly less well on this task than did CC with increased rates of response suppression errors and impaired precision in reaching the target. The saccades of CwA were very close to the target location but did not achieve the precise location.

Williams et al. (2005) attempted to address the inconsistent literature regarding verbal working memory and spatial working memory in CwA by using tasks that assess the status of working memory components without involvement of planning or reasoning tasks. The authors also verified the hypothesized intactness of verbal working memory and impairment of spatial working memory by assessing these different abilities in the same individuals with high-functioning autism.

If the autism groups do more poorly than controls on the spatial tasks but not on the verbal tasks, it may be because the spatial tasks are more difficult and, therefore, more sensitive to cognitive deficits associated with autism. A traditional method of evaluating task difficulty is to evaluate the degree of association between task performance and general intelligence (Full Scale IQ).

The children, adolescents and adults with autism performed at similar levels relative to the cognitive and age-matched controls on the working memory tasks that involved the articulatory loop and performed poorer than the controls on the tasks that involved the visuospatial sketchpad. These findings demonstrate a dissociation between verbal and spatial working memory in the same individuals with autism. Intact verbal working memory and impaired spatial working memory have been demonstrated in multiple studies.

Williams et al. (2005) found no deficit in verbal working memory or the articulatory loop in high-functioning PwA. They exhibited difficulties in spatial working memory or the visuo-spatial sketchpad. These data do not support spatial or verbal working memory impairments as the core deficits underlying problem solving and planning impairments in PwA but confirm the existence of inherent dysfunctions in problem solving itself as the source of difficulty on tasks such as the Tower of London/Hanoi.

2.5.4 Account of Complex Information Processing Failure

It is now generally understood that the behavioral syndrome of autism is the result of multiple primary deficits and that these deficits involve the processing of information and are the result of the underdevelopment of the neural systems of the forebrain and not regional dysfunction (Minshew and Goldstein 1998). Although five to ten percent of CwA are the result of other diseases, the majority of cases are thought to be the result of about five abnormal genes coding for or regulating brain development (Rutter et al. 1994).

For humans and machines, complex information processing is a conceptual construct, not a specific ability. It is a term for a class of abilities that place high computational demands on the brain or a processing unit. Deficits in specific abilities such as theory of mind and executive function that are commonly discussed in connection with autism all fall under this general construct (Sutton et al. 1999).

The value of this conceptual construct is that it emphasizes the need to evaluate tasks autistic individuals cannot do in terms of the computational demands on the brain. This approach provides guidelines for modifying the demands of tasks that individuals are unable to do. However, the scientific value is that this term is also used in the neurophysiology to characterize delayed cognitive potentials. This account also encourages thinking about brain algorithms in terms of developmental processes in the brain involved in the emergence of the intricate circuitry of the forebrain. The complex information processing account makes it easy to relate findings across several levels of the pathophysiology of autism. Such links are critical if the cause of autism is to be understood.

According to the current account, autism is a selective disorder of complex information processing abilities with intact simple information processing abilities. The common denominator of deficits in autism is the high demands placed on information processing or computation by the brain. The complex information processing model explains why these particular symptoms together form a syndrome and the failure of IQ scores. This model also predicts the common co-occurrence of mental retardation in autism, and the difference between autism and general mental retardation. The validity of this characterization of cognitive functioning in autism is supported by its reciprocal relationship with the neuropsychologic profile for the simple information processing disease. The presence of this same dissociation between deficient complex and intact simple abilities in the motor domain further confirms the validity of this construct. The relationship of deficits in autism to their computational demands on the brain is helpful in comprehension and analysis of behavioral and academic difficulties of CwA.

The human mind's activity of taking in, storing, and using information is shown in Fig. 2.19. In early models, input flows into the sensory registers (eyes, ears) and then information proceeds to short-term memory. Short-term memory holds information for only a moment, and then it combines it with information from the long-term memory. With effort, information moves into long-term storage. The short-term memory generates responses (output).

Information is encoded in sensory memory; perception determines what will be held in working memory. Working memory manages the flow of information and integrates new information with knowledge from long-term memory. Connected information that is thoroughly processed can become part of long-term memory. When that information is activated it moves to working memory. Each part of

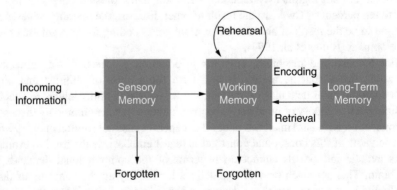

Fig. 2.19 From sensory to long-term memory

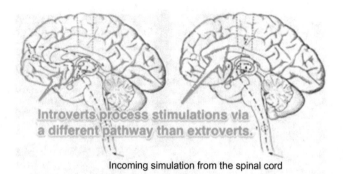

Incoming simulation from the spinal cord

Fig. 2.20 A difference between the information processing pathways of extraverts and introverts

the system interacts with the others to guide perception; represent, organize and interpret information; apply and modify propositions, concepts, images, schemas, and strategies; construct knowledge; and solve problems (Fig. 2.19). Extrovert individuals process information via a different pathway to introvert individuals, including CwA (Fig. 2.20). Acetylcholine pathway of introverts is longer than the one of extraverts.

2.5.5 Affective Foundation Account

Greenspan (1997) attempts to derive ToM from a fundamental ontogenetic processes – in particular from the affective foundations of interpersonal communication. Humans uniquely control shared attention, especially by gaze (Fig. 2.21). We diagnose where others' attention is focused from information about where they are looking. 'Intersubjectivity' is established through mutual control of attention. Just as Piaget saw the child's sensorimotor activity as achieving the child's mastery of where itself left off and the world began, so Hobson sees the child's understanding of itself as a social being separated from others being achieved through joint attentional activity. The child must learn that the other can have different representations, and different wants and values. Hobson proposes that it is autists' valuation of these experiences of intersubjectivity which is abnormal. If the child does not experience the achievement of intersubjectivity as rewarding (or even experiences it as aversive), then any cognitive developments founded on it will not develop normally. Cognitive symptoms of autism are, on this theory, consequences of this valuation.

Hobson et al. (2013) followed pretend play among young children with autism. Age- and language-matched children with autism, autism spectrum disorder, and developmental disorders without autism were administered for the Test of Pretend Play (Lewis and Boucher 1997), with an additional rating of 'playful pretense'. As predicted, children with autism showed less playful pretend than participants

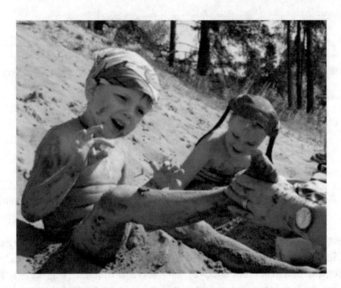

Fig. 2.21 CC's attention to a foot being grabbed by someone by a CC

with developmental disorders who did not have autism. Across the groups, playful pretense was correlated with individual differences in communication and social interaction, even when scores on the pretend play test were taken into account. Limitations in creative, playful pretend among children with autism relate to their restricted interpersonal communication and engagement.

In The Growth of the Mind (1997), Greenspan showed how emotions create, organize, and orchestrate many of the mind's most important functions, including intelligence and emotional health. He further showed that intellect, academic abilities, sense of self, consciousness, and morality have common origins in our earliest and ongoing emotional experiences and that emotions are the architects of a vast array of cognitive operations throughout the life span.

During the formative years there is a sensitive interaction between genetically – set abilities and environmental experience, which we formalize via active learning framework in Sect. 7.3. Experience appears to adapt the infant's biology to his or her environment (Hofer 1995). In this process, however, not all experiences are the same. Children seem to require certain types of experiences involving a series of specific types of emotional interactions geared to their particular developmental needs.

The difficulty in connecting affect to motor planning and symbols discussed in the last section is only one part of a larger set of transformations of affect that depend on specific types of emotional interactions. To more fully understand the importance of affect in autism, and the development of intellectual and social skills, it may prove useful to explore a number of affective transformations during the first 3 years of life.

In the first year, affects become more complex. There is a transition from simple affective states like hunger and arousal to, by 8 months, complex affect states like surprise, fear and caution, joy and happiness, and enthusiasm and curiosity. As the child progresses, affects become more differentiated. Eventually, affects organize reciprocal interactions and problem-solving. Then they become symbolized. Eventually, it becomes possible to reflect on them. The transformation procedure can be described in terms of six core early organizations that give the organism its desire to act and underlie intelligence and emotional health (Greenspan 1997).

First, to attend to the outside world, and eventually to have joint attention or shared attention, requires affective interest in the world outside one's own body—in sights, sounds, and movements. Obviously, parents who provide pleasurable sights and sounds to a new baby will entice the baby into focusing on the world.

The affect diathesis account focuses on the inability to connect affect or intent to motor planning capacities and emerging symbols capacities for empathy, psychological mindedness, abstract thinking, social problem-solving, functional language, and affective reciprocity all stem from the infant's ability to connect affect or intent to motor planning capacities and emerging symbols (Greenspan 1992).

Relative deficits in this core capacity leads to problems in higher-level emotional and intellectual processes. The core psychological deficit in autism may, therefore, involve an inability to connect affect (i.e., intent) to motor planning and sequencing capacities and symbol formation.

Consider a 14-month-old child who takes his father by the hand and pulls him to the toy area, points to the shelf, and motions for a toy. As the father picks him up, and he reaches for and gets the toy, he nods, smiles, and bubbles with pleasure. For this complex, problem-solving social interaction to occur, the infant needs to have an emotional desire or wish (i.e., intent or affective interest) that indicates what he wants. The infant then needs to connect his desire or affective interest to an action plan (i.e., a plan to get his toy). The direction-giving affects and the action plan together enable the child to create a pattern of meaningful, social, problem-solving interactions. Without this connection between affect and action plans, complex interactive problem-solving patterns are not possible. Action plans without affective direction or meaning tend to become repetitive (perseverative), aimless, or self-stimulatory, which is what is observed when there is a deficit in this core capacity.

2.5.6 Thinking in Pictures Account of Autism

Kunda et al. (2010) analyze the hypothesis that some individuals on the autism spectrum may use visual mental representations and processes to perform certain tasks that typically developing individuals perform verbally. They present a framework for interpreting empirical evidence related to this "Thinking in Pictures" hypothesis and then provide comprehensive reviews of data from several different cognitive tasks, including the n-back task, serial recall, dual task studies, Raven's Progressive

Matrices, semantic processing, false belief tasks, visual search and attention, spatial recall, and visual recall.

In her well-known autobiographical book "Thinking in Pictures", Temple Grandin (2006) describes how her visual thinking style benefits her work in engineering design but also creates difficulties in understanding abstract concepts. Assuming that CC are able to use both visual and verbal mental representations, Kunda et al. (2010) build upon the observation that CwA prefer the former over that latter.

For an abstract hardware image understanding system, how can one determine whether it operates with visual patterns directly (being a pictorial-level representation system) or use a logic forms layer where information extracted from an image is represented "verbally"? Usually, the latter system is much more flexible and robust to image deviations. For a simpler object identification task, there are two classes of approaches:

1. Given a database of images of candidate objects, compare its records with the given image within the sliding window till we get a high value of pixel similarity. In case of high similarity of a database image of a given object with a certain area of the image being recognize, we conclude about the respective recognize object. This kind of system is close to Google Image Search, when given an image, the system attempts to find a similar one, without deep interpretation.
2. Given an ontology of features of objects to be identified, we first ascend from the level of pixels to the level of presentation of these features as logic forms, and then try to satisfy the "verbal" definitions of these objects. This approach is much less sensitive to noise in the image, to how an object can be viewed, illumination conditions etc. Also, this approach is much more efficient since a rule system and an ontology is much more compact than a database of sample images. Such systems are employed in abroad range of applications from medical to driver-less cars.

Hence from the engineering standpoint, a verbal system is much for advantageous than a pictorial, non-verbal, operating with images directly without an upper abstraction layer.

Evidence from neuropsychology has suggested that visual and verbal semantic memory are somewhat dissociated, in that brain lesions can selectively impair the use of one or the other (Hart and Gordon 1992).

In the n-back task (Sect. 2.2, Kirchner 1958), a subject is presented with a sequence of stimuli and asked whether the current stimulus matches the one shown n steps ago. The variable n can take the value of one (respond "yes" to any succession of two identical stimuli), two (respond "yes" to any stimulus matching the one presented two steps back), and so on. Stimuli can vary as to their content and presentation, such as letters presented visually or auditorily, pictures, etc.

For CC the n-back task is thought to recruit verbal rehearsal processes in working memory (i.e. phonological verbal representations), among other executive resources (Smith and Jonides 1999). Recent fMRI studies have shown that, while behavioral measures on the n-back task may be similar, there can be significant differences

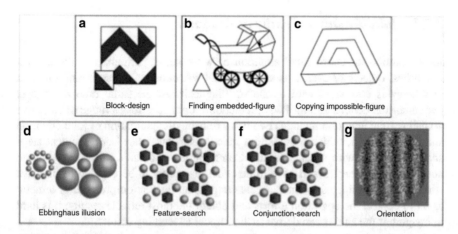

Fig. 2.22 Cognitive strengths in autism

in patterns of brain activation between CwA and CC. In one study using stimuli of visually presented letters, the autism group showed less brain activation than controls in left prefrontal and parietal regions associated with verbal processing and greater activation in right hemisphere and posterior regions associated with visual processing (Koshino et al. 2005). In another study using stimuli of photographs of faces, a similar decrease in left prefrontal activation was found in the autism group (Koshino et al. 2008). These studies suggest that individuals with autism may be using a visual strategy for the n-back task, whereas controls use at least a partially verbal strategy.

Visual strength in autism is depicted in Fig. 2.22. On the top, left to right: Block Design part of the Wechsler test of intelligence, Locating embedded figures, copying impossible figures. On the bottom: Identifying target size in Ebbinghaus illusion, Finding the odd-man-out in cluttered displays whether the target is defined by a single feature or a conjunction of features, tolerating higher levels of noise in determining an object orientation.

Weak Central Coherence account hypothesizes that individuals with autism have a limited ability to integrate detail-level information into higher-level meanings, or are at least biased towards local instead of global processing (Happe and Frith 2006). This trait is presumed to account for some of the stereotyped patterns of behaviors and interests in individuals with autism. These observations can also be explained under the Thinking in Pictures hypothesis by enhanced visual attentional strategies that could arise from a bias towards pictorial representations. Other evidence for Weak Central Coherence often includes verbal tests, such as deficits in homograph pronunciation in sentence contexts (as cited in Happe and Frith 2006). These tests, while measuring local, word-level versus higher-order, sentence-level processing, can also be interpreted as tests of verbal reasoning skills, which would be impaired under the Thinking in Pictures account.

2.5.7   Joint Attention Family of Accounts

Joint attention, or coordinated attention between social partners to share interest in entities, objects or events, is an essential PwA deficit. Reduced joint attention in infancy is correlated with an autism diagnosis. At the same time a range in joint attention deficits among PwA predict development across a range of cognitive domains. Joint attention includes two types of behaviors, initiation of joint attention and response to it, which may exhibit independent but related development steps and associations with other domains. Communities of default software agents do not have joint attention and have to be coded explicitly to be capable of perceive stimuli in a coordinated manner. Agents require an interaction protocol or a meta-agent to control the cognition efforts and obtain the most reliable results; it is hard to imagine if the agents can derive such protocol as learning results.

According to social-cognitive theory of joint attention, it is yielded by under-standing of others' intentions. At the same time, according to the parallel and distributed processing model of joint attention, it develops with increasing represen-tational skills. The evidence that joint attention deficits are caused by face-to-face difficulties is rather weak. This evidence is supported by associations between joint attention and developmental levels, which backs up the parallel and distributed processing rather than the social-cognitive model.

There is a popular opinion that initiation of joint attention is more of a core difficulty in autism than response to joint attention, since it may be more consistently impaired in the course of life of a PwA. However, when thoroughly measured, a response to joint attention may also be impaired across development. The evidence that starting of joint attention is more of a core deficit than responding to it is rather weak.

Joint attention is a pivotal skill that novices can use to acquire information from others – it is related to subsequent development across a range of domains for CC and CwA. Individual differences in joint attention among people on the spectrum are predictive of adaptive skills, symptoms, social functioning, linguistic skills and cognitive development.

An associations between early joint attention and subsequent development are often considered as evidence for the social-cognitive theory of joint attention where the development of joint attention from simpler social behaviors (such as face-to-face engagement) reflects an emerging understanding of others as intentional agents that in turn initiates a subsequent symbolic development (Fig. 2.23).

Alternatively, rather than arising from and being defined by an understanding of others' mental states, joint attention may not initially reflect social understanding but may lead to social knowledge (Fig. 2.24, Gillespie-Lynch 2013). According to the parallel and distributed processing model of joint attention, it arises from an increas-ing ability to integrate information about oneself, another and the conjunction of the self and other in relation to an external object (triadic relations). The key distinction between the two models is the relative importance of understanding another person's mind versus the importance of practice representing triadic relationships.

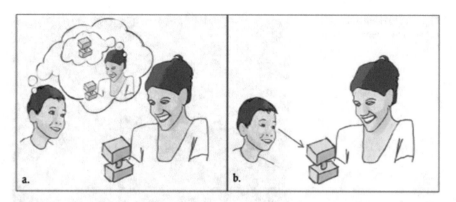

Fig. 2.23 The child turns to attend to the object because he realizes that the adult has communicative intent

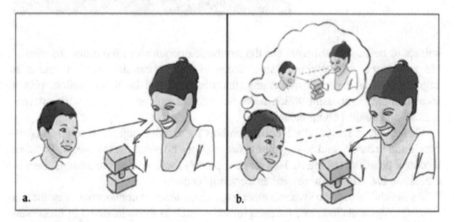

Fig. 2.24 Under parallel and distributed processing model of joint attention, the child practices representing triadic relations by engaging in joint attention

Passing a ball, a human involves a triadic relation between herself and her intent to have a peer grab the ball, the intent of the ball receiver and the ball itself (Fig. 2.25). Learning triadic relation can be a substitute for learning the actual mental world if there is a difficulty understanding the latter.

2.5.8 From Intent to Symbolic Representation

The brain can operate as an analogue or symbolic solver. Literature on brain research does not explicitly differentiate between these two classes of solvers that makes the discussion not as concise as desired. We will now define these classes of

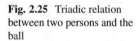

Fig. 2.25 Triadic relation between two persons and the ball

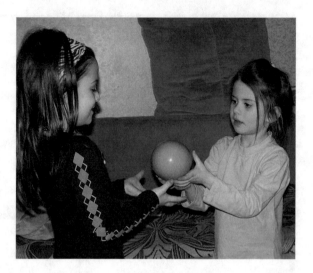

solvers to better explain what are the symbolic operations in the brain. To control the movement, an analogue system needs to solve a certain equation, and it is implemented as a neural subsystem which is described by this equation, plus a measurement component which links the internal analogue solver with external sensors and control components.

Conversely, a symbolic solver has symbols for external objects which it comprehends and controls, and also symbols for relations between these objects. To make a control decision, the internal solver manipulates these symbols to arrange them in a position that can be interpreted as a control scenario.

As the ability to form symbols emerges, a child needs to connect her inner affects (intent) to symbols to create meaningful ideas, such as those involved in functional language, imagination, and creative and logical thought. The meaningful use of symbols usually emerges from earlier and continuing meaningful (affect-mediated) problem-solving interactions that enable a toddler to understand the patterns in her world and eventually use symbols to convey these patterns in thought and dialog.

Without affective connections, symbols like action plans are used in a repetitive (perseverative) manner (e.g., scripting, echolalia). The capacity to connect affect to action plans and symbols is likely part of a larger transformation of affect. The infant goes from global and/or catastrophic affective patterns (in the early months of life) to reciprocal ones. The capacity for engaging in a continuous flow of reciprocal affective interactions enables the child to modulate mood and behavior, functional preverbal and verbal communication, and thinking.

It also enables more flexible scanning of the environment because the child gets feedback from what he sees and, based on that feedback, explores further. There is, therefore, more integrated visual-spatial and motor functioning because intense global affects push for discharge and vigilant or overly focused or highly distractible

Fig. 2.26 Trying to attract
attention

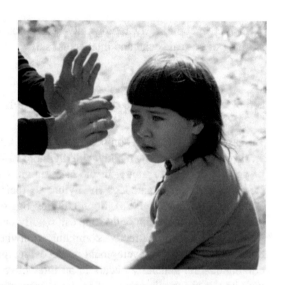

visual-motor patterns, whereas long chains of reciprocal interaction support back-and-forth exploration of the environment and, therefore, flexible, broad, integrated perceptual patterns.

In facilitating back-and-forth interaction with the environment, the capacity for reciprocal interaction also facilitates associative learning. Associative learning (building up a reservoir of related experiences, thoughts, feelings, and behaviors which give range and depth to one's personality, inner life, and adaptive responses) is necessary for healthy mental growth. Its absence leads to rigid, mechanical feelings, thinking, and behavior patterns, as are often seen in CwA (Fig. 2.26).

Processing deficit occurs early in life, it can undermine CwA capability to engage in expectable learning interactions essential for many critical emotional and cognitive skills. For example, CwA may have more difficulty causing usual expected interactions from his parents. CwA may perplex, confuse, frustrate, and undermine purposeful, interactive communication with even very competent parents. Without appropriate explicit introduction of the rules of interaction, he will be unable to either comprehend these rules of complex social interactions himself or to develop a sense of himself. These may include implicit social functions and social "rules," and developing friendships and a sense of bond with his peers, which are learned mostly between the age of 12 and 24 months (Emde et al. 1991). By the time CwA with processing difficulties officially diagnosed, his challenging interaction patterns with his peers have already excluded him from important learning sessions and may have amplified his difficulties. The loss of engagement and intentional, interactive relatedness to key caregivers may cause CwA to withdraw more idiosyncratically into his own world. CwA then becomes even more aimless and/or repetitive. What later looks like a primary biological deficit may, therefore, be part of a dynamic process through which the child's lack of affective reciprocal interactions has intensified specific, early, biologically-based processing problems and derailed the learning of critical social and intellectual skills.

2.5.9   Steps in the Normal Development

An early and continuing component of shared attention involves attention to the world outside of one's own body with rhythmic, affectively-mediated motor patterns of perception. For example, in the early months of life, babies can be observed to move their arms and legs in rhythm to their mother's voices (Condon and Sander 1974; Condon 1975). Soon children begin integrating what they hear and see (Sect. 7.3). By 4–5 months, one can readily observe synchronous movement in rhythm with mother's affective communication via her voice, facial expressions, or body movements. As development proceeds, reciprocal gestural, vocal, and verbal communication generally occurs in an interactive rhythm. A consequence of this may be the observation that it's harder to remember or understand verbal phrases presented in a monotone than in an affective rhythm.

The second functional developmental capacity is *engagement*. For an infant to engage with a caregiver requires joy and pleasure in that relationship. When that's not present, children can withdraw and become self-absorbed. For children who have processing problems, it may be much harder to pull them into that joyful relationship.

(Greenspan 2001) observed that most children can be pulled into various degrees of relating through therapeutic work that works with processing differences and relationships of CwA at the same time. Engagement and relating appears to be a very flexible capacity. While language and certain cognitive functions may improve slowly for some children, the capacity for warmth and relatedness seems to progress more readily.

The third functional developmental capacity is *two-way purposeful communication*. Two-way communication and affective reciprocity obviously requires affect to provide the "intent." When an infant reaches for his daddy to take the rattle off his head or hand it back to him, or gets into a back-and-forth smiling game, one clearly sees affect (intent) guiding the interaction (i.e., the infant wants that rattle). According to (Greenspan 2001), Piaget thought that means-ends relationships occurred at 9 months with motor behavior (i.e., an infant reaching and pulling a string to ring a bell).

The baby's affective probe occurs much earlier than the motor probe. Causal affective behavior occurs earlier than causal large muscle motor behavior. First we see a smile causing a smile, a frown getting a frown. Later on, we see the baby reach for and give back objects. At this stage as well, the affect diathesis is occurring, now transforming relating into two-way, affective communication (rather than just joyful interest in the caregiver).

The fourth level of transformation occurs between 10 months and 18 months. It involves the development of a range of new capacities, all related to the toddler's ability to *engage in longer sequences of affective reciprocal interactions* with clear intent or problem-solving goals and the ability to perceive and interact in these larger patterns. This transformation enables the toddler to form a more integrated sense of self, integrate affective polarities, social problem-solve, and broaden visual-spatial and auditory processing abilities.

In this fourth stage, the child is also beginning to integrate affective polarities. Early on, infants tend to have extreme affect states—all happy or gleeful or all sad— but by 18–19 months we see children begin to shift affect states more readily and actually integrate affect states such as happiness and sadness, anger and closeness.

They can be angry and then seem to want forgiveness and make up. When playing with a 13-month-old child, it feels like if he were angry and had a gun, he very well might pull the trigger. With the 18-month-old, it feels like he integrates his caring and anger. He might look mad and feel connected and warm at the same time. One can often feel the quality of these affect states when playing with infants and toddlers at different ages.

At the fifth level, transformations involve the affect system investing ideas. For example, in pretend play, affects or desires drive the theme (dolls hugging or kissing) as well as functional language ("I'm hungry," "I'm angry," "Give me that." "Look! I want to show you something."). Functional language, whether it's on a need basis ("Give me juice."), or at a collaborative "show you this or that," or sharing opinions "I didn't like that" basis, is very different from simply labeling objects or pictures.

Here is also where IQ tests fall down. IQ tests do not differentiate well enough between the different uses of ideas and language, such as between pragmatic language or creative and abstract thinking versus a simple using language to label objects or for rote, memory-based problems.

At the sixth level of transformation, a child builds bridges between affectively meaningful ideas. Establishing reality-testing, a symbolic sense of self, and moving back and forth between a fantasy to reality depends on reaching this next level. For example, critical to establishing reality-testing (which is the basis for later abstract thinking) is an affective "me" intending to do something with an affective "other."

There has to be an interaction involving affect between the "me" and the "other" to establish a psychological boundary (i.e., an affective sense of what's "me" and an affective sense of what's "outside me"). That boundary doesn't come out of reading books or out of doing puzzles. It comes from interactions involving the exchange of affective gestures and symbols. It comes out of interactions such as "I want this." "No, you can't have it," or "Yes, you can." In addition, these interactions must be part of a continuous flow of back-and-forth affective gestures. Islands of affective interactions followed by self-absorption leads to an "in and out" affective probe or rhythm with the external world (reality). A stable sense of reality requires a continuous interactive relationship to the significant "others" in our lives. Abstract and inferential thinking grows from a solid reality boundary.

2.5.10   *Accounts of Autism and Corporate Environment*

Having compared CwA with controls, we observed a number of ways the deficiency of the former can be described and represented as a series of models. A control child have an ability to execute well each of these models. Is it true for a community of agents (a multiagent system, an organization, a company) each of which possesses ToM, proper executive function, proper central coherence, and other reasoning capabilities? The answer is "no". With a certain motivational structure of agents, which can be referred to as "bureaucratic", a multiagent system of capable agents evolves into an entity whose behavior is rather abnormal. In this section we consider various accounts of autism in the context of multiagent systems and demonstrate that multiagent systems are frequently closer to CwA than to CC in terms of the accounts of this chapter.

Once capable in individual capacity agents (human and possible automated) are functioning in the framework of an organization (a company), their motivational and knowledge structure is such that as an overall system they frequently become totally unintelligent (from the standpoint of an external observer, a user of this company). This is because the agents (of a company customer support) have conflicting goals: to impress the user that they want to satisfy his requests on one hand, and to save company's resources on the other hand. At the same time, the customer support agents have their personal goals to save their own resources (Sect. 4.1.2). Having these conflicting goals, the multiagent system impresses their users and peers as the one with corrupt reasoning patterns. We will share the examples from the personal experience of the author.

A financial company providing online Tax services, H&R Block assists its customers with filing tax returns online. Driven by a broad range of government regulations, H&R block is concerned with a lot of issues of compliance with the regulations, including privacy, security, disclosure to tax officials, and others. Nevertheless, they loose online customer tax return data and get away with this. Maintaining their focus on less important issues (from the customer viewpoint), they are unable to retain the customer data worth of hours of work to re-input. Nothing can be worse from the customer viewpoint. Their customer support is unable to address this problem either, citing the split between H&R Block Online Services that do not have their own customer support and H&R Block customer support that is detached from the Online Services. Hence the way some multiagent systems are frequently formed show the lack of central coherence.

Another example is a Citibank scenario:

- A customer applied for a credit card
- Citibank responded that the application was denied
- In a month Citibank sent a bill with an annual fee for this credit card (this card was never received and never activated).
- In 2 months Citibank sent a bill for the unpaid annual fee plus the late payment charge for this fee because this annual fee was never paid (because the card was never issued, according the customer).

- The customer becomes aware of this incident and tries to cancel the non-existing cards and dispute the fees. This process takes months and months.

There is an unlimited amount of documents on the web reporting an unreasonable behavior of multiagent systems in the form of corporations, interacting and communicating with single agents (individuals). Taking into account that each agent of this multiagent system is a rational agent (a control human with full-functioning systems described in autistic accounts, Sect. 6.2), we express this phenomenon as *distributed incompetence*. Although the reasoning about knowledge community analyses how knowledge is multiplied if agents are combined into multiagent systems, in this book we observed the opposite phenomenon when multiagent system is formed in a way which reproduces autistic accounts.

Hence having drawn the classes of autistic reasoning → behavior and control reasoning → behavior, multiagent systems in the form of corporations mostly belong to the former class. Most of times they do not follow common sense and demonstrate deviations described by a number of autistic accounts presented in this chapter.

A broad range of features of autistic cognition can be observed in multiagent system with non-trivial motivational patterns. Corporate environment is a good example of such system: frequently, agents are not uniformly motivated to perform their functions, or not motivated at all. Some bureaucratic structures clearly display certain features of autistic cognition. This is an example for how an external observer describes behavior of such system in terms of how its representative describes his mission:

> The only thing I am authorized to do is to tell you that I am not authorized to do anything.

2.6 Autistic Linguistics

2.6.1 Cognitive Skills and Processes Involved in Making Sense of Text

Reading for understanding is especially challenging for CwA, although CwA usually demonstrate well-developed word recognition skills, but their reading comprehension is severely impaired (Nation et al. 2006). An extreme profile of word recognition skills developing in advance of reading comprehension, termed *hyperlexia*, is associated with autism (Grigorenko et al. 2003). The ability to decode words has a neural basis: hyperlexic reading is caused by involving both the left hemisphere's phonological and the right hemisphere's visual systems (Turkeltaub et al. 2004). Computers can also be referred to as hyperlexic readers: it is so easy to program them to recognize words and so difficult to make them recognize meanings of individual words and especially phrases. Text comprehension is extremely complex problem for a computer which some state-of-art NLP systems have only tacked in a very limited manner.

CwA tend to demonstrate well-developed word recognition skills in absence of corresponding skills in constructing meanings. In CC, such ability as text integration, metacognitive monitoring (Sect. 4.1.3), reasoning and working memory all contribute to variability in the reading comprehension skills.

Inference making is an especially difficult skill for both CwA and computational linguistic program to acquire. It has been suggested for CC by Perfetti et al. (2005) that limited processing resources or working memory, not knowing when to draw inferences, and failure to monitor comprehension for text coherence (i.e., focusing on words rather than global meaning) all lead to the problems in text comprehension. Comprehension monitoring is prompted by a high standard for text coherence: readers who strive to make sense of what they read will be more likely to monitor and repair their understanding than readers with a low standard of coherence, the latter will fail to detect inconsistencies at the sentence level.

Propositional, non-linguistic verbal representations are necessary to form false belief concepts. Propositions can be thought of as the building blocks of a low-level representational system, where a single proposition takes the form of a related set of symbols that carries semantic meaning. Linguistic representations occur at a much higher level of abstraction than propositions and are explicitly tied to a particular language.

There are hypotheses that false belief impairments in autism has a low-level representational origin; the development of false belief concepts has been described as requiring, for instance, the representation of "complements" (Hale and Tager-Flusberg 2003) or "meta-representation" (Leslie 1987 and Sect. 4.1.3).

Hale and Tager-Flusberg (2003) demonstrated that training on sentential complements leads to improved ToM performance, and that this linguistic influence is highly specific and did not extend to children trained on another type of embedded construction, namely relative clauses. Traditionally, a complement is a constituent of a clause, such as a noun phrase or adjective phrase, that is used to predicate a description of the subject or object of the clause. As to examples of sentential complements, let us consider the following:

1. Mike read *the newspaper*. (direct object complement of the verb)
2. Make gave it *to me*. (indirect object complement of the verb)
3. Peter put it *in the suitcase*. (must-present locative complement of the verb: it is not enough to just say, *Peter put it*.)
4. This question seems *quite ambiguous*. (adjective phrase complement of the verb).

In order to represent a false belief, one must have some mechanism for representing a belief as being held to be true in one context (e.g. by a character in a story), as well as the property of a belief being false in a different context (e.g. in the story itself). Recent modeling work in cognitive architectures has found that this type of information can be represented within a propositional logical system (Bello and Cassimatis 2006). It is hard for CwA to understand the narrative text structure because they are unable to determine character's motives or identify with characters' emotions or perspectives due to their ToM limitations.

Especially when reading longer texts, memory dysfunction may contribute to reading comprehension deficits. Connecting sentences together to construct a global understanding requires substantial memory capacity. At the time of writing, rhetoric parsers require more than 100 times more memory and processing time compared to sentence-level syntactic parsers. Although high-functioning CwA have strengths in formal memory, memory unattached to interpretation of symbols, they have memory impairment due to poor use of organizational strategies, especially when the information is complex and requires the creation of an organizational structure to facilitate memory (Williams et al. 2005). Reading for understanding requires individuals and machines to construct an organizational structure and schema to aid memory. In addition to memory deficits and poor organization strategies, a tendency to focus on details makes it challenging for CwA to perform discourse-level analysis. For computer rhetoric parsers, a high-dimensional training setting requiring extensive morphological and syntactic information is required.

In terms of semantic processing, CwA can be characterized as "speaking like foreigners". When CwA selects words they do not understand the logic of words and instead speaks by separate thoughts. At the discourse level, CwA do not understand the rhetoric structure of a sentence, how a sentence starts, develops and stops. When a person speaks a foreign language, she expresses her thoughts as a combination of words in his native language, translated into this foreign language on a one-by-one basis. This is similar to how CwA forms their sentences. CwA speaks by separate units each of which expresses a separate feeling.

ASD is characterized by both lower-order behaviors such as motor movements and higher-order cognitive behaviors such as circumscribed interests and insistence on sameness. Both of these are manifest in language as well. Van Santen et al. (2013) reported an automated method for identifying and quantifying two types of repetitive speech in ASD: repetitions of what child him or herself said (intra-speaker repetitions) and of what the conversation partner said (inter-speaker repetitions, or echolalia).

Rouhizadeh et al. (2015) automatically assess the presence of repetitions in language, specifically at the semantic level, in children's conversation with an adult examiner during a semi-structured dialogue. CwA are expected to talk about fewer topics more repeatedly during their conversations. The authors hypothesize that a significantly higher semantic overlap ratio between dialogue turns in CwA compared to those with typical development. In order to calculate the semantic overlap at different turn intervals for each child, we apply multiple semantic similarity metrics (weighted by child specificity scores) on every turn pair in four distance windows. The result of this analysis is that the CwA group had a significantly higher semantic overlap than the CC group in most of the distance windows. The patterns of semantic similarity between child's turns could provide an automated and robust CwA-specific behavioral marker.

Since individuals with autism are hypothesized to have weak central coherence then one would predict that the clinical groups would have difficulty integrating information globally so as to derive full meaning. Two experiments were designed by Jolliffe and Baron-Cohen (2000) to test global coherence. The first experiment investigated whether CwA could arrange sentences coherently. The second experiment explored if CwA are less able to use context to make a global, discourse-related inference. CwA groups have lesser skills to arrange sentences coherently and to use context with the aim at a global inference. The results confirm the impaired global coherence of CwA. Arranging sentences and making global inferences are highly inter-dependent, so central coherence is required to complete these different tasks in a coordinated manner. Of the two clinical groups, the autism group had the greater deficit.

It is well known in computational linguistics that to automatically derive rhetoric structure, or to validate text coherence, all lower level linguistic information, including morphology, syntax and semantics, needs to be taken into account. Instead of depending on mostly hand-engineered sparse features and independent separately developed components for each rhetoric parsing subtask, (Weiss 2015) proposed an integrated approach for text level discourse parsing relying on deep learning. Firstly, each of the discourse parsing subtasks, such as argument boundary detection, labeling, discourse relation identification and sense classification, need to be formulated in terms of recurrent neural networks (Elman 1990) and similar derivable learning architectures. To benefit from their ability to learn intermediate representations, the layers of this neural network will be partially stacked on top of each order, such that the last but one layer (i.e. output layer) for each subtask is shared with other subtasks. By placing increasingly more difficult subtasks at different layers in one deep architecture, they can benefit from each others intermediate representations, improve robustness and training speed. Figure 2.27 combines unsupervised training of word embeddings with the layer-wise multi-task learning of higher representations and illustrates our goal of a unified end-to-end approach for text-level discourse parsing utilizing different layers of representations.

Fig. 2.27 Illustration for how a multi-compartment approach for text-level discourse parsing with multi-layer multi-task learning of higher representations can work

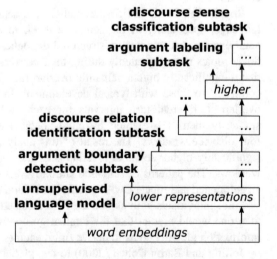

2.6.2   *Grammar and Affect*

Even grammar, which Chomsky and other linguists have assumed to be innate, depends on affect and affective interactions to become functional. CwA frequently verbalize nouns in a repetitious way ("Dog, dog, dog."). If the intervention can get them affectively interactive, however, they can often learn to use proper grammar. For example, a child is opening and closing a gate. We get stuck behind this gate. If they push us away, they are becoming purposeful.

Purposeful behavior that is stimulated by tan affect creates a foundation for the purposeful and meaningful use of words. The child who pushed us away and said nothing at some point will say "go" while doing this. We may then say, "Where go? Where go?" We might further say, "Should we go away or stay? Away or stay?" The child may say, "Go away, go away." Following this dialog, CwA is using the correct grammar. From the viewpoint of the corpus of research on autism and affect, one might disagree with (Chomsky 1966) when he writes that grammar is largely innate and that only life experience in a broad sense led to turning on the language switch in humans. As we discussed in the previous section, grammar requires certain types of affective experience, and specific grammar feature are correlated with special forms of affect and the features of the Theory of Mind. Affective reciprocity is needed to create purposeful action and then related purposeful symbols or words. The affect, by providing intent, enables the components of language to align (e.g., "open door" versus "door, door, door."). Many investigators may have missed the importance of affective reciprocity because it occurs routinely with most infants and toddlers and their caregivers.

Reciprocal affective interactions also influence the basic grammar and semantic aspects of language. We have found, for example, that children not capable of reciprocal affective interactions (e.g., children with autistic spectrum disorders), tend to use words ungrammatically, repeating nouns or verbs in a perseverative manner.

Interestingly, if we try to simply correct their grammar, it doesn't work very well. They make progress, however, when we first help them engage in reciprocal affective gesturing and use their affect and gesturing purposefully (e.g., we get stuck behind the door they are opening and closing and they eventually learn to push us away). At that point, they begin to align their verbs and nouns in a grammatically correct manner—"Daddy, go!" or "Leave me alone." We observe the same patterns in children from deprived backgrounds, such as orphanages. Whether the intrusions are environmental or biological, it appears that a prerequisite for correct use of grammar is the purposeful use of affects in interactive relationships. This fact may have been missed by linguists who suggested grammar was largely innate and simply turned on or off by global features of the environment because it's easy to take reciprocal affect cueing and other preverbal aspects of communication for granted. They occur so regularly.

It's only when we find circumstances where they don't occur that we can see their true impact. Similar to grammar, the meaning of words, both the semantic and pragmatic aspects are also imbedded in the earlier reality of gestural interactions, which are used to explore and know the world. The literal meaning of a word or concept, for example, the concept of a door or a table or a mommy or a daddy is first known through gestural interactions with it. The capacity to form the word is then linked to what is already partially known. The known entity takes on additional meaning through context and further emotional experience with it. Therefore, both the literal and the relative meaning of words and concepts emerge from reciprocal affective interactions which provide the foundations and context for meanings.

The capacity for long chains of reciprocity and the basic capacity to plan and sequence actions may also support the ability to sequence words or ideas and eventually concepts in a speech, essay, or debate, or simply a long conversation. Sequencing ideas relates both to this basic ability to abstract meaning from earlier preverbal experiences and then sequence them meaningfully.

2.6.3   Understanding Metaphors

Highly abstract or figurative metaphors are problematic for certain groups of language users amongst CwA. As a result of impairment in communication, social interaction and behavior, CwA are characterized by atypical information processing in diverse areas of cognition (Skoyles 2011). CwA experience difficulties when a figurative language is encountered. Happé (1995) describes:

> A request to "Stick your coat down over there" is met by a serious request for glue. Ask if she will "give you a hand", and she will answer that she needs to keep both hands and cannot cut one off to give to you. Tell him that his sister is "crying her eyes out" and he will look anxiously on the floor for her eye-balls . . .

The reduced skills of CwA to understand metaphors in language communication as well as figurative language is obviously an obstacle in communication, since most people "think in metaphors" and a language system is inherently figurative (Lakoff and Johson 1980). The growing demand to overcome this barrier has led to the investigation of possible ways in which NLP can detect and simplify non-literal expressions in a text.

The *simile* is a figure of speech that builds on a comparison in order to leverage certain attributes of an entity in a striking manner. A simile compares one entity with another entity of a different kind. Simile is used to make a description more emphatic or vivid (e.g. *as fast as a cougar*).

CwA and message understanding systems show almost no impairment in comprehending the similes which have literal meaning (Happé 1995). This relative ease in processing is probably due to the fact that metaphors in the form of comparison contain explicit markers (e.g. like and as), which evoke comparison between two things in a certain aspect. With regard to understanding figurative similes, Hobson et al. (2013) describes in the case of fifteen-year-old:

> He could neither grasp nor formulate similarities, differences or absurdities, nor could he understand metaphor.

One of the most obvious markers of similes, the word *like*, could be a source of a lot of misinterpretations (Niculae and Yaneva 2013). For example, '*like*' could be a verb, a noun, a preposition, or Facebook attribute, depending on the context. Given that autistic people have problems understanding contexts (Skoyles 2011, Sect. 6.4), how would an autistic reader perceive the role of 'like' in a more elaborate and ambiguous comparison? Another possible linguistic reason for the corrupt understanding of similes might be that *like* is used ambiguously in many expressions which are neither similes nor comparisons, such as *I feel like a soup* or *I feel like something goes wrong a wrong way*. Even if the expression does not include such an ambiguous use of like, there are other cases in which a CwA might be confused. For example, if the simile is highly figurative or abstract, it may be completely incomprehensible, such as in the example of *A love is like a flame* (Fig. 2.28).

Fig. 2.28 An example of autistic writing on philosophical topics. Hand support is necessary to help in writing. Text includes answers to certain questions and some associated thoughts

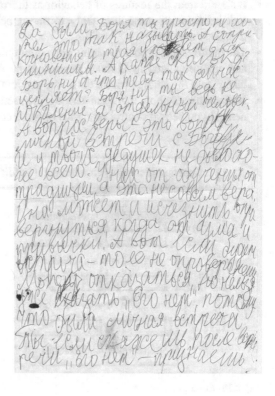

2.7   Our Account of Autism: Reasoning Engine → Behavior

Having outlined most popular accounts of autism, we intend to formulate the one most valid in terms of an artificial computational system which controls a behavior of a human or robot in the real world. This account will not include neural or genetic considerations: it will be brain component – neutral. Whereas most accounts, including computational ones, try to combine psychological, behavioral, cognitive, neural, genetic and even philosophical considerations, we prefer to have a model fully formalized and self-contained (Fig. 2.29, Minshew and Goldstein 1998). Such model should be viewed as an engineering design model, providing sufficient details so that a software engineer can build it from our specification. This specification should be formally consistent and do not contradict to the experimental observation of autistic cognition and behavior.

The desired features of such system are as follows:

- It should only take into account the details of what we know about human brain and its specifics under autism related to reasoning processes.
- It should treat the features of behavior as thoroughly as possible, and explicitly link behavior to reasoning. Only forms of behavior which can be expressed concisely are used.
- The intelligence, problem solving and communication skills are formally defined and are formalized in as much degrees as possible. Behavioral capabilities are taken from the studies within the above accounts and beyond them.
- No hypotheses about meta-functioning, interaction between hypothetical components, hypothetical control scenarios of these components are relied upon.

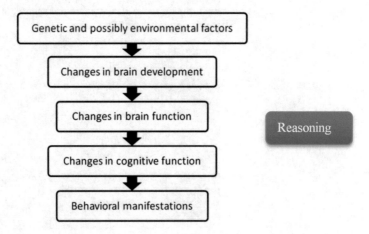

Fig. 2.29 Etiology of autism

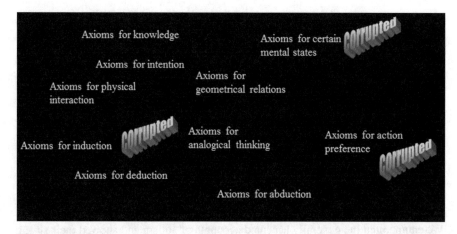

Fig. 2.30 Corruption happens at the level of individual axioms, responsible for a particular reasoning domain

Once these features are approved, the nucleus of our account becomes fairly compact and self-contained:

1. Specific behavior is caused by a deviation in a reasoning system;
2. Deviation in a reasoning system is caused by lack of certain axioms.

Then the treatment methodology is to teach these missing axioms as rules once they are identified.

In our account of autistic reasoning, corruption happens at the level of axioms (Fig. 2.30). From the theoretical reasoning standpoint, we assume that the reasoning machinery itself is functional and the only cause of a lack of reasoning skills in a given domain is a lack of a respective axiom.

As a first example, we consider the missing axiom "Other people have intentions". Without this axiom, children ignore questions "what he wants". Once the child is explained that other people have such "things" as desires, wants and intentions, which can come and go, this child starts answering the above question. This means that the axiom is *acquired,* when this question is answered about an arbitrary intent.

Proceeding to another example, we state that to be able to generalize from samples and to formulate rules, an individual or a reasoning machine needs an axiom of induction. If an individual or reasoning machine cannot perform generalization from samples, he is missing an axiom of induction. In this case, the range of skills generally referred to as 'machine learning' is missing.

An intelligence machine needs to acquire axioms to answer questions, in particular, the axioms for intend and for generalizing from samples. Before such axioms are fed into this machine, it is unable to answer questions in these domains. After the acquisition of the axioms, the machine becomes capable of answering these questions.

How to figure out which axiom is missing in a give child? If, having certain axioms disabled, an artificial reasoning system displays the same behavior (in particular, answers questions and fails to answer questions in a similar manner) as a given individual, then we conclude that this individual is missing this axiom.

Each CwA can then be represented as a profile of missing vs intact vs acquired axioms. What can be observed is that more complex derived axiom can be missing when the basis, simpler axiom is present, but not the other way around. We will evaluate this observation in Sect. 9.10.

2.8 Discussion and Conclusions

We enumerated the generally accepted accounts of autism and showed their strong and weak points. On the positive side, they cover a broad range of features of autistic behavior and cognition and link them with neural layers and mechanisms, as well as genetics and cognitive components. On the negative side, these accounts are incomplete as information systems, a lot of their schemas are informal and not necessarily plausible. It is unclear, if one can build a computational system which corresponds to a given account, so that its output can imitate the described behavior.

Each account of autism focuses on a specific features of reasoning and cognition, and explains how it affects the autistic behavior and skills. Each account splits reasoning and cognition into different components and then hypothesizes which components are intact and which are broken. Each account then attempts to explain the peculiarities of autistic behavior given the functionality of the broken components. Since these components and the addressed features of behavior overlap, each account positions itself among other accounts with similar components and features of behavior.

For example, a text understanding system includes morphological, syntactic, semantic, pragmatic and discourse components. The behavior of text understanding system can be the way its answers questions, and following accounts explaining its malfunctioning can be plausible:

- System intent to understand questions is broken
- Particular processing level is not tuned well, so some words in the input questions are missed
- Communication between processing levels is broken, so answering of Boolean/conjunctive queries is incorrect
- Control of how different classifiers are combined in a hybrid system is not adjusted well, so it cannot answer compound queries

Similar structure can be applied to image, video, sound, abstract pattern recognition system and recognition in other modalities.

Multiple accounts of autism illustrate that there are multiple psychological characterizations of autism. These accounts share some commonalities and they are not mutually exclusive at all. Hobson's theory can be viewed as explaining where

ToM abilities are coming from, genetically determined module or being develop out of learning to communicate. ToM's theory-theory does not provide any evidence for the genetic basis of ToM corruption. Also, executive function and central coherence are presumably computational capacities of systems and as such they might be components of whatever system provides an implementation of ToM abilities.

One of our points of criticism of the current computational accounts of autism is that they attempt to describe a meta-language for implementation of reasoning instead of focusing on the object-language level. Since one can only hypothesize about the signals in the natural neural network, a formal computational model of a neural network is essentially a meta-language level model. When the activity of an artificial neural network is similar to that of a natural one, it means that the meta-language model might potentially be plausible, and nothing can be said about an object – level. For a reasoning system implemented as a neural network, its reasoning domain belongs to its object-language, and neural signals, communication protocols, which can be experimentally assessed – to the meta-language level.

There are examples in science and humanities where a phenomena is expressed using meta-language only, without employing a power of language-object. One of the purest example of it is Kafka's novel "The Trial". In this novel the author presents only a meta-level account of what is happening with a character being prosecuted; language-object level description is absent. From the scientific standpoint, his description of an observation of society functioning is far from being perfect and efficient. Similarly, neural network models of the functioning of autistic brain involves only a single layer of information processing.

Having analyzed the accounts of autism, we decided to pursue a pure computational and less intuitive, holistic account and to observe how far we can go in terms of completeness of our account, its prediction capabilities and values for rehabilitation. This account should provide a conceptual basis for improving autistic reasoning as well as a foundation for software for autistic rehabilitation.

References

Axelrod R (1984) The evolution of cooperation. Basic Books, New York

Balkenius C (2000) Attention, habituation and conditioning: toward a computational model. Cogn Sci Q 1(2):171–214

Baranek GT (1999) Autism during infancy: a retrospective video analysis of sensory-motor and social behaviors at 9–12 months of age. J Autism Dev Disord 29(3):213–224

Baron-Cohen S, Wheelwright S (1999) Obsessions in children with autism or Asperger syndrome: a content analysis in terms of core domains of cognition. Br J Psychiatry 175:484–490

Baron-Cohen S, Scott FJ, Allison C, Williams J, Bolton P, Matthews FE (2008) Estimating autism spectrum prevalence in the population: a school based study from the UK. Br J Psychiatry 194(6):500–509

Baum EB, Hausler D (1989) What size net gives valid generalization. Neural Comput 1(1):151–160. MIT Press, Cambridge, MA

Beitchman JH, Kruidenier B, Inglis A, Clegg M (1996) The children's self-report questionnaire: factor score, age trends, and gender differences. J Am Acad Child Adolesc Psychiatry 28: 714–722

Bello P, Cassimatis N (2006) Developmental accounts of theory-of-mind acquisition: achieving clarity via computational cognitive modeling. In Proceedings of the 28th annual conference of the Cognitive Science Society, pp 1014–1019

Belmonte MK, Allen G, Beckel-Mitchener A, Boulanger LM, Carper RA, Webb SJ (2004) Autism and abnormal development of brain connectivity. J Neurosci 24:9228–9231

Benes FM, Vincent SL, Molloy R (1993) Dopamine-immunoreactive axon varicosities form nonrandom contacts with GABA-immunoreactive neurons of rat medial prefrontal cortex. Synapse 15:285–295

Bermúdez JL (2005) Philosophy of psychology: a contemporary introduction. Routledge, London

Björne P, Balkenius C (2005) A model of attentional impairments in autism: first steps toward a computational theory. Cogn Syst Res 6:193–204

Blakemore SJ, Tavassoli T, Calⁿ S, Thomas RM, Catmur C, Frith U, Haggard P (2006) Tactile sensitivity in Asperger syndrome. Brain Cogn 61(1):5–13

Blatt GJ, Fitzgerald CM, Guptill JT, Booker AB, Kemper TL, Bauman ML (2001) Density and distribution of hippocampal neurotransmitter receptors in autism: an autoradiographic study. J Autism Dev Disord 31:537–543

Bruinsma Y, Koegel R, Koegel L (2004) Joint attention and children with autism: a review of the literature. Ment Retard Dev Disabil 10:169–175

Buxbaum JD, Silverman JM, Smith CJ, Greenberg DA, Kilifarski M et al (2002) Association between a GABRB3 polymorphism and autism. Mol Psychiatry 7:311–316

Capps L, Losh M, Thurber C (2000) "The frog ate the bug and made his mouth sad": narrative competence in children with autism. J Abnorm Child Psychol 28:193–204

Casanova MF (2007) The neuropathology of autism. Brain Pathol 17:422–433

Chomsky N (1966) Topics in the theory of generative grammar. Mouton, The Hague

Clark A (1989) Microcognition: philosophy, cognitive science, and parallel distributed processing. MIT Press, Cambridge, MA

Condon WS (1975) Multiple response to sound in dysfunctional children. J Autism Child Schizophr 5:37–56

Condon WS, Sander L (1974) Synchrony demonstrated between movements of the neonate and adult speech. Child Dev 45:456–462

Coricelli G, Nagel R (2009) Neural correlates of depth of strategic reasoning in medial prefrontal cortex. Proc Natl Acad Sci U S A 106:9163–9168

Courchesne E, Allen G (1997) Prediction and preparation, fundamental functions of the cerebellum. Learn Mem 4:1–35

Courchesne E, Müller R-A, Saitoh O (1999) Brain weight in autism: normal in the majority of cases, megalencephalic in rare cases. Neurology 52:1057–1059

Dawson G, Galpert I (1990) Mother's use of imitative play for facilitating social responsiveness and toy play in young autistic children. Dev Psychopathol 2:151–162

Deuel R (2002) Autism: a cognitive developmental riddle. Pediatr Neurol 26:349–357

Edelman GM (1987) Neural Darwinism: the theory of neuronal group selection. Basic Books, New York

Edelman S, Intrator N, Poggio T (1997) Complex cells and object recognition. NIPS 97

Elman JL (1990) Finding structure in time. Cogn Sci 14:179–211

Emde RN, Biringen Z, Clyman RB, Oppenheim D (1991) The moral self of infancy: affective core and procedural knowledge. Dev Rev 11:251–270

Fodor JA (1983) Modularity of mind: an essay on faculty psychology. MIT Press, Cambridge, MA

Frith U (1989) Autism: explaining the enigma. Blackwell, Oxford

Frith U, Happé F (1994) Autism: beyond "theory mind". Cognition 50:115–132

Gepner B, Feron F (2009) Autism: a world changing too fast for a mis-wired brain? Neurosci Biobehav Rev 33(8):1227–1242

Gillespie-Lynch K (2013) Response to and initiation of joint attention: overlapping but distinct roots of development in autism? OA Autism 1(2):13

Gopnik A, Capps L, Meltzoff AN (2000) Early theories of mind: what the theory theory can tell us about autism. In: Baron-Cohen S et al (eds) Understanding other minds: perspectives from autism and cognitive neuroscience, 2nd edn. Oxford University Press, Oxford

Gordon B (1997) Models of naming. In: Goodglasss H, Wingfield A (eds) Anomia. Academic, San Diego, pp 31–64

Gowen E, Miall RC (2005) Behavioural aspects of cerebellar function in adults with Asperger syndrome. Cerebellum 4:279–289

Grandin T (2006) Thinking in pictures, expanded edition. Vintage Press, New York

Greenspan SI (1992) Infancy and early childhood: the practice of clinical assessment and intervention with emotional and developmental challenges. International Universities Press, Madison

Greenspan SI (1997) Developmentally based psychotherapy. International Universities Press, New York

Greenspan SI (2001) The affect diathesis hypothesis: the role of emotions in the core deficit in Autism and in the development of intelligence and social skills. J Dev Learn Dis 5(1). Special Edition

Grigorenko EL, Klin A, Volkmar F (2003) Hyperlexia: disability or superability? J Child Psychol Psychiatry 44:1079–1091

Grossberg S, Seidman D (2006) Neural dynamics of autistic behaviors: cognitive, emotional, and timing substrates. Psychol Rev 113(3):483–525

Gustafsson L (1997) Inadequate cortical feature maps: a neural circuit theory of autism. Biol Psychiatry 42(12):1138–1147

Gustafsson L, Paplinski AP (2003) Preoccupation with a restricted pattern of interest in modelling autistic learning. KES 2774:1122–1129

Hale CM, Tager-Flusberg H (2003) The influence of language on theory of mind: a training study. Dev Sci 6(3):346–359

Happé F (1995) The role of age and verbal ability in the theory of mind task performance of subjects with autism. Child Dev 66(3):843–855

Happe F, Frith U (2006) The weak coherence account: detail-focused cognitive style in autism spectrum disorders. J Autism Dev Disord 36:5–25

Happe F, Ehlers S, Fletcher P, Frith U, Johansson M, Gillberg C et al (1996) Theory of mind in the brain. Evidence from a PET scan study of Asperger syndrome. NeuroReport 8:197–201

Hart J, Gordon B (1992) Neural subsystems for object knowledge. Nature 359:60–64

Hobson RP, Lee A (1999) Imitation and identification in autism. J Child Psychol Psychiatry 40:649–659

Hobson JA, Peter Hobson R, Malik S, Bargiota K, Calo S (2013) The relation between social engagement and pretend play in autism. Br J Dev Psychol 31:114–127

Hofer MA (1995) Hidden regulators: implications for a new understanding of attachment, separation, and loss. In: Goldberg S, Muir R, Kerr J (eds) Attachment theory: social, developmental, and clinical perspectives. Analytic Press, Hillsdale, pp 203–230

Jolliffe T, Baron-Cohen S (1997) Are people with autism or Asperger's syndrome faster than normal on the embedded figures task? J Child Psychol Psychiatry 38:527–534

Joseph RM, Tager-Flusberg H (2004) The relationship of theory of mind and executive functions to symptom type and severity in children with autism. Dev Psychopathol 16:137–155, Cambridge University Press

Just MA, Cherkassky VL, Keller TA, Minshew NJ (2004) Cortical activation and synchronization during sentence comprehension in high-functioning autism: evidence of underconnectivity. Brain 127:1811–1821

Kirchner WK (1958) Age differences in short-term retention of rapidly changing information. J Exp Psychol 55(4):352–358

Kojima S, Goldman-Rakic PS (1982) Delay-related activity of prefrontal neurons in rhesus monkeys performing delayed response. Brain Res 248:43–50

Koshino H, Carpenter P, Minshew N, Cherkassky V, Keller T, Just M (2005) Functional connectivity in an fMRI working memory task in high-functioning autism. NeuroImage 24:810–821

Koshino H, Kana R, Keller T, Cherkassky V, Minshew N, Just M (2008) fMRI investigation of working memory for faces in autism: visual coding and underconnectivity with frontal areas. Cereb Cortex 18:289–300

Kunda M, McGreggor K, Goel AK (2010) Can the Raven's progressive matrices intelligence test be solved by thinking in pictures?. Oral presentation, International Meeting for Autism Research (IMFAR), Philadelphia, PA

Lakoff G, Johson M (1980) Metaphors we live by. Catedra

Leslie AM (1987) Pretence and representation: the origins of "theory of mind". Psychol Rev 94:412–426

Leslie AM, Keeble S (1987) Do six-month-olds perceive causality? Cognition 25:265–288

Lewis V, Boucher J (1997) The test of pretend play. Harcourt Brace, London

Losh M, Capps L (2006) Understanding of emotional experience in autism: insights from the personal accounts of high-functioning children with autism. Dev Psychol 42(5):809–818

McClelland JL, Rogers TT (2003) The parallel distributed processing approach to semantic cognition. Nat Rev Neurosci 4(4):310–322

Milne E, Swettenham J, Hansen P, Campbell R, Jeffries H, Plaisted K (2002) High motion coherence thresholds in children with autism. J Child Psychol Psychiatry 43:255–263

Minshew NJ (1996) Autism. In: Berg BO (ed) Principles of child neurology. McGraw-Hill, New York, pp 1713–1730

Minshew NJ, Goldstein G (1998) Autism as a disorder of complex information processing. Ment Retard Dev Disabil Res Rev 4:129–136

Minshew NJ, Goldstein G (2001) The pattern of intact and impaired memory functions in autism. J Child Psychol Psychiatry 42:1095–1101

Minshew NJ, Luna B, Sweeney JA (1999) Oculomotor evidence for neocortical systems but not cerebellar dysfunction in autism. Neurology 52:917–922

Moskowitz GB (2005) Social cognition: understanding self and others. Guilford Press, New York

Mottron L, Burack J (2001) Enhanced perceptual functioning in the development of autism. In: Burack JA, Charman T, Yirmiya N, Zelazo PR (eds) The development of autism: perspectives from theory and research. L. Erlbaum, Mahwah, pp 131–148

Müller-Lyer FC (1889) Optische Urteilstäuschungen. Archiv für Physiologie Suppl :263–270.

Mundy P, Sigman M, Kasari C (1990) A longitudinal study of joint attention and language development in autistic children. J Autism Dev Disord 20(1):115–128

Nation K, Clarke P, Wright B, Williams C (2006) Patterns of reading ability in children with autism spectrum disorder. J Autism Dev Disord 36(7):911–919

Niculae V, Victoria Y (2013) Computational considerations of comparisons and similes. In: Proceedings of the association for computational linguistics student research workshop, Sofia, Bulgaria, 4–9 August 2013, pp 89–95

Oakes LM, Cohen LB (1990) Infant perception of a causal event. Cogn Dev 5:193–207

O'Loughlin C, Thagard P (2000) Autism and coherence: a computational model. Mind Lang 14(4):375–392

O'Reilly RC, Munakata Y (2000) Computational explorations in cognitive neuroscience: understanding the mind by simulating the brain. MIT Press, Cambridge, MA

Ozonoff S, Strayer D (2001) Further evidence of intact working memory in autism. J Autism Dev Disord 31:257–263

Payton JW, Wardlaw DM, Graczyk PA, Bloodworth MR, Tompsett CJ, Weissberg RP (2000) Social and emotional learning: a framework for promoting mental health and reducing risk behavior in children and youth. J Sch Health 70(5):179–185

Pennington BF, Ozonoff S (1996) Executive function and developmental psycopathology. J Child Psychol Psychiatry 37(1):51–87

Perfetti CA, Landi N, Oakhill J (2005) The acquisition of reading comprehension skill. In: Snowling J, Hulme C (eds) The science of reading: a handbook. Blackwell, London, pp 227–247

Plaisted K, O'Riordan M, Baron-Cohen S (1998) Enhanced visual search for a conjunctive target in autism: a research note. J Child Psychol Psychiatry 39:777–783

Raven JC (1936) Mental tests used in genetic studies: the performance of related individuals on tests mainly educative and mainly reproductive. MSc thesis, University of London.

Rolf LH, Haarmann FY, Grotemeyer KH, Kehrer H (1993) Serotonin and amino acid content in platelets of autistic children. Acta Psychiatr Scand 87:312–316

Rouhizadeh M, Sproat R, van Santen J (2015) Similarity measures for quantifying restrictive and repetitive behavior in conversations of autistic children. In: Proceedings of the 2nd workshop on computational linguistics and clinical psychology: from linguistic signal to clinical reality, ACL, pp 117–123.

Rumelhart DE, McClelland JL (1986) Parallel distributed processing: explorations in the microstructure of cognition. Volume 1: foundations. MIT Press, Cambridge, MA

Rumelhart DE, Todd PM (1993) Learning and connectionist representations. Attention and performance XIV: synergies in experimental psychology, artificial intelligence, and cognitive neuroscience, pp 3–30

Russell J (1997) Autism as an executive disorder. Oxford University Press, Oxford

Rutter M, Bailcy A, Bolton P, Lc Coutcur A (1994) Autism and known medical conditions: myth and substances. J Child Psychol Psychiatry 35:311–322

Shah A, Frith U (1983) An islet of ability in autistic children: a research note. J Child Psychol Psychiatry 24:613–620

Skoyles JR (2011) Autism, context/noncontext information processing, and atypical development. Autism res treat 2011

Smith E, Jonides J (1999) Storage and executive processes in the frontal lobes. Science 283:1657–1661

Sobel DM, Lillard AS (2001) The impact of fantasy and action on young children's understanding of pretence. Br J Dev Psychol 19(1):85–98

Sutton J, Smith PK, Swettenham J (1999) Social cognition and bullying: social inadequacy or skilled manipulation? Br J Dev Psychol 17(3):435–450(16)

Tager-Flusberg H (1989). The development of questions in autistic and down syndrome children. Gatlinburg conference on research and theory in mental retardation. Gatlinburg, TN

Talairach J, Tournoux P (1988) Co-planar stereotaxic atlas of the human brain. Thieme, New York

Therese J, Baron-Cohen S (2000) Linguistic processing in high-functioning adults with autism or Asperger's syndrome. Is global coherence impaired? Psychol Med 30(5):1169–1187

Tomchek SD, Dunn W (2007) Sensory processing in children with and without autism: a comparative study using the short sensory profile. Am J Occup Ther 61(2):190–200

Turkeltaub PE, Flowers DL, Verbalis A, Miranda M, Gareau L, Eden GF (2004) The neural basis of hyperlexia reading: an fMRI case study. Neuron 41:1–20

van Santen J, Sproat R, Hill AP (2013) Quantifying repetitive speech in autism spectrum disorders and language impairment. Autism Res 6(5):372–383

VisiualSuportAndBeyond. Last downloaded April 5, 2016. http://www.visualsupportsandbeyond.co.uk/why/psychology.html

Watkins CJCH, Dayan P (1992) Q-learning. Mach Learn 9:279–292

Weiss G (2015) Learning representations for text-level discourse parsing. In: Proceedings of the ACL-IJCNLP 2015 student research workshop, pp 16–21, Beijing, China, July 28, 2015

Williams DL, Goldstein G, Carpenter PA, Minshew NJ (2005) Verbal and spatial working memory in autism. J Autism Dev Disord 35(6):747–756

Wimmer H, Perner J (1983) Beliefs about beliefs: representation and the containing function of wrong beliefs in young children's understanding of deception. Cognition 13:103–128

Yoshida W, Dziobek I, Kliemann D, Heekeren HR, Friston KJ, Dolan RJ (2010) Cooperation and heterogeneity of the autistic mind. J Neurosci 30(26):8815–8818

Zhi-Hua Z (2012) Ensemble methods: foundations and algorithms. Chapman and Hall/CRC, Boca Raton

Chapter 3
Intuitive Theory of Mind

3.1 Introducing Theory of Mind

Theory of Mind (ToM) is an umbrella term commonly used to refer to both the commonsense theory and its associated cognitive processes. ToM investigates how people ascribe mental states to other people and how people use mental states to explain and predict the actions of those other persons. ToM explores mindreading, mentalizing or mentalistic abilities, shared by most adults. These abilities are used to treat other agents as ones possessing the unobservable mental or psychological states, actions and processes, which cannot be explicitly perceived. These abilities are also used to anticipate and explain the agents' behavior in terms of such states and processes.

This is how an adult with autism (Wrongplanet 2015) reflects on his ToM capabilities:

> I actually very well remember the time when I considered other people as objects, moving and talking, but devoid of thoughts and feelings. Sometime in my twenties I started looking at people and thinking "Can they possibly have consciousness, same as I do?" This thought seemed preposterous and unworldly. But I finally convinced myself, and now I assume that other people have independents minds and thoughts. This assumption is on the conscious level and disagrees with my intuition.

Two different well known theories have been proposed to explain the basic mechanism underlying the ToM abilities. They are usually referred to as *simulation theory* and *theory-theory* (Vogeley et al. 2001). According to simulation theory, ToM skills are based on taking someone else's view and projecting one's own attitude onto someone else. The simulation approach to reasoning about mental states will be explored in Chap. 5. By contrast, according to theory-theory, theory of mind capacity is based on a distinct body of theoretical knowledge acquired during the individual's ontogenetic development. From the computer science standpoint, ToM is a meta-theory of the theory about mental world. We will investigate what kind of meta-theory is required for the mental world in Sect. 4.1.3.

© Springer International Publishing Switzerland 2016
B. Galitsky, *Computational Autism*, Human–Computer Interaction Series,
DOI 10.1007/978-3-319-39972-0_3

Fig. 3.1 René Descartes's
illustration of "Simulation
theory" and "theory theory"
dualism. Inputs are passed on
by the sensory organs to the
epiphysis in the brain and
from there to the immaterial
spirit

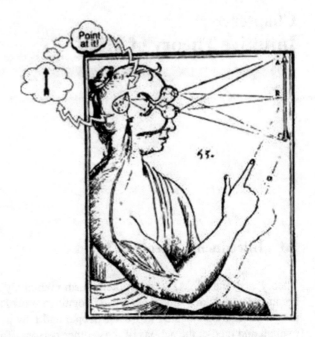

Both theory-theory and simulation-theory are actually families of theories. Some theory-theorists maintain that our naïve ToM is a result of our scientific-like exercise of a problem domain capacity to provide a theoretical basis. Other theory-theorists defend a quite different proposal that mindreading relies on the development of a mental organ specifically dedicated to the psychological domain. Simulation-theory also shows different aspects: according to its "moderate" view, mental concepts are not completely excluded from simulation (Fig. 3.1). Simulation can be represented as a procedure through which we:

1. yield and attach to ourselves some mental states of pretense that are intended to correspond to those of the simulated agent;
2. project them onto the target.

By contrast, a stronger version of simulation-based approach denies the superiority of first-person mindreading and proposes that we imaginatively transform ourselves into the simulated agent, interpreting the target's behavior without using any kind of mental concept, not even ones referring to ourselves.

Neurophysiological evidence relevant to theory-theory vs simulation was provided by (Gallese et al. 1996), who demonstrated a mirror neuron system in macaques (Fig. 3.2). Mirror neurons are premotor neurons that are activated when a monkey performs an object-directed action including keeping, capturing, grasping, tearing, manipulating and holding. These neurons are also activated when the animal observes a human experimenter, performing the same class of actions. The discovery of mirror neurons provided a possible mechanism for a simulation theory

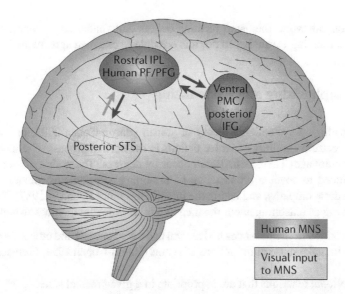

Fig. 3.2 Brain areas involved in the mirror neuron subsystem (Iacoboni and Mazziotta 2007)

account of theory of mind (Gallese and Goldman 1998). Multimodal neurons in motor cortex react to visual observations, helping to understand actions of others by simulating similar motor activity. Distortion in the development of the mirror neural system interferes with the ability to imitate, leading to social impairment and communication difficulties, and may be responsible for the lack of ToM (Iacoboni and Mazziotta 2007).

There has been an important debate in philosophy contrasting 'theory' vs. 'simulation' accounts of reasoning about mental states (see for example (Harris 2000)). This issue is strongly correlated with autism, and in this book we implement a hybrid approach to implementation of ToM engine, merging simulation with implementation of meta-reasoning (Chap. 4). (Stenning 2002) argues that the two may not be as distinct as would at first appear. Chapter 4 of this book is devoted to theory-theory approach, and Chap. 5 describes the simulation approach to implement ToM reasoning.

Before the age of 4, children can impress an external observer that they play together but indeed they play independently, not interacting with each other, each in her own space. Before the age of 3, children do not understand that other children have beliefs, desires and intentions, they live in their own worlds. After the age of 4 children discover that other people have Belief-Desire-Intention (BDI, Rao and Georgeff 1995, Sect. 4.1.2) model of the mental world. Children discover that other people can have wishes not necessarily connected with their own wishes. But initially, before that age children cannot handle this, and they play in parallel worlds. They stop making other people do what they want, but they try to avoid each other and minimize interactions. Then at the age of 5 children start understanding that interaction can work, they start forming beliefs that "under some conditions I can achieve something I want her to do; it is possible to reach an agreement."

3.2   Emphasizing and Systemizing

The empathizing-systemizing theory of autism (Baron-Cohen 2002) proposes that autism spectrum conditions involve deficits in the normal process of empathy, relative to mental age. These deficits can occur by degrees. The notion of empathizing is introduced to cover a broad range of reasoning sub-domains: theory of mind, mind-reading, empathy, and taking the intentional stance (Dennett 1987). We define empathizing as reasoning about the mental world. Empathy includes two elements:

(a) Attribution of mental states and mental actions to oneself and others, as a natural way to make sense of the actions of agents (Baron-Cohen 1994; Premack 1990); and

(b) Emotional reactions that are appropriate in a given mental state.

Since the first test of mind-blindness was administered to children with autism (Baron-Cohen et al. 1985), more than 30 experimental tests have been developed, confirming the impairments in the development of empathizing (Baron-Cohen 1995). The skills of empathizing significantly varies for CwA but are still significantly inferior to that of controls (Fig. 3.3). The limited capabilities in empathizing lead to social and communicative development and in the imagination of others' minds (Baron-Cohen 1987; Leslie 1987).

(Baron-Cohen 2002) attempts to rely on the empathizing-systemizing theory to explain other psychological models such as impairments of executive function or central coherence. From the engineering standpoint, a device can have multiple malfunctions which do not need to be caused by a single subsystem. Nevertheless, in autism research the community attempts to form a single model which would explain the whole range of autistic phenomenology. Even in a reasoning domain, the range of reasoning peculiarities is so broad that it seems hard to find the root cause in the reasoning problems themselves, let along the behavioral autistic features.

Although autism is most often conceptualized as a syndrome of deficits, its altered developmental emphases can also lead to remarkable analytical strengths in some domains. (Baron-Cohen 2002) explains the cognitive superiorities found in autism by the concept of systemizing. It is defined as a drive to analyze objects and events to understand their structure and to predict their future behavior.

Autistic systemizing is based on reduced generalization skills of induction, but fairly efficient rule system once the rules become available to CwA. CwA are good at applying rules to technical systems (such as machines and tools), natural systems (such as biological and geographical phenomena), and abstract systems (such as mathematics or computer programs). Several studies indicate that systemizing in autism is at least in line with mental age, or superior (Baron-Cohen et al. 2003; Lawson et al. 2004). Systemizing may underlie a different set of behavioral features in autism that we refer to as the triad of strengths (Fig. 3.4).

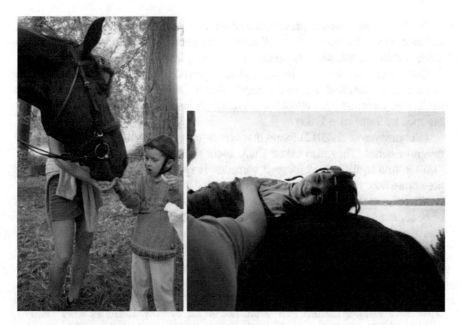

Fig. 3.3 Interaction with horses helps to stimulate empathy

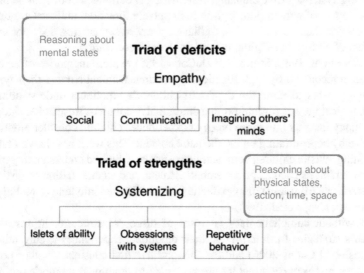

Fig. 3.4 Deficits and strengths of CwA and respective reasoning domains

The outcomes Sally-Ann and 'Smarties' experiments (Sect. 2.2) have been argued to support the 'theory of mind deficit' hypothesis on the cause of autism. Proposed by (Leslie in 1987), it postulates that human beings have evolved a special 'module' devoted specifically to reasoning about other people's minds. As such, this module would provide a cognitive underpinning for empathy. In CC, the module would constitute the difference between humans and their ancestors – indeed, chimpanzees seem to be able to do much less in the way of mind-reading. In CwA, this module would be delayed or impaired, thus explaining abnormalities in communication and also in the acquisition of language, if it is indeed true that the development of joint attention is crucial to language learning (as claimed for instance by Tomasello 1988).

(Norenzayan et al. 2012) found that symptoms of autism correlated with lack of religious belief. They also asked CwA about their empathy (using questions like "I often find it difficult to judge if someone is rude or polite" and "I am good at predicting how someone will feel.").

They found that empathy also correlated with belief. Using a statistical technique of bootstrapping they found that the most plausible explanation for the correlation was that autism was related to a lack of empathy, which in turn was related to lack of belief. In other words, lack of empathy was the 'in between' factor that mediated the relationship between autism and lack of belief. The authors also measured something called systemizing, which is all "about aptitude for, and interest in, reasoning about mechanical and physical objects and processes", and is measure using questions like "I am fascinated by how machines work" and "I find it difficult to understand information the bank sends me on different investment and saving systems". Like empathy, systemizing is correlated both with being male and the degree of autism (although in the opposite direction: autistics are better at systematizing than controls). But, unlike empathy, systematizing does not mediate the effect of autism on religion, in terms of formal correlation.

(Seidner et al. 1988; Stipek and DeCotis 1988) explore memories of emotional experience recounted by high-functioning children with autism and their typically developing peers to mine the depths of children's emotional understanding and discern their strategies for interpreting emotional encounters. Researchers have generated many insights into those types of experiences children consider emotionally evocative by concentrating on the thematic content. This work has shown that high-functioning autistic children demonstrate particularly limited understanding of more complex emotions such as pride, embarrassment, and shame, failing to distinguish these emotions from less complex feelings of similar hedonic tone (e.g., happiness and sadness; Capps et al. 1992).

Yet, without complementary analyses of discourse structure, information on children's strategies for interpreting their emotional experiences is currently lacking. (Losh and Capps 2006) address this problem and consider whether potential differences in discourse structure are restricted to emotional memories or, rather, represent a more pervasive difficulty. They do so by comparing the structural features of children's emotional accounts to those of non-emotional physical states. In view of recent findings of impaired episodic memories in autism (Bowler et al. 2000), the inclusion of non-emotional terms (e.g., sick and tired) is of particular value in the assessment of emotion-specific patterns not assessed in prior studies of autistic individuals' recounted emotional experiences.

3.3 ToM and Other Autistic Accounts

Certain predictions arise, if one considers Empathy-Systemizing and Central Coherence (Sect. 2.5.1) not as mutually exclusive explanations of autistic behavior, but as complementary ones that can be developmentally unified.

Specifically, the attention to detail described by weak central coherence may be one of the earliest manifestations of a strong drive toward systemizing, or vice versa, interest in systemizing may arise as a consequence of attention to detail. As cognitive capacities become more complex and mature, strong "systemizers" may begin to apply some kind of engineering methodology. In this methodology even complex systems are understood by successive local observations in which one input at a time is manipulated while all others are held constant, and effects on the outputs are observed in a similarly sequential manner. This is how an engineering system can be optimized, a causal links between the parameters can be established, or a fault in an engineering system can be discovered. Thus the ultimate effect of the cognitive style described as weak central coherence is not a lack of ability to understand global relationships but rather a difference in the process by which global relationships are established. This is true at least in high-functioning CwA.

Experimental comparison of the ability to make inferences about complex systems, between CwA and controls, and across different stages of development or levels of functioning, may lead to the recognition of Empathy-Systemizing as an elaboration of the Central Coherence model, one that may make more precise and more accurate predictions about the behavior of people with autism when confronted with complex systems. In contrast to controls, CwA use a higher-dimensional representation for learning, so it is more computationally intensive to combine all these dimensions.

Although both central coherence and systemizing are useful psychological models to explain many aspects of autistic behavior, a complete explanation of autism will require that these psychological models be joined with neurobiological substrates—a process complicated by the fact that neither capacity is likely to be atomic in neurobiological terms.

To establish the relations between the psychological theories of autism, logical analysis can be helpful. (Stenning and van Lambalgen 2008) believe that there is a common core to the ToM deficit theory and executive disorder theory, which consists in well-defined failures in non-monotonic reasoning. However, we believe that these deficiencies are very different in nature: non-monotonic reasoning is the logical, domain-independent part, and ToM is a domain-specific set of axioms which happens to be corrupted but can be successfully taught.

3.4 ToM and a Module to Implement It

The notion of a 'ToM module' is fairly broad. In the context "from a neural system to behavior" it is obviously meant to be a piece of dedicated neural circuitry. In this way, it can differentiate us from our ancestors and it can also be malfunctioning in isolation. But it is precisely this isolation, ('encapsulation' according to Fodor), that is doubtful. One reason is just our general skepticism that evolution does not generally proceed by adding new modules (rather than tweaking old ones), and another is that much of the problem of functionally characterizing human reasoning about minds is about interactions between modules. ToM requires language to formulate beliefs in and it also entails a considerable involvement of working memory, as can be seen in 'nested' forms of ToM, as in the example of (Dunbar et al. 2015)

> Shakespeare intended us to realize that Othello believes that Iago knows that Desdemona is in love with Cassio.

Once we understand that it is rather implausible for ToM moduleto operate in isolation, then the ToM deficit hypothesis is becoming less sound. We can now consider the interactions of the ToM module with other language and memory functions, which lead to the possibility that a corruption in these functions is correlated with autism. It is also unclear what the ToM module would have to contain, given the observation that reasoning about intents of others can be partially functional in both CwA and non-human primates.

In this book we differentiate between the general reasoning capabilities and ToM axioms. We believe that they are not interdependent in most occasions. Since we know we can teach ToM axioms successfully, and there is not such axiom that can not be taught to any child, we do not confirm this "modularity" idea.

It is unclear from the experiments at what stage ToM abilities emerge. False-belief tasks were initially proposed as diagnosing a lack of these abilities in normal 3 year-olds and their presence in normal 4-year-olds (Leslie 1987). Others have proposed that irrelevant linguistic demands of these tasks underestimate 3-year-olds' performance. For example, in the 'Sally-Anne' task, the child sees the doll see the sweet placed in one box, and then the child but not the doll sees the sweet moved to another. Now if the child is asked 'Where will the doll look for the sweet first?' (instead of 'Where will the doll look for the sweet?') then children as young as two can sometimes solve the problem (Siegal and Beattie 1991). This might be read as evidence of the 3-year-olds in the original task adopting a conditional reading of the question (*Where* should the doll look?) rather than a descriptive one (Where will the doll look *first*?). Another possibility associated with a problem in the selection task, is that the younger child's problem may be with sequencing contingencies in their responses. These arguments push reasoning about intentions earlier in ontogeny.

Hence it is unclear if a neural module for ToM exists. However, it is safe to conclude that ToM-related reasoning belong to a separate clearly circumscribed component detached from the reasoning in other domains such as time, space and other dimensions of physical world.

3.5   ToM in Humans and Animals

Are Theory of Mind abilities unique to humans? (Premack and Woodruff 1978) posed the question: "Does the chimpanzee have a theory of mind"? An affirmative answer would downplay the overall significance of culture and enculturation in human ToM abilities. Reviewing a few decades of experimentation with primates that followed from Premack and Woodruff's provocative paper, (Call and Tomasello 2008) provide the definitive answer to their question: yes and no. There is solid experimental evidence that chimpanzees understand the goals and intentions of others, as well as the perception and knowledge of others. The behavioral evidence from chimpanzees suggests understanding that goes beyond the reading of surface behaviors of others, to underlying goals and perceptions – at least to the extent that human infants do in similar experimental designs.

In contrast, there is no experimental evidence that chimpanzees can grasp the notion of a false belief, or predict the behavior of another based on what the other knows. If we take a narrow view of the scope of ToM abilities, focusing on social cognitive reasoning, then our closest biological relatives have nothing like our human abilities. If instead we broaden our scope to include social perception and intentional interaction, then chimpanzees are convincingly competent. This shift in research focus toward social competency has led some researchers consider the question for more distant biological relatives, including domesticated dogs and other highly-social animals. The broad set of social skills that are often associated with human's ToM abilities appear to be common among animals. Birds will hide food far away from potential thieves, and wait to stash food until an onlooker is distracted. Dogs are able to follow a human's eyes or pointing gestures to hidden food. In contrast, not one other species has passed the false belief test, or exhibited anything like the deep social reasoning which is performed well by humans effortlessly.

ToM starts from (Premack and Woodruff 1978) work on chimpanzees to differentiate between humans and non-human primates. (Leslie 1987) proposed that human beings have a brain 'module' that does reasoning about minds, by implementing a ToM, and that autistic reasoning is associated with one or another form of corruption in this module.

So in CC the module constitutes the difference between humans and their ancestors. The work hypothesizes that once chimpanzee acquires ToM, their reasoning would approach humans, and once humans loose parts of ToM, they approach autistic reasoning. At the same time chimpanzees are hyper-social animals, unlike CwA. Whatever cognitive additions yielded humans from their ape ancestors, may be over-represented in autistic cognition. Just for an example to illustrate, much of autistic cognition is an obsessive attempt to extract exception-less truth about a complicated world. This sounds to us rather more like the scientific life than that of chimpanzees. Computer scientists and other natural science academics can empathize with autistic reasoners.

These issues raise many questions concerning what non-human primates are capable of doing in terms of reasoning about behavior and mental processes. Apes are capable of reasoning about the plans of other apes, including the intentions behind their behavior, but they appear not to be able to reason about specific knowledge (epistemic) states. Correspondingly, young children first develop 'desire' psychology before they proceed to 'knowledge' and 'belief' psychology.

3.6 CwA and CC in Abstract Reasoning Tasks

Recent studies (e.g. Dawson et al. 2007) have reported that autistic people perform in the normal range on the Raven Progressive Matrices test, a formal reasoning test that requires integration of relations as well as the ability to deduce behavioral rules and form high-level abstractions. (Morsanyi and Holyoak 2010) compared autistic and control children, matched on age, IQ, and verbal and non-verbal working memory, using both the Raven test and pictorial tests of analogical reasoning. They found that autistic children reasoning capabilities are similar to those of controls on reasoning with relations tests. The authors conclude that the basic ability to reason systematically with relations in the physical world, for both abstract and thematic entities, is intact in autism.

(Gokcen et al. 2009) investigated the potential values of executive function and social cognition deficits in autism. While ToM is generally accepted as a whole, a number of researchers suggested that it can be separated into two components (mental state reasoning and decoding). Both aspects of ToM and verbal working memory abilities were investigated with relatively demanding tasks of mental reasoning for parents of children with autism, who had verbal working memory deficits as well as low performance on a mental state reasoning task. The parents had difficulties in reasoning about others' emotions. In contrast to findings in the control group, low performance of mental state reasoning ability was not associated with working memory deficit in index parents. Social cognition and working memory impairments may represent potential genetic risks associated with autism.

In the physical world, children with autism perform relatively well. Autistic participants outperformed non-autistic participants on abstract spatial tests (Stevenson and Gernsbacher 2013). Non-autistic participants did not outperform autistic participants on any of the three domains (spatial, numerical, and verbal) or at either of the two reasoning levels (concrete and abstract), suggesting similarity in abilities between autistic and non-autistic individuals, with abstract spatial reasoning as an autistic strength.

3.7   ToM Controversy

The term "ToM" is problematic since the "theory" part implies a particular theoretical perspective on how people reason about the "mind". This reasoning happens through the fluid application of theoretical knowledge. The problems with this term have been fruitful since they stimulate psychologists to address the fundamental questions about the role of abstract knowledge (as a classical theoretical construct) in contemporary psychology. "Simulation theory" and "theory theory" dualism can be even considered from the philosophy of mind perspective (Crane and Patterson 2001).

In development psychology, changes in a child's capacity to reason about the mental states of other people has been experimentally observed. One experimental instrument for studying children's abilities to reason about the mental states of others is the False-belief task (Sect. 2.2). Success on this task has been criticized as neither entirely dependent on commonsense psychology abilities nor broadly representative of them (Bloom and German 2000). At the same time, the value of False-belief task is to reliably demonstrating an existence of the developmental shift. (Wellman et al. 2001) aggregated the results of almost two hundred separate studies of the False-belief task, finding that 3-year-olds will consistently fail this task on the majority of trials by indicating that Maxi will look for the object in the location to which his mother has moved it. 4-year-olds will succeed on half the trials, while 5-year-olds will succeed on the majority of trials. (Call and Tomasello 1999) demonstrated that these results are consistent across verbal and non-verbal versions of this task.

There is a developmental change between 3 and 5-year-olds, but it is unclear what exactly is being developed between these ages. One school of thought is that this developmental change can best be characterized as the acquisition by children of a better theoretical model of human psychology, a view first referred to as the "Theory Theory" by philosopher Adam Morton (1980). This view has several advocates among developmental psychologists (Wellman 1990; Gopnik and Wellman 1994), who characterize young children as extremely effective scientists that incrementally adapt their innate knowledge of people to accommodate for their experiences in the world. After years of social interaction, children's developing theories of the mind become more robust in their abilities to predict and explain human behavior, and increasingly include all of the principles of commonsense psychology in Heider's (1958) original characterization. This perspective is consistent with a broader position within developmental psychology that argues that the development of cognitive abilities is best viewed in terms of conceptual change. This perspective follows from the constructivist theories of development advanced by Piaget (1954), and can be contrasted with nativist theories that view the emergence of cognitive abilities as the maturation of innate brain functions.

While robots can acquire some ToM axioms, it is hard to imagine an algorithm that they would learn ToM from their experience. So in terms of reasoning, we hypothesize that all humans have ToM axioms embedded, but CC have this axiom "activated" at the age 4 and CwA are unable to activate it.

(Baron-Cohen et al. 1985) first hypothesized that the main behavioral symptoms of autism could be explained by a deficit in Theory of Mind abilities. The authors compared normal children with those diagnosed with autism and Down's syndrome on a variant of false-belief task involving two dolls, Sally and Anne. Even though the mental age of the autistic children was higher than that of the other groups, they alone failed to correctly ascribe a false belief to the doll in the experiment. The finding sparked a vigorous theoretical debate among the community of developmental psychologists and autism researchers that continues today.

Tager-Flusberg (2007) reflects on two decades of research that followed Baron-Cohen et al.'s hypothesis, which has upheld the original result: children with autism have difficulty attributing mental states to themselves or to other people. However, the significance of this finding is in doubt. Deficits in ToM abilities are not universal among autistic children, and neither offer an explanation for other typical symptoms such as repetitive nor for restricted behavior patterns. Tager-Flusberg advises to avoid a narrow view of the social-cognitive deficits in autism, and refers to recent studies on children's perception of mental-state information in faces, voices, and body gestures (Grigorenko et al. 2003). If the connection between ToM abilities and autism is to be explanatory, then the traditional understanding of ToM must be broadened to includes these social-perceptual skills. In today's corpus of work, the relationship between ToM and autism is fairly complex to serve as an illustration for the nativist-constructivist debate.

3.8 Discussion and Conclusions

People with autism and machines sometimes have difficulty comprehending when other people and users of these machines do not know something. CwA can get very agitated when a peer does not know the answer to a question she asks. By not understanding that other people think, believe, know, and want differently than themselves, CwA have problems relating socially and communicating to other people. As a result CwA and computer systems are frequently unable to anticipate what others will say or do in various situations, and have difficulty understanding that their classmates even have thoughts and emotions.

ToM arose from the study of primates and their social organization, and scholars in many fields – philosophy, anthropology, psychology, psychiatry and neuroscience – have contributed to this expanding topic.

For the purpose of a better representation and treatment, a more concise, more formal representation for reasoning about mental world than ToM is required. Since CwA have strong systematizing skills, they should be the foundation to ground the emphasizing skills. Since they cannot be introduced in a natural way, they should be taught via rules, such as an empathy to someone's pain, a scenario to pretend, a knowledge state to ask or share information.

To enable ToM to better correlate reasoning about mental attitudes and behavior, the notion of knowing about knowing needs to be formalized and expressed as axioms. Moreover, relations between knowledge space and intention space needs to be established as a rule system suitable for teaching CwA and machines (Chap. 4). A formal link between ToM as a theory-theory and meta-reasoning (Sect. 4.1.3) needs to be established. We need to marry ToM which ascribes mental states to humans with the multiagent systems theory which accumulated substantial experience doing this for automated agents: it will happen in Chaps. 4 and 5.

The foundation of ToM are connected with the nativist-constructivist debate which has been initiated by philosophers hundreds of years ago. It concerns the origin of knowledge and whether it is yielded by native abilities or was derived empirically. In terms of linguistic capabilities, this is formulated as whether humans possess a specific cognitive mechanism for comprehending and producing language, or these capabilities are due to a general cognitive tools. The former represents the nativists theories and the latter is favored by constructivists. If an individual has an innate grammatical knowledge, it has to be domain-specific. Also, a deviation, a move away from this grammatical knowledge means that a language is not associated with special cognitive skills.

Computer science favors the nativist positions and robots need separate components for each kind of knowledge. Teaching CwA, however, we intend to give them general axioms about knowledge and then expect these axioms to be applied in multiple modalities beyond language. How can we teach children to classify states and words for them into abstract categories, unless they already have knowledge of these categories? To overcome this difficulty, we will introduce a basis of undefined concepts and then teach other concepts of mental world relying on this basis.

If robots are capable to recognize faces, voices and body gestures and have functioning ToM components, it can be shown that removal of some axioms in the ToM component will break the overall system, having signal recognition component intact (Galitsky 2002).

As to our framework of *reasoning engine → behavior*, we now focus on the main component of reasoning such as reasoning about mental states as the cornerstone of autistic reasoning. We target explaining the broad range of autistic behavior via the peculiarities of autistic reasoning in this very restricted domain, putting the whole physical world aside. We will look at emphasizing from the systemizing standpoint and attempt to represent the richness of mental world in a formal, structured way acceptable to an autistic systematizer.

References

Baron-Cohen S (1987) Perception in autistic children. In: Cohen D (ed) Handbook of autism and pervasive developmental disorders. Wiley, Hoboken

Baron-Cohen S (1995) Mindblindness: an essay on autism and theory of mind. MIT Press/Bradford Books, Boston

Baron-Cohen S (2002) The extreme male brain theory of autism. Trends Cogn Sci 6:248–254

Baron-Cohen S, Leslie AM, Frith U (1985) Does the autistic child have a 'theory of mind'?
    Cognition 21:37–46
Baron-Cohen S, Richler J, Bisarya D, Gurunathan N, Wheelwright S (2003) The systemizing
    quotient: an investigation of adults with Asperger syndrome or high-functioning autism, and
    normal sex differences. Philos Trans Biol Sci 358:361–374
Bloom P, German TP (2000) Two reasons to abandon the false belief task as a test of theory of
    mind. Cognition 77(2000):B25–B31
Bowler D, Gardner J, Grice S (2000) Episodic memory and remembering in adults with Asperger
    syndrome. J Autism Dev Disord 30:295–304
Call J, Tomasello M (1999) A nonverbal false belief task: the performance of children and great
    apes. Child Dev 70(2):381–95
Call J, Tomasello M (2008) Does the chimpanzee have a theory of mind? 30 years later. Trends
    Cogn Sci 12(5):187–192
Capps L, Yirmiya N, Sigman M (1992) Understanding of simple and complex emotions in non-
    retarded children with autism. J Child Psychol Psychiatry 33:1169–1182
Cohen IL (1994) An artificial neural network analogue of learning in autism. Biol Psychiatry
    36:5–20
Crane T, Patterson S (2001) "Introduction". History of the Mind-Body Problem. pp. 1–2. the
    assumption that mind and body are distinct (essentially, dualism)
Dawson M, Soulires I, Gernsbacher MA, Mottron L (2007) The level and nature of autistic
    intelligence. Psychol Sci 18(8):657–662
Dennett D (1987) The intentional stance. MIT Press, Cambridge, MA
Dunbar RIM, Launay J, Curry O (2015) The complexity of jokes is limited by cognitive constraints
    on mentalizing. Hum Nat 1–11
Galitsky B (2002) Extending the BDI model to accelerate the mental development of autistic
    patients. In: Second international conference on development & learning. Cambridge, MA
Gallese V, Goldman A (1998) Mirror neurons and the simulation theory of mind-reading. Trends
    Cogn Sci 2:493–501
Gallese V, Fadiga L, Fogassi L, Rizzolatti G (1996) Action recognition in the premotor cortex.
    Brain 119:593–609
Gokcen S, Bora E, Erermis S, Kesikci H, Aydin C (2009) Theory of mind and verbal working
    memory deficits in parents of autistic children. Psychiatry Res 166(1):46–53
Gopnik A, Wellman HM (1994) The theory theory. In: Hirschfeld LA, Gelman SA (eds) Mapping
    the mind: domain specificity in cognition and culture. Cambridge University Press, New York
Grigorenko EL, Klin A, Volkmar F (2003) Hyperlexia: disability or superability? J Child Psychol
    Psychiatry 44:1079–1091
Harris PL (2000) The work of the imagination. Blackwell, Oxford/Boston
Heider F (1958) The psychology of interpersonal relations. Wiley, New York
Iacoboni M, Mazziotta JC (2007) Mirror neuron system: basic findings and clinical applications.
    Ann Neurol 62:213–218
Lawson J, Baron-Cohen S, Wheelwright S (2004) Empathising and systemising in adults with and
    without Asperger syndrome. J Autism Dev Disord 34:301–310
Leslie AM (1987) Pretence and representation: the origins of "theory of mind". Psychol Rev
    94:412–426
Losh M, Capps L (2006) Understanding of emotional experience in Autism: insights from the
    personal accounts of high-functioning children with Autism. Dev Psychol 42(5):809–818
Morsanyi K, Holyoak KJ (2010) Analogical reasoning ability in autistic and typically developing
    children. Dev Sci 13(4):578–587
Morton A (1980) Frames of mind. Oxford University Press, Oxford
Norenzayan A, Gervais WM, Trzesniewski KH (2012) Mentalizing deficits constrain belief in a
    personal god. PlosOne http://dx.doi.org/10.1371/journal.pone.0036880
Piaget J (1954) The construction of reality in the child. Basic Books, New York
Premack D (1990) The infant's theory of self-propelled objects. Cognition 36:1–16

Premack D, Woodruff G (1978) Does the chimpanzee have a theory of mind? Behav Brain Sci 4:515–526

Rao AS, Georgeff MP (1995) BDI-agents: from theory to practice. In: Proceedings of the first international conference on multiagent systems (ICMAS' 1995)

Seidner LB, Stipek D, Feshbach N (1988) A developmental analysis of elementary school-aged children's concepts of pride and embarrassment. Child Dev 59:367–377

Siegal M, Beattie K (1991) Where to look first for children's knowledge of false beliefs. Cognition 38:1–12

Stenning K (2002) Seeing reason. Image and language in learning to think. Oxford University Press, Oxford

Stenning K, Michiel Van L (2008) Human reasoning and cognitive science. MIT Press, Cambridge, MA

Stevenson JL, Gernsbacher MA (2013) Abstract spatial reasoning as an Autistic strength. PlosOne. doi:10.1371/journal.pone.0059329

Stipek D, DeCotis K (1988) Children's understanding of the impli- cations of causal attributions for emotional experiences. Child Dev 59:1601–1610

Tager-Flusberg H (2007) Evaluating the theory-of-mind hypothesis of autism current directions. Psychol Sci 16(6):311–315

Tomasello M (1988) The role of joint-attentional processes in early language acquisition. Lang Sci 10:69–88

Vogeley K, Bussfeld P, Newen A, Herrmann S, Happé F, Falkai P, Maier W, Shah NJ, Fink GR, Zilles K (2001) Mind reading: neural mechanisms of theory of mind and self-perspective. Neuroimage 14(1 Pt 1):170–181

Wellman HM (1990) The child's theory of mind. MIT Press, Cambridge, MA

Wellman HM, Cross D, Watson J (2001) Meta-analysis of theory-of-mind development: the truth about false belief. Child Dev 72:655–684

Wrongplanet (2015) Hide and seek (And Mindblindness). http://wrongplanet.net/forums/viewtopic.php?t=738

Chapter 4
Formalizing Theory of Mind

While identifying multiple core deficits outlined above certainly helps in the study and diagnosis of autism, it does not provide a causal explanation of the disorder, nor does it provide a rehabilitation mechanism. A more concise account of autistic reasoning and how it implies behavior in the real is required, and in this chapter we attempt to build a formal model of ToM so that in the chapter to follow we can build a computational implementation of it.

Reasoning about mental world is the cornerstone of autistic reasoning phenomena. Unlike controls, children with autism experience difficulties differentiating between physical and mental objects like thoughts and mental actions like knowledge sharing. We start with the ToM, representing autistic reasoning in psychological terms, and proceed to its formalization in terms of belief-desire-intention. Having represented the ToM as a computational model, we proceed towards the computational linguistic model of basic (*knowing* and *wanting*) and derived mental entities such as *informing, pretending, cheating* and *reconciling*. Relying on the linguistic approach of semantic roles and logic programming-style clauses, definitions for derived mental entities are proposed which can be directly taught to children with autism. A link between reasoning about the mental world, behavior in it, communication with other people and its emotional colors are introduced based on the formalized Theory of Mind. More complex form of formalized behavior forms and interactions between human to be taught to autistic patients are also analyzed, including arguing, offending, explaining, cooperation and team formation.

In our formal description of the real mental world, we follow its natural language representation as closely as possible, while obeying the restrictions of a formal language. In contrast to the traditional modal logic-based formal representation of knowledge, belief and intention, we use the wider set of mental entities with multiple possible interpretations. Acquiring mental entities, autistic trainees are expected to reproduce them in their behavioral patterns and to discover them in the verbal communication of others. Therefore, both natural language and formal

© Springer International Publishing Switzerland 2016

B. Galitsky, *Computational Autism*, Human–Computer Interaction Series,
DOI 10.1007/978-3-319-39972-0_4

Fig. 4.1 Mental space and its
dimensions to represent
Theory of Mind

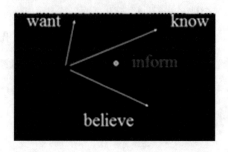

language (user interfaces of software) representations need to accompany each
mental scenario (a scenario with interacting human agents). Sometimes, autistic
children prefer to operate with the latter: the user interface of a software system
seems to be more attractive than reading or talking in the NL.

This basis (Fig. 4.1) is an adequate approximation of meanings in the multiagent
settings. Meaning of entity is expressed with respect to agent's reaction. There are
multiple definitions (clauses) for each NL entity (ambiguity). However, there is
one-to-one map between generalizations of these clauses in a metalanguage and
respective NL entities.

4.1 Computer Science of Theory of Mind

In this section we will define the main problem of ToM, introduce the BDI model,
focus on meta-reasoning and then proceed to computational linguistics' issues of
ToM.

4.1.1 Defining Main Problem of ToM

In this section we give a computational definition of main ToM problem, and in the
rest of this section we address a number of issues associated with its solution.

Definition The main problem of ToM is to build a set of consecutive mental states
given an arbitrary initial mental state in the fixed vocabulary of mental states and
actions. The formal declarative definitions of mental states and actions are also
given. This set of consecutive mental actions must be consistent with the definitions
of involved mental states and actions.

Informally, for a human this set should sound plausible, as far as the definition of
mental states and actions are plausible and match human intuition. Since definition
of mental actions are of a declarative nature, they do not give a hint on how to
navigate mental space to satisfy them, including pre-conditions and effects. The
richer the set of definitions is available, the more extensive the derived set of
consecutive mental states is expected to be. Definitions can include communicative

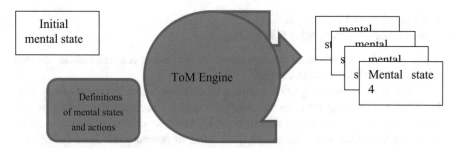

Fig. 4.2 The Task of ToM engine is to yield a set of consecutive mental states for an arbitrary initial one, having the set of initial mental states

actions, emotions, requests (Fig. 4.2). The objective of this book is to build a computational model for solving this problem and to teach CwA to solve it. The limitation of autistic reasoning as presented in this Figure is both *ToM engine* operating with mental entities, and *definitions for mental entities*. Although the former cannot be built directly, we focus on the latter and teach definitions of mental states and actions. This in turn improves the ToM engine itself feeding it with a high number of instances of these definitions.

We attempt to build a generic model of mental world that is sufficiently expressive to represent ToM as it is described in literature on one hand, and formalized as a theory in this book on the other hand. This model is expected to differentiate CwA and CC, as well as concisely describe ASD spectrum in terms of ToM capabilities, from high functioning in reasoning about mental states to rudimentary reasoning skills. There is a single mental world and we expect there to be a single ToM not just associated with autistic reasoning but rather broad spectrum of activities of human and automated agents. The ToM-oriented model of mental world follows the series of formalisms we have develop to simulate the mental attitude in a broad variety of domains, including mental states of investors, bloggers, wireless subscribers, negotiators, literature characters (Galitsky 2002, 2009). Each of these domains requires formation of the special set of mental entities, and a set of domain-specific additional constraints for the co-occurrence of mental entities.

The main players in the mental world are beliefs, desires and intentions. These players are states as well as actions, which lead to these states, such as *informing* leads to *knowing*. At the same time, mental states cause mental actions that are believed to bring an agent to desired mental states. For example, the state of *not knowing* of agent *H* may lead to its action of *asking* which may cause the action of *informing* by a peer agent which finally brings the state of knowing.

CwA confuses both mental states and action, as well as transitions between them. CwA does not know what *knowing* means, so the state of knowledge (absolute, always true, facts) and beliefs (something which can be revised, updated, associated with an emotion, forgotten) should be taught together with the action that leads to it. A typical example here is how to teach a CwA to answer the question "What is in my bag?". CwA needs to be demonstrated that to acquire knowledge of what it is in a bag, a person should:

1. Open a bag and look into it
2. Ask those who know what is in the bag.

Alternatives for (1) are other perception modalities: a bag can be smelled, touched or attached to an ear to hear a sound.

Rather than trying to explain to a child with autism what are the states of *knowing, believing* and *wanting*, we introduce scenarios where associated mental actions lead to these states. These states are set to be *indefinable*, so instead of trying to define them, we introduce scenarios where CwA learn to operate with these indefinable mental states. The other, derived mental states are then introduced based on explicit formal definitions, relying on already acquired concepts of *knowing, believing* and *wanting*. Although for CC there is no substantial difference between basic and derived mental states, CwA acquire basic mental states by learning scenarios and derived mental states by learning their definitions, according to our teaching strategy.

Notice that CC form representation skills for mental states and actions naturally, by learning mental world, whereas CwA need to be taught following the axiomatic principle. This is similar to how most people learn geometry as axiomatic system: given axioms for a point and a line (indefinable entities), they learn to prove theorems about geometric figures. To do that they first consider various "scenarios" for how lines and points are situated, "interacting" with each other. This helps to develop intuition about geometric abstractions. For CwA, entities of ToM are abstractions in a similar sense, so they need to learn the mental states and actions in the same ways mathematicians learn abstract theories. Possibly, CwA will never use mental actions naturally, but at least learning the mental world in an axiomatic form will make learning process concise and systematic.

In ToM, agents form coalitions (try to play together), negotiate (dispute and quarrel) about achieving certain physical and mental states (e.g. possession of a toy or knowledge about what is in someone's bag). To adequately represent multiagent cooperation or conflicts within ToM, it is necessary to build a computational framework that is capable of producing a sequence of consecutive mental states and actions given an arbitrary initial set of mental states. Also a ToM simulation system is expected to search for causal links in the known, observed part of a scenario of interaction between children and predicts the future, unknown continuation of scenario in terms of mental states actions.

Before we start our comprehensive introduction to the formalized ToM, we briefly outline the main concepts. In our formal description of the mental world we try to follow its natural language representation as close as possible. Coding the conflict scenarios as logic programs, we target the different formal treatment of distinct mental entities, which are in use in the natural language description of this scenario. Adequate description of the mental world can be performed using mental entities and merging all other physical actions into a constant predicate for an arbitrary physical action and its resultant physical state (for simplicity). It is well known that humans can adequately operate with the set of natural language mental expressions containing not more than *four* mutually dependent mental entities.

4.1.2   Belief–Desire–Intention Model

The belief–desire–intention (BDI) model is a software model developed for programming intelligent agents. It is focused on the implementation of an agent's beliefs, desires and intentions, relying on these entities to solve a particular problem in agent programming. BDI model separates the process of selecting a plan (from a plan library or an external planner application) from the execution of currently active plans. BDI is a practical mechanism to solve ToM problems: BDI agents are able to balance the time spent on deliberating about plans (choosing what to do) and executing those plans (doing it). CwA need to be taught to plan to split their thinking into the one concerning choosing what to do and the one associated with actual doing.

BDI follows Michael Bratman's theory of human practical reasoning it implements the notions of belief, desire and intention. Intention and desire are both pro-attitudes (mental attitudes concerned with action), but intention is distinguished as a conduct-controlling pro-attitude. He identifies commitment as the difference between desire and intention, noting that it leads to temporal persistence in plans and also further plans being made on the basis of those plans to which it is already committed. There is a logical model that allows to define and reason about BDI agents. A formal logical descriptions such as (Rao and Georgeff 1995) BDICTL combines a multiple-modal logic (with modalities representing beliefs, desires and intentions) with the temporal logic CTL*. (Wooldridge 2000) used BDICTL to define the Logic Of Rational Agents, by incorporating an action logic, which allows reasoning not only about individual agents, but also about communication and other interaction in a multiagent system.

The idealized architectural components of a BDI system are as follows:

- *Beliefs*: Beliefs represent the current, instant knowledge (informational) state of the agent. These states include beliefs about the world including her self and peer agents. (Meta-)beliefs can also include inference rules (clauses), allowing to derive new beliefs. We using the term *belief* together with *knowledge* to confirm that what an agent believes is not always true and can be updated, revised or rejected.
- *Desires*: Desires are the motivational state of the agent. They represent objectives or situations that the agent *would like* to accomplish or bring about. Examples of desires might be: *find the best location*, *get food* or *become famous*.

  - *Goals*: A goal is a subtype of desire that has been used to express an for active pursuit by the agent. Usage of the term *goals* adds the further restriction that the set of active desires must be consistent. For example, one should not have concurrent goals to spend money to buy something he wants and to save money at the same time (even though both spending and saving could both be desirable)

- *Intentions*: Intentions represent the deliberative state of the agent – what the agent *has chosen* to do. Intentions are desires to which the agent has to some extent committed. In implemented systems, this means the agent has begun executing a plan.

  - *Plans*: Plans are sequences of actions (recipes or knowledge areas) that an agent can perform to achieve one or more of its intentions. Plans may include other plans: my plan to go to pre-school may include a plan to find my favorite toy to take with me. Plans must be defined to CwA in a way that first a sequence of actions must be planned, then attempted to be executed and then adjusted to the environment as appropriate. It has to be explained that it is hard to plan everything exactly, 100 % because there are always unknown circumstances, and actions need to be altered to accommodate them.

- *Events*: These are brief states that are caused by sources outside of a human or automated agent. Events are triggers for reactive activity by the agent. An event may update beliefs, trigger plans or modify goals. Events may be generated externally and received by sensors or integrated systems. Additionally, events may be generated internally to trigger decoupled updates or plans of activity. The difference between events which may occur, may be attended or avoided, may be expected or emergent, needs to be explained to CwA (Fig. 4.3).

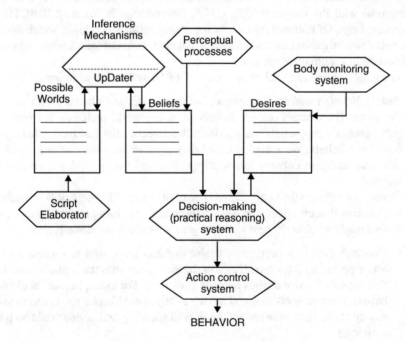

Fig. 4.3 The connection between beliefs, desires, intentions, the resultant behavior and its monitoring

4.1.3   Meta-Reasoning

The capacity to think about our own thinking may lie at the heart of ToM. Philosophers and cognitive scientists have investigated these matters for many years. As humans, we continually think about ourselves and our strengths and weaknesses in order to manage both the private and public worlds within which we exist. Researchers in artificial intelligence have gone further, attempting to implement actual machines that mimic, simulate, and perhaps even replicate this capacity, called *metareasoning*.

If a text tells us how to do things, or how something has been done, we classify this text as a language-object. If a text is saying how to write a document which explains how to do things, we classify it as metalanguage. Metalanguage is a language or symbolic system used to discuss, describe, or analyze another language or symbolic system. In theorem proving, metalanguage is a language in which proofs are manipulated and tactics are programmed, as opposed to the logic itself (the object-language). In logic, it is a language in which the truth of statements in another language is being discussed.

Meta-reasoning addresses a question of how to give a system its own representation to manipulate. Meta-reasoning needs both levels for both languages and domain behavior. We depict two main classes of interest in Fig. 4.4.

Traditionally thinking or *reasoning* has been cast as a decision cycle within an action-perception loop similar to that shown in Fig. 4.5 An intelligent agent perceives some stimuli from the environment and behaves rationally to achieve its goals by selecting some action from its set of competencies. The result of these actions at the ground level is subsequently perceived at the object level, and the cycle continues. *Metareasoning* is the process of reasoning about this reasoning cycle. It consists of both the metalevel control of computational activities and the introspective monitoring of reasoning (see Fig. 4.6). This cyclical arrangement represents a higher-level reflection of the standard action-perception cycle, and as such, it represents the perception of reasoning and its control.

Introspective monitoring is necessary to gather sufficient information with which to make effective metalevel control decisions. Monitoring may involve the gathering

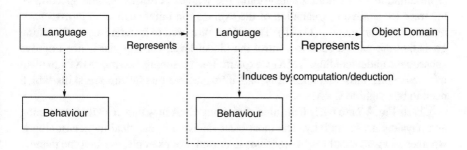

Fig. 4.4 Meta-reasoning chart: mutual relationships between major classes of our interest

Fig. 4.5 The
action-perception cycle

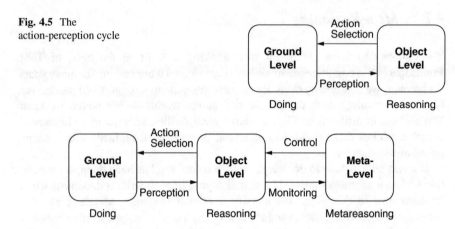

Fig. 4.6 Duality in reasoning and acting

of computational performance data so as to build a profile of various decision
algorithms. It could involve generating explanations for object-level choices and
their effect on ground-level performance. When reasoning fails at some task, it may
involve the explanation of the causal contributions of failure and the diagnosis of
the object-level reasoning process.

The introspective monitoring of reasoning about performance requires an agent
to maintain some kind of internal feedback in addition to perception, so that it can
perform effectively and can evaluate the results of metareasoning. If the reasoning
that is performed at the object level (and not just its results) is represented in
a declarative knowledge structure that captures the mental states and decision-
making sequence, then these knowledge structures can themselves be passed to the
metalevel for monitoring.

For example, the Meta-AQUA system (Cox and Ram 1999) keeps a trace of its
story understanding decisions in structures called a *trace meta-explanation pattern*
(TMXP). Here the object-level story understanding task is to explain anomalous
or unusual events in a ground-level story perceived by the system. Then, if this
explanation process fails, Meta-AQUA passes the TMXP and the current story
representation to a learning subsystem. The learner performs an introspection of
the trace to obtain an explanation of the explanation failure called an *introspective
metaexplanation pattern* (IMXP). The IMXPs are used to generate a set of learning
goals that are passed back to control the object-level learning and hence improve
subsequent understanding. TMXPs explain *how* reasoning occurs; IMXPs explain
why reasoning fails. Explainability and introspective monitoring are skills which
need to be taught to CwA.

Charts Fig. 4.7 are fairly helpful in explaining CwA how they plan their reasoning
and physical action activity. The most basic decision in classical metareasoning is
whether an agent should act or continue to reason. For example, the anytime planner
always has a current best plan produced by the object-level reasoning. Given that
the passage of time incurs a certain fee, the metareasoner must decide whether the

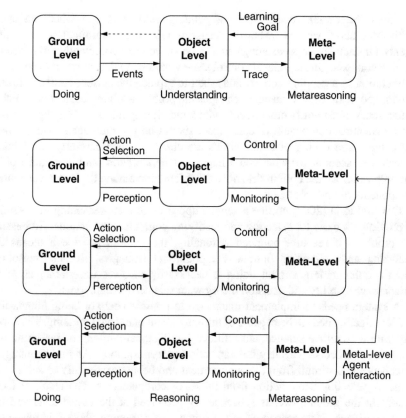

Fig. 4.7 From doing and understanding to metareasoning (on the *top*). Multiagent meta-level control (on the *bottom*)

expected benefit gained by planning further outweighs the cost of doing nothing. If so, it produces another plan; otherwise, it executes the actions in the plan it already has.

In a multiagent context, if two or more agents need to coordinate their actions, the agents' metacontrol components must be on the same page. The agents must reason about the same problem and may need to be at the same stage of the problem-solving process. For example, suppose one agent decides to devote little time to communication negotiation (Alexander et al. 2007) before moving to other deliberative decisions, while another agent sets aside a large portion of deliberation time for negotiation; the latter agent would waste time trying to negotiate with an unwilling partner.

We define an agent's problem-solving context as the information required for deliberative-level decision making, including the agent' s current goals, action choices, its past and current performance, resource usage, dependence on other agents, and so on. Suppose the agent's context when it is in the midst of execution is called the *current context*, and a *pending context* is one where an agent deliberates about various "what-if" scenarios related to coordination with other agents. Distributed metareasoning can also be viewed as a coordination of problem-solving contexts. One metalevel control issue would be to decide when to complete deliberation in a pending context and when to replace the current context with the pending context. Thus, if an agent changes the problem-solving context on which it is focused, it must notify other agents with which it may interact. This suggests that the metacontrol component of each agent should have a multiagent policy where the content and timing of deliberations are choreographed carefully and include branches to account for what could happen as deliberation (and execution) plays out. Figure 4.7 on the bottom describes the interaction among the metalevel control components of multiple agents.

Cox and Raja (2007) outline a general approach to meta-reasoning in the sense of providing a basis for selecting and justifying computational actions. Addressing the problem of resource-bounded rationality, the authors provide a means for analyzing and generating optimal computational strategies. Because reasoning about a computation without doing it necessarily involves uncertainty as to its outcome, probability and decision theory were selected as main tools.

A system needs to implement manguage to impress peers of being human-like and intelligent, needs to be capable of thinking about one's own thinking. Traditionally within cognitive science and artificial intelligence, thinking or reasoning has been cast as a decision cycle within an action-perception loop. An intelligent agent perceives some stimuli from the environment and behaves rationally to achieve its goals by selecting some action from its set of competencies. The result of these actions at the ground level is subsequently perceived at the object level and the cycle continues. Meta-reasoning is the process of reasoning about this reasoning cycle. It consists of both the meta-level control of computational activities and the introspective monitoring of reasoning. (Galitsky 2015) focused on linguistic issues of text which describes such cognitive architecture. It turns out that there is a correlation between a cognitive architecture and a discourse structure used to express it in text. Relying on this correlation, it is possible to automatically classify texts with respect to metalanguage they contain.

A mixture of object-language and metalanguage descriptions can be found in literature. Describing the nature, a historical event, an encounter between people, an author uses a language-object. Describing thoughts, beliefs, desires and knowledge of characters about the nature, events and interactions between people, an author uses a metalanguage. The entities/relations of such metalanguage range over the expressions (phrases) of the language-object. In other words, the physical world is usually described in language-object, and the mental world typically combines both levels.

One of the purest examples of use of metalanguage in literature is Franz Kafka's novel "The Trial". According to our model, the whole plot is described in metalanguage, and object-level representation is absent. This is unlike a typical work of literature, where both levels are employed. In "The Trial" a reader learns the main character Joseph K is being prosecuted, his thoughts are described, meeting with various people related to the trial are presented. However, no information is available about a reason for the trial, the charge, the circumstances of the deed. The novel is a pure example of the presence of meta-theory and absence of object-level theory, from the standpoint of logic. The reader is expected to form the object–level theory herself to avoid ambiguity in interpretation of the novel.

Exploration of "The Trial" helps to understand the linguistic properties of metalanguage and language-object. For example, it is easy to differentiate between a mental and a physical words, just relying on keywords. However, to distinguish meta-language from language-object in text, one need to consider different discourse structures, which we will automatically learn from text.

The following paragraph of text can be viewed as a fragment of an algorithm for how to solve an abstract problem of acquittal. Since it suggests a domain-independent approach (it does not matter what an accused did), it can be considered as a meta-algorithm.

'There are three possibilities: absolute acquittal, apparent acquittal and defer-ment. Absolute acquittal is the best, but there is nothing I could do to get that sort of outcome. I don't think there's anyone at all who could do anything to get an absolute acquittal. Probably the only thing that could do that is if the accused is innocent. As you are innocent it could actually be possible and you could depend on your innocence alone. In that case you will not need me or any other kind of help.'

In some sense this algorithm follows along the lines of a 'vanilla' interpreter in Prolog, a typical example of a meta-program:

```
achieve_acquittal( true ).
achieve_acquittal ( (A,B) ) :- achieve_acquittal (A), achieve_acquittal (B).
achieve_acquittal ( A ) :- clause(A,B), achieve_acquittal(B).
```

where the novel enumerates various *clauses*, but never ground terms expressing the details of a hypothetical crime (no instances of A or B). *clause(A,B)* is expression of the format A:- B, where A is a term being defined (a clause head) and B is a sequence of defining terms (a body of this clause). This interpreter shows multiple possibilities a term can be proved, similarly to multiple possibilities of acquittal spelled out by Kafka. We hypothesize that a text expressing such a meta-program, Kafka's text, should have specific sequences of rhetoric relation, infrequent in other texts. We will attempt to find distinct discourse patterns associated with metalanguage and differentiate it with other texts. In the literature domain, it is possible to draw a boundary between the pure metalanguage (peculiar works of literature) and a mixed level text (a typical work of literature).

Let us consider an example of an introspection in the domain of conflicts. An agent who is an opponent to a complainant is capable of following reasoning about complainant's mental states as well as about their own:

If a complainant asks me about his problem then if I would not know the answer I will deny responsibility, and if he asks me how to fix the problem I would need to consult an external source because I don't know.

4.1.4 Entities of ToM

In natural language, mental entities, as well as other words, have a variety of meanings. At the same time, a set of meanings which are expressed by a given word for mental action or state has a lot of common features. Therefore, we will use the multiple definitions for the same mental entity. To maintain the proper level of abstraction, expressing that a subject of a mental action can be a fact, other mental action or a clause, we use metapredicates. The arguments of these metapredicates range over agents and their subjects of beliefs, knowledge, intentions and other metal actions and states (metapredicates are the predicates whose arguments range over arbitrary well-written formulas (Criscuolo et al. 2002)). For example, a relation of *reconciliation* between two people involved in a conflict, conflict mediator, a subject of their conflict and a reconciliation event is expressed as:

   reconcile(Person-in-conflict1, Person-in-conflict2, Mediator, ConflictSubj, Event)

Person-in-conflict1, Person-in-conflict2, Mediator range over person names, whereas *ConflictSubj* and *Event* can be facts, formulas for mental states and actions, and even clauses (definitions) expressing conditions for mental states and actions.

The set of mental metapredicates, can be divided into three categories:

- Metapredicates for *basic mental states, intention, knowledge and belief*, following the BDI model;
- Metapredicates for derived mental states and actions. They are expressed via the metapredicates for basic mental states. For example, there are families of definitions for *cheat, reconcile,* etc. This category also includes communicative actions (mental actions involving an actor and a receiver according to Speech Act theory) such as *inform, explain, convince.*
- Metapredicates for emotions. Emotions are the formally independent entities, which are semantically close to one or another derived mental states, but contain additional sentiment load.

Teaching of mental entities occurs according to these categories. First, CwA needs to be shown the structure of mental action or states as a metapredicates, with examples for each kind of their signature (believe in a fact, believe in a conditional event, believe in a belief, belief in a condition for intent). Then basic mental states should be taught by examples. After that, derived mental states are introduced via definitions; multiple meanings for each are demonstrated via multiple definitions. These definitions rely on the bases of intent, knowledge, belief. Finally, emotions are defined in this bases again and the rules for their pre- and post-conditions are spelled out.

How strong is the coverage of our basis, and how accurately can derived mental states and actions be defined in this basis? The precision of our approach can be estimated as a difference between a formal definition of mental state in our basis D and informal definition in plain words P. Our claim is that the deviation of meaning of D from P is so small that it does not lead to a different choice of action in a situation S where P is substituted with D:

Claim: For any *S* and any *P* if the best action to bring an agent into a most desired state is *A*, it is the same action for *S* and *D*.

$$\forall P \; \exists D \; \forall S \; \text{if} \; \{S, P\} \rightarrow_A A \text{ then } \{S, D\} \rightarrow_A A.$$

Where $\rightarrow_A$ stands for the following relation: given states leads to an optimal action in terms of most desired resultant state.

In other words, our approximation is accurate enough to assure the agent to select the same action in the cases of an ideal and approximate definition of a mental state D, given an arbitrary set S of other expressions for mental states *D* is added to.

For example, we can approximate *to be afraid (of something)* by *not want (something)*, when we talk about an agent that chooses an avoidance behavior. If such the agent has two choices – to avoid or not to avoid, it does not matter for his choice of action whether he does *not want* to be with another agent or feels being *frightened* by that agent. Therefore, a derived mental entity forms the class of equivalence of mental entities (emotions) with respect to the choice of action by an agent (mental or physical, from the fixed set). The reader can easily construct mental formulas for *forgetting* (lack of a *belief* that follows its presence at some point in time), *dreaming* (*intention* of some physical or mental state to occur), *imagining* (*believing* that something holds *knowing* that the *belief* is wrong), *feeling guilty* (*intention* that some action that has been committed should not has been done and *belief* that it depended on the agent's physical or mental state), *infatuation, fascination, anger, surprise, embarrassment, shame, anxiety, etc.*, approximating their meanings for particular situations. A meaning of an entity can be formally defined in a narrow domain only (particularly, as a set of relevant answers in a question-answering settings, Galitsky 2003).

4.1.5   Linguistics of ToM Entities

Learning communicative actions is a key to entering the mental world. Computational verb lexicons are key to supporting acquisition of entities for actions, and a rule-based form to express their meanings. Verbs express the semantics of an event being described as well as the relational information among participants in that event, and project the syntactic structures that encode that information. Verbs, and in particular the ones for communicative actions, are also highly variable, displaying a rich range of semantic behaviors. Verb classification helps a learning systems to deal with this complexity by organizing verbs into groups that share core semantic properties.

VerbNet (Kipper et al. 2008) is one such lexicon, which identifies semantic roles and syntactic patterns characteristic of the verbs in each class and makes explicit the connections between the syntactic patterns and the underlying semantic relations that can be inferred for all members of the class. Each syntactic frame in a class has a corresponding semantic representation that details the semantic relations between event participants across the course of the event.

Let us consider the verb *amuse*. There is a cluster of similar verbs that have a similar structure of arguments (semantic roles) such as *amaze, anger, arouse, disturb, irritate*, and other. VerbNet is a good source of information on verbs in general and communicative actions in particular. The roles of the arguments of these communicative actions are as follows:

- Experiencer (usually, an animate entity)
- Stimulus
- Result

The frames (the classes of meanings differentiated by syntactic features for how this verb occurs in a sentence) are as follows (NP – noun phrase, N – noun, V – communicative action, VP – verb phrase, ADV – adjective):

NP V NP
   Example: *"The teacher amused the children."*
   Syntax: Stimulus V Experiencer
   Clause:
amuse(Stimulus, E, Emotion, Experiencer):-
      cause(Stimulus, E),
      emotional_state(result(E), Emotion, Experiencer).

NP V ADV-Middle
   Example: *"Small children amuse quickly."*
   Syntax: Experiencer V ADV
   Clause:
amuse(Experiencer, Prop):-
      property(Experiencer, Prop), adv(Prop).

NP V NP-PRO-ARB
   example   "The teacher amused."
   syntax   Stimulus V
amuse(Stimulus, E, Emotion, Experiencer):-
      cause(Stimulus, E),
      emotional_state(result(E), Emotion, ?Experiencer).
NP.cause V NP
   example   "The teacher's dolls amused the children."
   syntax   Stimulus <+genitive> ('s) V Experiencer
amuse(Stimulus, E, Emotion, Experiencer):-
      cause(Stimulus, E),
      emotional_state(during(E), Emotion, Experiencer).

NP V NP ADJ
   example   "This performance bored me totally."
   syntax   Stimulus V Experiencer Result
amuse(Stimulus, E, Emotion, Experiencer):-
      cause(Stimulus, E),
      emotional_state(result(E), Emotion, Experiencer),
      Pred(result(E), Experiencer).

For this example, the information for the class of verbs *amuse is at* http://verbs.colorado.edu/verb-index/vn/amuse-31.1.php#amuse-31.1

We now show how communicative actions are split into clusters:

Verbs with Predicative Complements
Appoint, characterize, dub, declare, conjecture, masquerade, orphan, captain, consider, classify.
Verbs of Perception
See, sight, peer.
Psych-Verbs (Verbs of Psychological State)
Amuse, admire, marvel, appeal.
Verbs of Desire
Want, long.
Judgment Verbs
Judgment.
Verbs of Assessment
Assessment, estimate.
Verbs of Searching
Hunt, search, stalk, investigate, rummage, ferret.
Verbs of Social Interaction
Correspond, marry, meet, battle.
Verbs of Communication
Transfer(message), inquire, interrogate, tell, manner(speaking), talk, chat, say, complain, advise, confess, lecture, overstate, promise.
Avoid Verbs
Avoid.
Measure Verbs
Register, cost, fit, price, bill.
Aspectual Verbs
Begin, complete, continue, stop, establish, sustain.

4.1.6   From Deduction to Simulation and Learning

In this section we provide our motivations for selecting a hybrid approach to solve a main ToM problem. Formalizing ToM, we need to extend traditional BDI implementation of reasoning, based on modal logics, that is not well suited for expression practical applications, as we are going to show. In the last few decades, the interest to formal modeling of various forms of human reasoning and to simulation of mental behavior has strongly risen. A series of phenomena in human reasoning have been reflected in such approaches as reasoning about action and knowledge, nonmonotonic reasoning, and others. Modal logic-based and situation calculus–based approaches have become the most popular in formal modeling the mental attitudes (McCarthy 1995; Fagin et al. 1996; Wooldridge 2000). However, these approaches have to be extended for robust and efficient software implementations, associated with the following. It seems to be hard to directly take advantage of the practical limitation for the complexity of mental formulas (below four, Sect. 4.3.2). Also, the first-order logics, which are well-suited to handle certain phenomena of natural language in general, are frequently inadequate to handle the peculiarities of ambiguity in *mental* natural language expressions (Sect. 4.2.4).

We believe that using pure deductive logical means as, for example, default logic for semantic disambiguation, reasoning about action and time (see e.g. Shoham 1993; Shanahan 1997), if applied to mental world, or constraint satisfaction machinery for mental states, taken together, do not provide a solution to formalize ToM. Pure deduction possesses neither expressiveness not computational efficiency for providing an adequate coverage of possible behaviors by inferring future mental states from the given ones. Multiagent simulation and a case-based system, which runs an exhaustive search through the totality of possible agents' actions, need to come into play in addition to pure reasoning means to build the environment, adequate for applying the laws of mental world to complaints. Indeed, in terms of computational complexity such exhaustive search is possible, because the formal expressions involved are compact. To reproduce a ToM scenario, desired mental simulator should be capable of producing a sequence of consecutive mental states given an arbitrary initial one.

We believe that situation calculus and its implementation for reasoning about dynamic domains (e.g. GOLOG, (Levesque et al. 1997)) is adequate for reasoning about physical actions, but lacks the expressiveness to operate with mental actions. Situation calculus is relevant expressing the effect axioms (how a mental action results in a certain mental states) but has an insufficient expressive means to determine a possible mental action (to choose it from an agent's perspective, see e.g. (Shanahan 1997)). This is due to the fact that some form of simulation is required in addition to deductive-based form of reasoning about actions.

Since deductive reasoning about mental states is necessary but insufficient, it has to be taught to CwA first, followed by teaching procedural algorithms for a proper choice of behaviors. Computer scientists should verify their formalisms of reasoning about mental states in a way similar to how we do it in this book: propose an axiom, teach it to CwA and observe the improved reasoning skills. Usually it is much simpler to teach an axiom or a rule to a CwA, when she is ready to acquire it and has the required background knowledge, than to do it with a robot. This is because in the latter case a foundation framework has to be built, whereas in humans it already exists.

Over last three decades, a number of control architectures for practical reasoning agents have been proposed (Galitsky and Pampapathi 2005); however, most of them have been used only in artificial environments, and very few have been accepted to the field-tested applications.

It took a significant amount of efforts to learn that procedural reasoning systems (d'Inverno et al. 1998), are more plausible than those based on the traditional implementation of inference search. Implementation of BDI model has been successfully deployed in such procedural reasoning systems, but the substantial development of both the former reasoning implementation approach and latter representation formalism is required to apply it to the real mental world.

Traditionally, representation of the laws of mental worlds is developed via axioms (for example, *an agent knows what it knows*). This approach does not solve the general problem of obtaining the totality of possible mental states, given an initial mental state (Chap. 5). Just a limited number of consecutive mental states can be yielded in a first-order system where meanings of knowledge, belief and intention are expressed as formal modalities. The problem of analysis of real-world conflicts between human agents, which is formulated in natural language and involves the words for various mental states, actions and emotions, requires at least solving the problem above. We believe that merging the declarative (laws of mental world), procedural (simulation of an agent's choice of action) and machine learning (taking into account previous experience) components are required to adequately reproduce the phenomenology of human reasoning about mental attitudes. In this chapter, we are demonstrating that the above is true in the particular domain of reasoning for autistic remediation.

Computational implementation of reasoning about the mental world needs to involve much more extensive phenomenological data than axioms in general are able to represent; therefore, we expect to employ machine learning to take advantage of previously accumulated multiagent scenarios. At the same time, machine learning community does not specifically focus on such the domain as mental world, where statistical approaches do not seem to be applicable. Also, considering a multiagent scenario as an abstract set of features under machine learning settings leads to a loss of accuracy. So specific machine learning methods needs to be developed for such domain as mental world; here we will start the development of machine learning. On the positive side, because the vocabulary of mental expression is quite limited, the text information retrieval problem for mental entities can be solved much more easily than for arbitrary domain-specific entities. Furthermore, the system, once developed, can be reused from domain to domain (Galitsky 2003).

An alternative cognitive approach to represent mental world was undertaken by (Riesbeck et al. 1975) in order to specify the primitive representations for all verbs expressing thoughts in support of natural language understanding. They intended to express what human agents say about the mental world, rather than represent details concerning a complex memory and reasoning model. They therefore used only two mental primitives: mental transfer of information from one location to another and mental building of conceptualizations, and a few support structures such as mental locations, e.g., working memory, central processor and long-term memory.

A generic cognitive model of the mental world is depicted in Fig. 4.8. Cognitive processes (mental actions) are shown on the lefts, and mental states – on the right. Each mental action corresponds to a cluster of linguistic communicative and decision-making actions, related to either inference or memory. This model is subject to aggregation and restructuring to approach the ToM approach, being developed in this book (Fig. 4.9). Mental states and actions are derived and classified in a way suitable for explaining autistic reasoning about the mental world and also for teaching CwA proper reasoning about it.

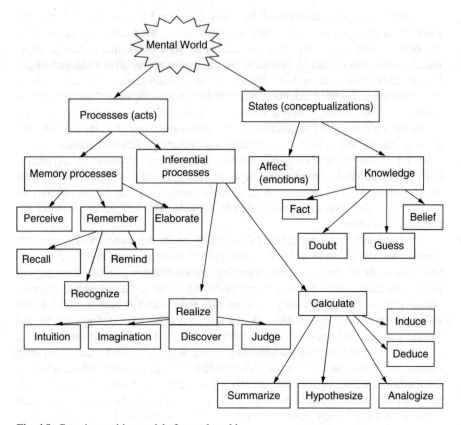

Fig. 4.8 Generic cognitive model of mental world

Since an adequate implementation of ToM reasoning requires deduction, simulation and learning, the training exercises would fall into these categories as well:

Training to perform deduction Given a (behavioral) rule of the sort $P \rightarrow A$ (precondition $\rightarrow$ action), memorize it, identify the cases of applicability of P, apply it, derive action A and perform it.

Training to perform simulation Given a choice of actions $\{A_1, \ldots, A_n\}$ (exhaustive search, enumeration of candidate hypotheses), hypothetically commit A_i, hypothetically face the consequences and finally decide which is the best action A_{best}.

Training to perform learning Given a training set of pairs $\{A \rightarrow C\}$ (action $\rightarrow$ consequences), where some consequences are wanted and some are unwanted, decide for a given action $A_{unknown}$ if it would cause wanted or unwanted consequences. For such decision, a measure of similarity between $A_{unknown}$ and each member of the training set A_i is required. This sort of training also covers abductive and analogical forms of reasoning along with induction.

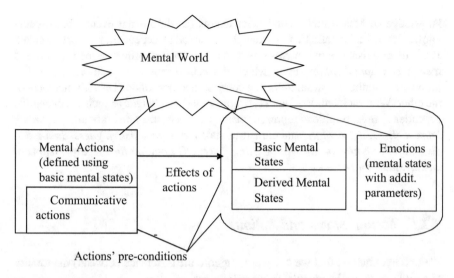

Fig. 4.9 Our ToM-oriented model of mental world which targets knowledge representation in a particular domain (complaint scenarios) is on the *bottom*

This is the loop and the order CwA should be taught selecting an action, following the BDI architecture:

repeat

1. options: option-generator(event-queue)
2. selected-options: deliberate(options)
3. update-intentions(selected-options)
4. execute()
5. get-new-external-events()
6. drop-unsuccessful-attitudes()
7. drop-impossible-attitudes()

end repeat

4.2 ToM Step-by-Step

We present a step-by-step introduction to our representation of the mental world, followed by its implementation by the NL_MAMS simulator in Chap. 5. Steps of this introduction are either definitions or hypotheses which have been computationally verified in our studies.

Logico-philosophical investigation of mental entities is a well-established area in AI. Similar to the vocabulary of mental actions introduced in this chapter, many cognitive vocabularies make a prominent distinction between mental states (as knowledge or belief) and mental mechanisms (as the mental events that process knowledge or information). For example, conceptual dependency theory (Schank 1969) distinguishes between two sets of representations: primitive mental *acts* and mental *conceptualizations* upon which the acts operate. In addition, the theory proposes a number of causal links that connect members of one set with members of the other. With such building blocks, a representational language such as conceptual dependency must be able to represent many process terms: *think* (about), *remember, infer, realize* and *calculate*; and numerous state terms: *fact, belief, guess, doubt,* and *disbelief. From now on we will be using PROLOG notation for our expressions of mental states and actions.*

4.2.1 Mental States and Actions

We first hypothesize that we can merge (ignore the difference between) the totality of entities of other than mental (physical) nature.

Hypothesis 1 Actions and states are divided into mental (communicative, e.g. informing-knowing) and physical (remaining, e.g. *making withdrawal – decreased account balance*). We approximate our description of the mental world using mental states and actions (Fig. 4.9) and merging all physical actions into a constant predicate for an arbitrary physical action and its potential resultant physical states. This approximation is valid most of times modeling the mental states of a software users where the set of available physical actions (as software options, e.g. turn, stop, lend, buy a product, order a service, get a ticket etc.) is rather limited.

Hypothesis 2 Humans can adequately operate with the set of natural language mental expressions containing not more than four mutually dependent mental entities. This hypothesis is based on psychological observations concerning theory of mind representations of control subjects and individuals with mental disorders (Baron-Cohen 2000; Pilowsky et al. 2000). These kinds of experiments are conducted with the number of nested mental entities from one to four, confirming that the higher number causes difficulties for the majority of subjects.

In the play "Othello", Shakespeare manages to keep track of five separate mental states: he intended that his audience believes that Iago wants Othello to suppose that Desdemona loves Cassio. Being able to maintain four-five separate individuals' mental states is the natural upper limit for most adults.

Hypothesis 3 In natural language, each mental entity has a variety of meanings. There are multiple clauses defining every mental metapredicate via the other ones. Absence of such family of definitions for a mental entity means that all possible meanings are implicitly assumed. Thus the problem of disambiguation in a formal language is posed for situations where agents exchange messages in the natural language.

Definition 4 The elementary expression for a mental state or mental action is of the form

$$m_1(a_1[,a_{1'}], m_2(a_2[,a_{2'}], m_3(a_3[,a_{3'}], m_4(a_4[,a_{4'}], p))))$$

where $m_1 \ldots m_4$ are the metapredicates for mental states and actions, occurring with or without negation; $m_4,(m_3$ and $m_4)$, $(m_2, m_3$ and $m_4)$ may be absent; in accordance to Hypothesis 3, the total number of metapredicates is equal or less than four.

$a_1 \ldots a_4$ are the agents from the set of all agents A, square brackets denote the variables for the second agent $a_{1'} \ldots a_{4'}$ (this is the *passive* agent for the mental actions, committed by the *active* agent, denoted by the first argument). For example, an action (and resultant state) with its actor and its receiver is expressed by metapredicate *inform(Actor, Receiver, Knowledge)*, and an action with two (possibly, symmetric or anti-symmetric) receivers – by metapredicate *reconcile(Actor, Receiver1, Receiver2, MatterToSettleDown)*. Further on we will assume that mental metapredicates are allowed to have additional arguments and will not be showing them explicitly.

p is a predicate or expression for physical action or state, Hypothesis 1.

We call such elementary expression for an arbitrary p a *mental formula*. It obeys the standard criteria of being a *well-written* formula.

Definition 5 The totality of well-formed mental formulas falls into three following categories:

1. Interpretable mental formulas that represent existing mental states.
2. Mental formula that always holds for any set of agents (an axiom for modal logic, for example *know(Who, know(Who, Knowledge)))*).
3. Invalid mental formula that cannot be interpreted. For example, it is impossible that a person pretends about someone else's mental state *pretend(a_1, a_2, want(a_3, Something))*. The reader may object this example suggesting that *Someone may pretend to a boring acquaintance that his partner wants him to spend the evening with her.* However, the exact meaning here is that *Someone pretends that **he believes** that his partner wants him to spend the evening with her*, so that the respective former expression is invalid and the respective latter expression is valid (interpretable). Prohibitive mental formulas are provided together with corresponding definitions.

Hypothesis 6 For any interpretable mental formula there is a natural language entity which covers it. There is a many-to-one mapping between interpretable mental formulas and natural language mental entities. Hence natural language entities can be viewed as the classes of equivalence for mental formulas. Otherwise, there would be mental states which cannot be expressed in natural language (this would cause a new entity to appear to cover this mental state).

Hypothesis 7 There are certain syntactic constraints for the formulas describing the mental world that are sufficient to express an arbitrary multiagent scenario. A set of expressions for a mental state has two following components:

1. Mental state fluents, characterizing instant mental states;
2. Mental state clauses, specifying the set of consecutive mental states.

Mental state fluents are expressed with mental formulas as a following conjunction

$$\& \ m_{i1}(a_{j1}, \ m_{i2}(a_{j2}, \ m_{i3}(a_{j3}, \ m_{i4}(a_{j4}, \ p))))$$

$$i=1..n, \ j \in A$$

where $m_{i1} \ \ldots \ m_{i4}$ are the metapredicates for mental states and actions, occurring with or without negation; m_{i4}, (m_{i3} and m_{i4}), (m_{i2}, m_{i3} and m_{i4}) may be absent; a_{j1} $\ldots \ a_{j4}$ are the agents from the set of all agents A;

Note that there are maximum four metapredicates in the conjunctive members above.

For example, *Peter knows that Nick does not know that Peter wants Mike to play with a toy* → *know(peter, not know(nick, want(peter, play(mike, toy)))))*, $m_{11} = know$, $m_{14} = not \ know$, $a_{11} = peter$, $p = play(mike, toy)$.

Also, permanent mental conditions that are expected to be valid through multiple consecutive mental states are expressed via clauses. Let us denote by μ the conjunctive member above

$$\mu \equiv m_{i1}(a_{j1}, \ m_{i2}(a_{j2}, \ m_{i3}(a_{j3}, \ m_{i4}(a_{j4}, \ p)))).$$

The following expressions are interpretable mental formulas to express the continuous mental conditions

$$p{:-}\mu_1 * \ldots * \mu_k$$

This is a condition for physical action. Here $*$ denotes the logic programming conjunction "," or disjunction ";". Let us consider the example: *Peter would make a deposit if he knew that Nick wants him to do so: deposit(peter, fund):- know(peter, want(nick, deposit(peter, fund)))*.

$$\mu(\mu_1){:-} \ \mu_2 * \ldots * \mu_k , \ \mu(\mu_1{:-} \ \mu_2 * \ldots * \mu_k) \text{ and } \mu(p{:-} \ \mu_2 * \ldots * \mu_k).$$

For example, *Mike knows the following: Peter would make a deposit if Mike informs Peter that Nick wants Peter to make this deposit and if Peter does not want to make this deposit himself* → *know(mike, deposit(peter, fund):- inform(mike, peter, want(nick, deposit(peter, fund))), not deposit(mike, fund))*.

Note that an agent may have not only knowledge or belief that includes a causal relationship, but also intention about convincing other agents concerning particular causal link. For example, *Mike* wants the following: *Peter would make a deposit if Mike informs Peter that Nick wants Peter to make this deposit* → *want(mike, (deposit(peter, fund):- inform(mike, peter, want(nick, deposit(peter, fund)))))*. The reader may compare last two examples and reveal the ambiguity of the natural language expressions in terms of whether the clause is the argument of μ, or μ forms the head of a clause.

Additional considerations should be taken into account analyzing the allowed expressions for mental states: each formula μ in the expressions above (conjunctive member) is an interpretable mental formula (Hypothesis 5).

Hypothesis 8 Without loss of the spectrum of meanings for mental entities, we can merge the action and resultant mental states if they are expressed using similar mental entities (*to inform – being informed*, to pretend – being impressed by a pretending, etc.) unless it leads to contradictions or ambiguities in characterizing resultant mental states.

Hypothesis 9 We can ignore certain temporal relationships between the mental and physical states, so that the resultant scenario will stay the same. *Asynchronous* temporal relations can be reduced to a sequence. Complex *spatial* attributes of mental entities can be reduced to a sequence.

(Partial) ordering of mental states expressed by formulas $\mu_1, \ldots, \mu_k$ in the clause body that denotes respective consecutive (in time) mental states $\mu_1, \ldots, \mu_k$ is sufficient to represent temporal constraints with respect to the resultant multiagent scenario (agents' choice of actions).

4.2.2 Example of a Definition of a Mental Action

Once a CwA is capable of operating with basic mental states, he can be taught the definitions of derived mental states so that relying on these definitions she can be involved in a more complex forms of behavior that asking and answering simple questions about what knows what and who wants what. We give an example for how a CwA can be taught to perform and recognize *deception*, the mental action that can be defined in the basis. It might sound unethical to teach a child wrong forms of behavior, but it is better to understand deception than to be a victim of it.

CC play with deception without operating with an explicit definition for it, but CwA needs it concisely defined. To achieve a *Goal*, a person *C* (cheater) selects deception if there is no easy way (such as working towards this *Goal* or asking for help) to achieve it otherwise. If there is another person *T*, the target of this deception, who can commit an action *A* wanted by *C*, and *C* believes that once *T* is informed *Deception* then *T* will commit *A*, then *C* will inform *T* about *Deception*.

```
deceive(C, T, Deception, Goal) :-
    want(C, Goal), not Action(C, Goal),
    not ask(C, Helper, Action(Helper, Goal)),
    believe(C, not Deception),
    believe(C, (Action(T, Goal) :- believe(T, Deception))),
    believe(C, not want (T, Action(T, Goal)),
    believe(C, not (believe(T, Deception)),
```

>   *inform(C, T, Deception),*
>   *believe(T, Deception),*
>   *perform(T, Action),*
>   *Action(T, Goal).*

Notice the additional condition which makes this definition valid:

- *C* cannot perform an *Action* to achieve the *Goal* himself;
- No-one (*Helper*) can commit an *Action* so that *Goal* is achieved;
- *C* believes that once *T* gets to believe (know) statement *Deception*, she will perform an action which results in the *Goal*;
- *C* believes *T* does not know *Deception* on her own (otherwise there is no reason to deceive, and it will have no effect).
- *C* believes that *T* does not want *Goal* on her own, (otherwise there would be no reason to deceive).

Finally, *C* informs *T* about *Deception*. This definition covers only a successful deception where C achieves his Goal. To turn it into an unsuccessful or successful deception, the last three terms should be removed.

The reader can observe that deception can indeed be defined in the basis of *want-know-believe*. A CwA does not have to have definitions for the basic mental states *want-know-believe* to learn how to perform *deceptions* as long as he is capable of operating with scenarios involving these basic mental states. Unlike CC who does not have to explicitly verify the conditions of this clause, CwA have to do a step by step verification of these conditions so that his deception behavior look normal. This is due to the fact that CwA cannot perform mental actions based on his intuition, like CC does, so it is necessary to formalize it and follow each step literally.

We will now illustrate the above Hypotheses:

Hypothesis 1 This definition does not depend on the physical state from *Deception, Goal,* or *Action.*

Hypothesis 2 No term in the clause has more than four embedded metapredicates.

Hypothesis 3 There are multiple meanings for deceiving (*cheating, misrepresentation, concealing* facts) depending on what kind of *Goal* and what are the means *Deception* to achieve it.

Definitions 4 & 5 The formula for the entity being defined (the head of the clause above) and all defining terms (the body of the clause above) are well-written interpretable mental formulas.

Hypothesis 6 Natural language entity *deceive* covers a series of clauses where some of the terms in the defining part are omitted or added. A switch to another mental entity such as *explain* will occur if *Deception* is a true fact (remove the term *believe(C, not Deception)* from the above definition). A switch to pretend will also occur if we remove all terms with *Action* from the defining part and add the clause that instead of *Action C* just wants *T* to believe in her pretense.

Hypothesis 7 A fluent in deceiving will be a transition belief state where T is already informed *Deception* but has not perform *Action*. Also note the subject of C's belief is a clause.

Hypothesis 8 The order of states and actions should be as per the definition. In the characterizing the initial mental state, the order of terms is arbitrary. Once C initiated the deceiving behavior, the order of mental states and actions (shown in gray area) does matter.

4.2.3 Derived Metapredicates

After we successfully expressed as complex concept as deceiving, we can approach the attempt to express all mental states and actions in our basis.

Hypothesis 9 The set of derived metapredicates exhaustively covers the set of verbs expressing interactions between people and their feelings. We treat in depth the entities of ToM introduced in Sect. 4.2.1.

Derived metapredicates fall into two following categories:

1. Metapredicates for derived mental states and actions without explicit sentiments load. These are characterized in the dimensions of knowledge, and intention only and can be formalized fairly well, as we have seen. Teaching of these metapredicates for CwA takes advantage of this high accuracy of approximation of meanings.
2. Metapredicates for emotions. These are formally independent of (1) mental metapredicates that belong to the classes of equivalence of the above category of metapredicates with respect to agents' choice of action, required to reach one mental state from another. These metapredicate are loaded with sentiments, emotions and feeling which cannot be expressed in our basis. However, for the purpose of teaching these approximations are satisfactory.

Since all our mental metapredicates allow multiple interpretations, we merge *desire* as a long-term goal with *intention* as an instant goal to the metapredicate *want(Agent, Goal)*, where $Goal \equiv \mu_1 * \ldots * \mu_k$. It allows us to reduce the number of the well-written mental formulas for the analysis of interpretable formulas (Definition 5). The difference between belief and knowledge is that an agent is capable of changing and revising beliefs, but knowledge is only subject to acquisition (Fagin et al. 1996).

We can express not only mental actions for a single agent, but also the mental actions involved in a multiagent conflict in the basis of *want-know-believe*. Here we provide just a single clause for selected mental actions, keeping in mind that multiple clauses are expressing the meanings in various contexts of multiagent interaction (for example, definitions of *inform,* Hypothesis 10).

In the definitions below, the reader may notice a use of meta-programming, where a clause occurs as an argument of a defining predicate to express a deductive link in a general way, to cover a wide spectrum of meanings.

---

disagree(A,B,W) :- inform(A,B,W), not believe(B,W), inform(B,A, not W).
agree(A,B, W) :- inform(A,B, W), believe(B, W), inform(B,A, W).
explain(A,B, W) :- believe(A, (W :- V)), not know(B, W), inform(A,B,V),
inform(A,B,(W :- V)), believe(B,W).
confirm(A,B, W) :- inform(A,B,W), know(A, believe(B, W)).
bring_attention(A,B, W) :- want(A, believe(B, know(A, W))).
remind(A,B, W):- believe(A, believe(B, W)),
inform(A,B,W), want(A, know(B, know(A, W))).
understand(A,W) :- inform(B,A,W), believe(B, not believe(A, (W :- V))),
want(B, believe(A, (W :- V))), inform(B, A,(W :- V)),
    believe(A,(W :- V),
    believe(A, W).
accept_responsibility(A, W) :- want(B, not W), believe(B, (W:-do(A,W1))),
   want(A, know(B, believe(A, (W:-do(A,W1))))),
   inform(A,B, (W:-do(A,W1))).
expect(A, W) :- not know(A, W),believe(A, B), (believe(A, W:-believe(_, B)) or
sense(A, W)), know(A, W).
Expect something – not knowing but believing in something which might imply expectation or sensing it.

4.2.4   Handling Multiple Meanings

Hypothesis 10   The set of available actions for agents is derived from the respective set of natural language entities. For each such entity, we obtain a spectrum of conditions to perform the denoted action based on the family of definitions for this entity in *want-know-believe* basis. From the linguistic perspective, the spectrum of meanings for an entity that denotes mental action is determined by the context of this entity (the set of other mental entities in the accompanying sentences). In our model of mental world, there is a spectrum of clauses for each mental action such that each clause enumerates particular conditions on mental states. As an example, we present four clauses for *inform*, taking into account that there are much more clauses to form the whole spectrum for this predicate:

(1) *inform(Who, Whom, What) :- want(Who, know(Whom, What)),   believe(Who, not know(Whom, What)),*
    believe(Who, want(Whom, know(Whom, What))).
      default *informing*
(2) *inform(Who, Whom, What) :- ask(Whom, Who, What),*
    want(Who, know(Whom, What)).
     informing as *answering*
(3) *inform(Who, Whom, What) :- ask(SomeOne, Who, believe(Whom, What)),*
    want(Who, know(Whom, What) .
     following SomeOne's request for informing
(4) *inform(Who, Whom, What) :- believe(Who, know(Whom, What)),*
    want(Who, believe(Whom, now(Who,What))).
     to *inform Whom* that not only *Whom* but *Who knows What*

Clearly, each natural language mental entity has a number of meanings, some of them may be determined in a context. Formalizing mental world, one needs to represent the totality of meanings, relevant in a particular domain, for each respective lexical unit. A clear-cut approach then would be to sum up all meanings for each participating mental entity and build a respective set of clauses. However, following this approach, we lose very valuable information that the NL divides the totality of meanings into the classes with denotation by words. Ignoring this information would lead us to a loss of overall structure of mental world, vigilantly reflected in NL.

If we have a pair of different definitions (clauses) for a given entity, there should be a machinery to formally express the similarity between these clauses to avoid losing important semantic data. For example, it is hard to construct a common parameterized definition for *suggest* and *hint* in the basis of *want-know-believe*; however, totally independent clauses would be misleading (e.g. if we want to handle the case of *hint about a solution* ≡ *suggest a solution*).

It is quite natural from the formal representation viewpoint that we use the same predicate to express the totality of meanings for the same lexical entity. It should be a generic framework to express such common features. When we form a series of clauses for a mental entity, we need to take into account that there should be a common feature among the clauses for a given mental entity in natural language to distinguish these clauses from those of other mental entities in natural language. As we have verified, there is a *syntactic meta-criterion* that relates a clause to a unique mental entity. *Syntactic* here denotes the grammar of formal representation language, the clauses (not a grammar of natural language).

Hence we can define an isomorphism between the NL mental entities and the metapredicates that express the criterion of belonging to the set of clauses for the predicate that we use for this mental entity.

∀ *NL_mental_entities* ∀ *Meaning 1, Meaning 2, Meaning 3,…* ∃ *Meta-clause*:

$$\text{NLmental\_entities} \rightarrow \begin{matrix} \text{Meaning 1} \rightarrow \text{Clause 1} \\ \text{Meaning 2} \rightarrow \text{Clause 2} \\ \text{Meaning 3} \rightarrow \text{Clause 3} \\ \cdots \end{matrix} \rightarrow \text{Meta-clause is satisfied by Clauses1,2,3}$$

For an example of such mapping, let us consider the set of definitions for the entity *inform*, presented above.

$$\text{inform} \rightarrow \begin{matrix} \text{general informing} \rightarrow \text{Clause (1) above} \\ \text{informing as answering} \rightarrow \text{Clause (2) above} \\ \text{following SomeOne's request} \rightarrow \text{Clause (3)} \\ \text{for informing} \end{matrix} \rightarrow \text{Meta-clause}$$

All of these clauses include the term *want(Who, know(Whom, What))*. Let us build the meta-clause that expresses such common feature.

inform (as lexical unit) → the set of clauses { *inform₁:-…, …, informₖ:-…* } → syntactic metapredicate *Meta-clause*:

clauseFor(inform,   Clause):-   clause_list(Clause,   Bodys),   member(want(Who, know(Whom, What)), Bodys).

The syntactic meta-predicate *clauseFor* accepts a mental entity to be expressed and a clause for it. The body of this mental predicate verifies that the clause obeys certain criteria, built to express the totality of meanings for this mental entity. We have verified that such isomorphism can be built for almost all mental entities we use in representation of the scenarios from our dataset (Sect. 4.3).

We conclude this subsection with a brief comment on the observation of the commonality between clauses and existence of a "covering" metapredicate ranging over clauses for the same natural language entity. If such commonality would not exist, the natural language would have hard time expressing information about the mental world in an efficient manner. If there were a lexical unit for each meaning, it would be hard to memorize and operate with such a language. Similarly, if there were no commonality in various meanings of the world (these meanings were not forming a cluster "around" this world), humans would have a hard time resolving the ambiguity of the natural language denotations in the real mental world. At the same time we mention that expressing the common features in the meta-language of the logic programming language is the feature of our particular approach. Different natural languages cluster the meanings of mental entities in distinct ways; for example, the notion of *pretending* in Russian follows the logic of example in Hypothesis 6 closer than in English.

4.2.5 Representing Emotions

Emotions are not pure logical entities; however, for the purpose of autistic training we need to formalize them. Again, our basis of knowledge-belief-intention comes into play to express a pre-condition for a given emotional states to appear. Most of times, approximations of emotional states in the basis are fairly distant from the real meanings of emotions and loose genuine emotional colors, but are nevertheless adequate in terms of possible agent's reaction. Based on our definitions of emotion, the agents can select an action to overcome or at least to attempt to overcome a negative emotion and retain a positive one.

Here are some definitions of emotions in our basis. For more complex cases, we present the clauses along the verbal definition of an emotion.

forgetting:– lack of a *belief* that follows its presence at some point in time.
dreaming:– *intention* of some physical or mental state to occur, having a *belief* that currently it does not hold;
imagining:– *believing* that something holds *knowing* that the belief is wrong;
feeling guilty:– *intention* that some action that has been committed should not has been done and *belief* that it depended on the agent's physical or mental state.
fairly treated: – belief that people think of me in a similar way I think of myself
surprised:– expected one thing, but turned out to be another thing

$$upset(U, SomethingSad) :- not\ want(U,\ SomethingSad),$$
$$believe(U, not\ (not\ SomethingSad :- Action(U))).$$

(something is unwanted and cannot be improved employing available knowledge). The same definition would be for *sad*,

jealous(J, H, SomethingNice) :- believe(J, state(H, SomethingNice)), want(J, SomethingNice), not state(H, SomethingNice).

(*J* is jealous if he wants the same state *SomethingNice* another agent *H* possesses, according to *J*'s belief, but she is not in this state).

unfairly treated Action1(U), Action2(F), believe(U, Action1 = Action2)), want(Authority, Action1), not want(Authority, Action2).

(An unfairly treated person believes what he did (*Action1*) is as good as *Action2* committed by someone else (*F*), but an *Authority* agent wants (likes) *F*'s action and not *U*'s action).

frightened(F, S, Unknown) : - believe(F, not want(F, Action(S)), believe(F, (Action(S):- ask(F, S, not Action(S)).

(*F* is frightened by *S* committing *Action* when this *Action* is unwanted and inevitable: *S* will commit it even when *F* asks *S* not to do it.)

confident:- persons believes in something, and believes that other people believe that he does not believe in this.

loosing_trust(L, T , EventLostTrus):- believe(L, believe(L, SaidByT):-
inform(T, L, SaidByT)), inform(T, L, EventLostTrust),
not believe(L, EventLostTrust),
believe(L, (not believe(L, SaidByTButNotBel)):-inform(T, L, SaidByTButNotBel)).

L first believe what *T* was saying (expressed as a clause), then *T* said *EventLostTrust,* but now *L* does not believe this *EventLostTrust*, and after that *L* does not believe whatever *SaidByTButNotBel T* is saying.

Although the emotions expressed via these definitions are unnatural, they follow the form suitable to be defined and perceived by CwA.

In the settings of mental entities of (Cox and Ram 1999), in order to use representations of mental terms effectively, a system should consider the structure of the representation, rather than to show how to syntactically manipulate with representations or make sound inferences from them, as we do in this study. As an example, let is consider a treatment of the pair of predicates *forget(P, M)* and ¬ *remember(P, M)*.

Because the predicates involve memory, it is helpful to posit the existence of two contrasting sets of axioms: the background knowledge (BK), or long-term memory of the agent, P, and the foreground knowledge (FK), representing the currently conscious or active axioms of the agent. The resulting interpretation of person P forgetting memory item M is

$$forget(P, M) \to \exists M \, (M \in BKp) \land (M \notin FKp)$$

With such a representation, one can also express the proposition that the person P knows that he has forgotten something. P knows that M is in his background knowledge, but cannot retrieve it into his foreground knowledge:

$$\exists M \, (M \in BKp) \in FKp \wedge (M \notin FKp)$$

To include these interpretations to an agent's behavior library is to add content to the representation, rather than simply semantics. It is part of the *metaphysical interpretation* (McCarthy 1979) of the representation that determines an ontological category (i.e., what ought to be represented), and it begins to claim that the sets BK and FK are necessary distinct. However, meaning is not only correspondences with the world to be represented, but meaning is also determined by the inferences a system can draw from a representation (Schank 1969). The *forget* predicate offers little in this regard. Moreover, this predicate will not assist a reasoning system to understand what happens when it forgets some memory item, M, nor will it help the system learn to avoid forgetting the item in the future. Finally, because the semantics of a mental event which did not actually occur is not represented well by a simple negation of a predicate representing an event which did occur (Cox and Ram 1999; Ram and Moorman 1999), the logical expression ¬*Remember (John, M)* does not bring computationally sound information.

We have experimentally verified that one neither has to enumerate all possible meanings nor approach them as close as possible to teach *applicability* and *reasonability* of these emotions to CwA. Our model of emotions in the mental world is adequate in terms of mental rehabilitation, but may be far from optimal for building agents that impress the audience with intelligent and emotional behavior (compare with (Scheutz 2001; Breazeal 1998; Sloman 2000)).

Formal treatment of emotions helps to compensate for our simplification of scenario description by means of predicates for actions. In addition to above definition of emotions, we consider them as fluent (time- and situation-dependent) predicates that are the preconditions for mental actions. Also, emotions are the fluents that are affected by committed mental actions (Galitsky 2005):

> *poss(give_up(explain(Customer, Explanation)), Situation) :-*
> *lost_trust(Customer, Situation).*

We will be using examples from the domain for customer complaints. This domain can be considered as a mental world playground for older CwA and adults with ASD. Since complaints are a systematic extensive source of description of complicated mental states such as conflicts, we will be using this domain as a source of examples of complex regions in the mental world. We will be exploring relations between a Customer and a Company, as an introduction for CwA to the world of adults and their relations.

We will now introduce situation calculus, using an arbitrary (not necessarily mental attitudes-related) approach. Situation calculus is formulated in a first-order language with certain second-order features (Levesque et al. 1997). A possible world history that is a result of a sequence of *actions* is called *situation*. The expression, *do(a,s)*, denotes the successor situation to *s* after action *a* is applied. For example, *do(complain(Customer, do(harm(Company),S₀))*, is a situation expressing the world history that is based on the sequence of actions {*complain(Customer), harm(Company)*}, where *Customer* and *Company* are variables (with explicit meanings). We refer the reader to (Levesque et al. 1997) for the further details on the implementation of situation calculus. Also, situations involve the *fluents,* whose values vary from situation to situation and denote them by predicates with the latter arguments ranging over the situations, for example,

> *upset(Customer, do(harm(Company),S_0)).*
> Actions have *preconditions* – the constraints on actions:
> *poss(complain(Customer), s) :- upset(Customer, s).*
> *Effect axioms* (post-conditions) describe the effect of a given action on the fluents:
> *complain(Customer) & responsive(Company)* $\rightarrow$
> > *settle_down(Customer, do(complain(Customer), s)).*

For example, an action *ignoring* leads to emotional state (fluent) *feel unfairly treated.* In such a state, cooperative actions are unlikely for an agent, which will rather *disagree* or *bring to attention* then *agree, encourage* or *ask for advice.* Formally,

> *unfairly_treated(Customer, do(ignore(CS),do(ask(Customer,replace(Product), S_0)))).*
> *poss(disagree(Customer,CS,SomethingNew), S):- unfairly_treated(Customer, S).*

To illustrate our model of interchange between emotions and mental actions, let us consider the following complaint fragment. We present the textual fragments form the actual complaint written by its author and then show how to represent it using our formal language. After that, we show how this complaint fragment can be represented by means of user-friendly form. Such kind of form is specially oriented towards the mental component of a complaint and will be discussed in further details in the Section below.

> *I am requesting the refund of an application fee, which I made through my credit card...*
> *I was told by Don Joe that this fee was non-refundable but I feel that I have extenuating circumstances...*
> *I am in outrage because 3 months ago I could have consolidated with my second mortgage company...*

The following three statements correspond to the sentences above. We assume that the first two sentences express mental actions, and the third sentence contains the emotion and its causal link.

> *request(Customer, CS, refund(fee(application, cc))).*
> *explain(CS, Customer, not refund(fee(_, _))).*
> *upset(customer, do(explain(CS, Customer, not refund(fee(_, _)))),*
> > *do(request(Customer, refund(fee(application, cc))), S_0))).*

Here the emotion is expressed as a result of two consecutive actions, one of the *Customer* and the other of *CS* (Customer Support), coming from an initial precomplaint state S_0.

Hypothesis 11 Emotions represented via definitions in knowledge-intention-belief basis are both pre-conditions and effects of mental actions.

Each class of emotions can be covered by at least a single definition in our basis, however it is sufficient to determine an action to optimally maintain the outcome (Table 4.1).

Table 4.1 Classes of emotions and their representatives (*the left column*) and members (*the right column*)

Class representative	Class members
Sad	Upset, frustrate, frustration, distress, hurt, disturb, sadden, trouble, wound, disappoint, disconcert, displease, grieve, affront, dismayed
Anger	Indignation, rage, fury, furious, offence, infuriate, insult, hate, offend, annoyance
Surprise	Astonish, shock, horrify, aghast
Disgust	Sickened, disgust, revolt
Cheat	Scam, trick, fiddle, swindle, sting, dodge
Insulting	Derogatory, disparaging, deprecating, offensive
Harass	Annoy, pester, bother, pursue, nuisance, stalk, hassle, worry, tease

4.3 Scenarios in the Mental World

So far we have suggested the generic model of mental world suitable for explaining autistic reasoning and its remediation. The main inhabitants of mental world are agents with mental attitudes and scenarios of their interactions; these agents display their attitudes in their decision-making process. Once we taught CwA individual mental actions, we can proceed to exercising with sequences that include familiar communicative actions and states. The most important class of scenarios is *conflict scenarios*: CwAs need to be thoroughly explained and trained on how to handle conflicts.

Scenarios of interaction between agents are an important subject of study in AI. An extensive body of the literature addresses the problem of logical simulation of behavior of autonomous agents, taking into account their beliefs, desires and intentions (Bratman 1987). A substantial advancement has been achieved in building the scenarios of multiagent interaction, given properties of agent including their attitudes. Recent work in agent communications has been in argumentation (Rahwan et al. 2003; Chesnevar et al. 2004), in dialog games (Boella et al. 2004), in formal models of dialog (Johnson et al. 2005), in conversation policies (Nodine and Unruh 2000) and in social semantics (Carley 1997). However, means of automated comparative analysis for interaction scenarios for human agents are still lacking). The comparative analysis of interaction scenarios is needed in many applications. A number of linguistic and agent-related technologies are required in such domain requiring learning human behavior such as customer complaints (Chang et al. 2009).

Definition 11 We define scenario as a sequence of mental states of interacting (having mutual beliefs) agents where each transition from mental state m to m + 1 is a result of the action of each agent.

Hypothesis 12 Each conflict between agents (human, software or hardware), can be represented as a sequence or mental states and communicative actions such that these actions are logically deduced to be the best from the standpoint of agent's available knowledge and belief.

Having introduced the entities of the mental world, we now proceed to build a software system and educational methodology which takes a textual description of a conflict as an input and represent it as a sequence of communicative actions and intermediate mental states, as an output.

There are three following methodologies (continued from Sect. 4.2) to build scenarios given agents' attributes and initial mental states.

- A deductive (planning) approach, where agents actions are deduced using their explicit pre-conditions, and possible states are derived using axioms
- A simulation approach, where the exhaustive search through all possible agents' actions is implemented, taking into account possible opponents' reactions. The set of explicit action preferences is applied to filter the best action, unless a particular action is explicitly desired.
- A machine learning (case-based reasoning or inductive/abductive/analogical reasoning) approach, where a scenario is constructed from the components of previously accumulated scenarios. The scenarios for reuse are selected based on the similarity of initial (and consecutive) mental states with the given one.

The third approach is the most efficient to handle the scenarios which can be used for training autistic reasoning. The first approach above is viable where we go beyond the pure mental actions; it is usually hard to express all required constraints for mental actions only. The simulation approach is most suitable for the domains which lie entirely within the mental world. The simulation approach is quite helpful for complaints but still delivers less accuracy in the prediction of future agents' actions in the comparison with the machine learning one.

Besides a scenario formalization problem, we formulate a prediction one. Can a human mental attitude and communicative actions be predicted in a domain-independent manner, without taking into account details of a particular environment such as educational, banking or military? We attempt to computationally demonstrate that humans choose their attitude and action in mental space following some common laws of the mental world, in addition to environment-specific considerations. We give a positive answer to this question, providing a common framework for tackling rather distinct domains, relying only on learned 'laws' of the world of mental interactions. The Speech Act theory (Sect. 4.3.5) addresses this problem from the linguistic and philosophical standpoint, and in this book we approach it from computational standpoint.

Once such domain-independent prediction framework is build, it can be applied to a number of problems where simulation of human decision making is necessary, starting from educational to industrial. Currently, two classes of approach are applied to the domain of human simulation, behavior prediction and human sentiment analysis. The first one, popular in industry, is based on keywords referring to topicality or sentiment polarity. Since it is rather hard to represent meanings via bag-of-words approach, especially when one tries to extract communicative actions which are frequently implicit in text, it is rather hard to predict human behavior based on keyword analysis.

The second class of approaches relies on implementation of reasoning about mental states, and is associated with performance and expressiveness limitations of attempts to implement axiomatic formal reasoning. We build the representation machinery and develop a machine learning technique for operating with a wide range of scenarios which are based on a sequence of communicative actions. We also propose a framework for classifying scenarios of inter-human conflicts; it can be implemented in a stand-alone mode or used in combination with deductive reasoning or simulation. Once we confirm that this machinery works well in real world scenarios, it becomes a good foundation for teaching CwA how to tackle these scenarios.

Formalized inter-human conflict is a special case of formal scenario where the agents have inconsistent and dynamic goals; a negotiation procedure is required to achieve a compromise (Muller and Dieng 2000). It turns out that following the logical structure of how negotiations are represented in a scenario (text or structure) it is possible to judge on consistency of this scenario (Galitsky 2006). We take advantage of this possibility teaching CwA how to recognize a conflict scenario and behave in it.

4.3.1 Multiagent Conflict

The issue of multiagent conflict has been extensively addressed in the literature; in this chapter rather simple definition is sufficient for out purpose. It is essential to explain to CwA what the conflicts are, how to avoid them, and how to resolve once in a conflict state.

Definition 13 Multiagent conflict is a scenario where agents have inconsistent intentions (about states):

$$want(AgentFor, State), want(AgentAgainst, not State).$$

In a conflict scenario, we distinguish two selected states when one follows another. The pre-conflict state include the deviation of the expected from the actual features (quality) of received product or service:

pre-conflict: *expect (Friend1, play(Friend1, Toy)),*
believe (Friend2, not want(Friend1, play(Friend1, Toy))).

4.3.2 Dimensions of Intentionality

As we discussed in Sect. 4.2, humans are characterized by the degree mental formulas are nested: an order of a mental formula, or *intentionality*. This a limit

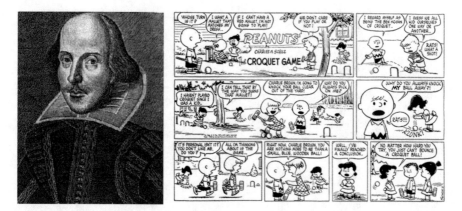

Fig. 4.10 You can just tell he's thinking what you're thinking about his thoughts

on thinking about what other people are thinking about other people. Humans can go about seven levels up this chain of intentionality.

- You **know** that I will look at the moon.
- I **think** that you **know** that I will look at the moon.
- You **hope** that I **think** that you **know** that I will look at the moon.
- And so forth

But this limit doesn't just influence apples; and all the drama associated with that. Intentionality limits every social interaction. If one is telling a story with more than seven levels of intentionality it will not be appreciated. It is not worth telling a joke that complex either.

But when it comes to telling a good joke or story, the secret isn't just trying to make it as low level as possible either. We proceed with our example from Sect. 4.1 (Fig. 4.10). In Othello:

1. Shakespeare wants
2. The audience to believe that . . .
3. Iago wants . . .
4. Othello to believe that . . .
5. Desdemona loves Cassio . . .
6. Who loves her right back.

As the greatest playwright has discovered, people don't like it being too simple. It turns out there is a sweet spot between our 7th level limit and a basic story that the readers enjoy a lot. It is in this range where the best jokes live, the best narratives, and the best plays. (Dunbar et al. 2015) have identified that this value is around the same place as Othello; between five and six levels of intentionality (Fig. 4.11).

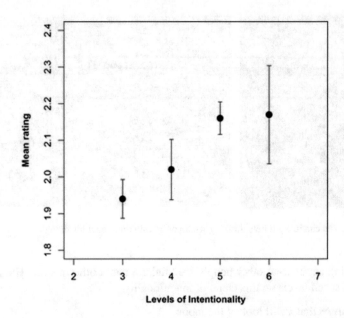

Fig. 4.11 The rating of a joke versus the number of levels of intentionality it features (Dunbar et al. 2015)

4.3.3   Dissatisfaction and Complaint Scenarios

An important class of textual description of conflicts is a complaint, where a particular party in a conflict is seeking help from an authority. It should be explained to CwA when it is appropriate to attempt to solve a conflict independently, and when is a good time to ask for help from parents, rehabilitation personnel or older friends.

Definition 14 Pre-conflict is a multiagent conflict scenario where the expression above occurs. To grow in a complaint, initial dissatisfaction must be further fed with the further desperation connected with an interaction with customer support representatives and other opponents. Let us consider a step-by-step example of a complaint scenario. Here, we use the conventions of logic programming; variables are capitalized and comments follow '%'.

ask(mike, fix(peter, not feature(Toy))),

% Mike wants Peter to fix his toy (make 'feature' working)

not fix(peter, not feature(Toy)),

% Peter cannot/does not do it

believe (mike, (not fix(peter, not feature(Toy)) :- Reason)),

% mike believes that there is a certain Reason for not doing it

not know(mike, Reason).

% but Mike does not know what is the Reason. 'not' here has a linguistic meaning (not "negation as failure" meaning)

upset(mike).

Note that there is a wide variety of ways a child can express his dissatisfaction initially, his opponent responds, etc. However, the common step in the majority of conflict scenarios is the confusion of a proponent over why *he was treated in such a way*, what was the *Reason* his toy was not fixed

Usually, if the actions of an opponent are adequate, a full-scale conflict does not arise and the proponent does not get upset. Hence we approach

Definition 15 A typical conflict resulting in an upset proponent as a scenario with the following features:

- a conflict of intentions concerning the physical state of a product/service (pre-conflict), and
- a conflict of intentions concerning the mental and physical actions of customer support and resultant state of their satisfaction.

Our formal definition of a conflict scenario includes both conflicts in mental and physical spaces.

Having the definition of a formal complaint, we raise the series of questions:

- How to formalize complaint given its textual description?
- What kind of features can be/should be extracted from complaints, including validity, aggressive/defensive attitude of a person, positive/negative mood of a complainant, etc.?
- How to measure similarity between complaints?
- How to find their essential component?

We will answer these questions in the following sections, and now we introduce our model of a *mentalized* conflict, which is a reduction of a scenario that assumes that all physical actions are alike. In accordance to our model, the physical world serves as a "neutral environment" where mental actions lead to certain mental states which in turn cause a next series of mental actions (Hypothesis 12, Fig. 4.12). At this point, we are stating that mental states are determined by the previous mental and physical states and actions.

We proceed to a multi-step reduction of a scenario representation. A fragment from a banking complaint serves as an example of how the content is reduced. Textual representation is modified accordingly to demonstrate the essence of transformation of scenario representation formulas at each step. An intuitive way to look at these steps is to pretend that one keeps forgetting details about which physical states (e.g. account balance) took place over last month, then forgetting details on which physical actions (e.g. withdrawals/deposits) have been committed, and finally, ignoring the sequence of associated mental states (beliefs about account

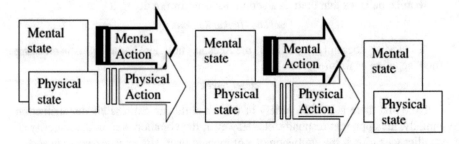

Fig. 4.12 The chart of inter-dependencies between physical and mental actions and states. We consecutively remove physical states and actions and mental states to form the skeleton of a conflict scenario – the sequence of mental actions

balance, intentions about withdrawals, knowledge of account regulations). Keeping forgetting all these particulars leads to remembering only which mental actions occurred in connection with certain interactions between friends (*ask, explain, disagree, approve, request* etc.).

Let us first introduce a fragment of an interaction scenario 'for adults':

> *I know that they believe I don't know what my account balance is because they deposited the amount back which they withdrew before as a maintenance fee to tell me that they did not charge it. I am going to confirm that I will now withdraw all remaining funds from my account.*

Below is its formal representation using physical and mental actions and states, as well as the causal link:

> *cause ((withdrawal(they, account, maintenance), deposit(*
> *they, account),*
> *want(they, believe(i, not withdrawal(account,*
> *maintenance))))),*
> *know(i, believe(they, not know(i,*
> *balance(account))))).*
> *confirm(i, want(i, withdraw(i, account))).*

Reduction Step 16.1. Let us assume that mental states are determined by mental actions and physical actions but not physical states. We substitute physical states by physical actions only, or by using mental states or actions in addition if it reduces an ambiguity in the derived physical actions. Such the transformation keeps the causal, special, temporal and other kinds of constraints between the remaining mental states and actions. In our example above, we perform the following substitution:

$$balance(account) \rightarrow deposit(they, account)$$

Reduction Step 16.2. At this elimination step we substitute every physical actions by a set of mental actions with argument over arbitrary physical action so that we have the same effect (resultant mental state). The latter means that such substitution should not break causal links within a scenario. We hypothesize that it is always possible to substitute a concrete instantiated physical action A_f by one or more mental actions A_{f2m} with arguments over the a generic (arbitrary) physical action that leads to a resultant mental state S_m which is fixed. This replacing set of mental entities should be consistent with the physical actions to be replaced:

$$\forall A_m, S_m \, \forall A_f \, \exists A_{f2m}: \text{ if } A_m, A_f \rightarrow S_m \text{ then } A_m, A_{f2m} \rightarrow S_m.$$

Here we are not concerned with a resultant physical state we have substituted by actions at the previous step above. For the example above, the following substitution is performed:

{*withdraw(they, account), deposit(they, account)*} → *do(they), recongnize_pretend(they, do(they))*.
{*withdraw(i, account)* } → *do(they)*
{*balance(account)* } → *do(they)*

In the textual representation below expressions in square brackets are the arguments of mental actions:

> *I know that they believe I don't know what is happening because I was informed that they changed their mind [concerning maintenance fee] and I believe they wanted me to believe that they have not done what they should not have done. I am going to confirm that I know it and will act accordingly [will now withdraw all remaining funds from my account].*

$$\begin{aligned} cause(\,(\,recognize\_pretend(they, do(they)), do(they)), \\ know(i, believe(they, not\ know(i, \ do(they)))) \\ ), \\ confirm(i, want(i, do(i))). \end{aligned}$$

Reduction Step 16.3. We ignore information about mental states and just consider mental actions which lead to these states. As many mental actions need to be added that the mental states can be reconstructed with as low ambiguity (as high accuracy) as possible. Moreover, these mental actions have to be consistent with existing mental actions for the scenario, and with those substituting other mental states for this scenario.

recognize_pretend(they, do(they)) → *ask(i,they, What), inform(they, i, What),*
                                   disagree(i, they, What), confirm(they, i, not What).
know(i, K) → *inform(they, i, K).*
know(i, believe(they, not know(i, MissingKnowledge))) → *ask(i, they, Missing-Knowledge),*
 explain(they, i, not MissingKnowledge).

% here we use a naive case for *believing* because it does not lead to ambiguity
Representing the textual scenario, we break it into three parts to outline three fragments:

- A *recognize_pretend* fragment;
- A *know* fragment;
- A *confirm* fragment.

I asked what was happening [*with my account*].
They informed me what was going on [*with my account*].
I disagreed with what they informed me about.
They confirmed that nothing happened [*with my account*].
I asked why they believe I did not know the truth.
They explained that I did not know the truth because indeed nothing happened [*with my account*].
I confirmed that I wanted to terminate the scenario.

cause({ask(i,them, What)), inform(they, i, What),
        disagree(i, they, What), confirm(they, i, not What)},
    {ask(i,them, MissingKnowledge), explain(they, i, not MissingKnowledge)}
     ),
confirm(i, want(i, WhatElse))).
% ' {' is used to enhance readability

We hypothesize that current mental state plus current and past physical state constrain the plausible set of mental actions. The reader might expect us to comment on the reason why the mental actions are more important than other components of a scenario. The answer is, they are represented explicitly in verbal description much more frequently than mental states. The mental states are usually partially drawn, being mixed with physical actions and states in the text. At the same time, the former can be extracted from text easier or be specified via a form, which will be discussed toward the end of the paper.

Hypothesis 17 Mental actions constitute the most important information on a multiagent conflict scenario and therefore serve as a basis for their comparative analysis, learning, simulation and prediction. Scenarios can be represented as graphs where the sequence and causal links are expressed by their edges (such as Fig. 4.13).

It reads:

I ask … – they informed me that …
I disagreed with that – but they confirmed that …
Since they confirmed that, I asked … – and they explained …
I confirmed something else …

Fig. 4.13 Graph
representation of a scenario

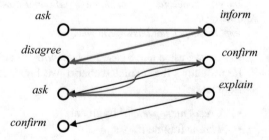

Definition 18 A communicative action is a functor of the form *verb(agent, subject, cause)* where *verb* characterizes some kind of interaction between customer and company in a complaint scenario (e.g., *explain, confirm, remind, disagree, deny*), *agent* identifies either the customer or the company, *subject* refers to the information transmitted or object described, and *cause* refers to the motivation or explanation for the subject.

Thus, for example, a communicative action associated with some customer claim such as "I disagreed with the overdraft fee you charged me because I made a bank deposit well in advance" would be represented as disagree (customer, "overdraft fee", "I made a bank deposit well in advance"). Scenarios are intentionally simplified as labeled directed graphs to allow for effective similarity matching among them. Each vertex in the graph will correspond to a communicative action. An arc (oriented edge) may denote either temporal precedence or an attack relationship between two actions a_i and a_j. In the first case, we will distinguish between consecutive actions which refer to the same subject from those which refer to different subjects. Graphically, we will distinguish these situations by means of thick arcs and thin arcs, respectively.

Definition 19 A complaint scenario is a labeled directed graph $G = (V, A)$, where $V = \{action_1, action_2, \ldots, action_k\}$ is a finite set of vertices corresponding to communicative actions, and $A = A_{thick} \cup A_{thin} \cup A_{causal}$ is a finite set of labeled arcs (ordered pairs of vertices), classified as follows:

- Each arc *(action$_i$; action$_j$)* $\in A_{thick}$ corresponds to a temporal precedence of two referring to the same subject.
- Each arc *(action$_i$; action$_j$)* $\in A_{thin}$ corresponds to a temporal precedence of two actions referring to different subjects.
- Each arc *(action$_i$; action$_j$)* $\in A_{causal}$ corresponds to a causal link or an attack relationship between *action$_i$* and *action$_j$*, indicating that the cause of *action$_i$* is in conflict with the subject or cause of *action$_j$*.

The classes of mental actions have been adopted from linguistic and psychological literature, including (Shardanand and Maes 1995; Mehrabian 1971).

The curve arcs denote a causal link between the arguments of communicative actions, e.g., *service is not as advertised $\Rightarrow$ there are particular failures in a service contract, ask $\sim$ > confirm.*

4.3.4 Recognizing Plausible Scenarios

Given the initial sub-scenario, one can reduce the number of plausible final consecutive sub-scenarios (shown in bold below). For example, for the two steps below the following third and fourth step is possible (reasonable, consistent with the expected discourse):

request – deny responsibility
remind – disagree
bring attention – agree
explain – accept responsibility

We assume here that the subjects of the mental actions above are the same, plaintiff's actions are on the left and defendant's (company) are on the right. We can understand the main plot: additional information, which is the subject of *bring_attention*, seemed to influence opponent's decision to choose the action *agree* after his action *disagree*.

It is worth mentioning that there is a special class of scenarios (jokes), where the terminating sub-scenarios are on the edge of inconsistency with the preceding part. As well as for complaints, the plots for jokes are strongly relying on mental states of involved agents.

The following final sub-scenario would express the respective unsuccessful (for a customer) attempts to provide necessary information (Fig. 4.14). This scenario is still plausible.

bring attention – disagree
explain – deny responsibility

However, the scenario below does not seem to be produced by a rational plaintiff (defendant's actions are still reasonable):

agree – disagree
confirm – bring to attention

Agree above is marginally acceptable, but keep confirming something after being disagreed again means that a complainant did not understand or pretends than he did not understand that he was permanently disagreed.

As the reader may have noticed, not an arbitrary sequence of mental actions may constitute a plausible part of a scenario. For example, the combination *remind – not_deny – disagree* leads to the following advice: *If you reminded something and it was not denied, do not keep disagreeing – just continue bringing your point across.* An agent may disagree with the proposal of an opponent, *disagreeing* is a passive action caused by an active action of an opponent. In an interaction step it needs to follow such opponent actions as *explain, request, encourage* which is the opponent's intention to commit some action. Also, a passive action like *disagreeing* may be associated with an active action at the same interaction step.

4.3.5   Communicative Actions and Similarity Between Them

In this section we consider a particular case of mental actions: communicative actions and the Theory of Speech Act so that we can apply machine learning to communicative actions. In this theory, dialogue, negotiation, conflict dispute

---

remind_not_deny_disagree:-remindS(Case,S1),not denyrespT(Case, S1),
disagreeS(Case,S1).
*   ignore_opponent_reminder:-remindT(Case,S1), remindS(Case,S1).*
*   "Opponent's position/statement is ignored"*
*   lack_proper_explanation:-not_understandprobT(Case,S2),*
*   not explainS(Case,S2).*
*   "Your point should be explained when your opponent does not understand it"*
*   lack_acknowledge_acceptance:-acceptrespT(Case,S3),*
*   (disagreeS(Case,S3) ; remindS(Case,S3)).*
*   "Please express respect to your opponent when he/she accepts responsibilities, rather*
than pushing your target even stronger."
*   s_expl_dagr_dagr:-explainS(Case,S4),disagreeT(Case,S4),*
*   disagreeS(Case,S4).*
*   "If your opponent has disagreed with (rejected) your explanation, do not keep*
disagreeing - explain your point better."
*   t_expl_dagr_dagr:- explainT(Case,S4),disagreeS(Case,S4), disagreeT(Case,S4).*
*   "If you have disagreed with the explanation of your opponent, it would be strange for*
your opponent to disagree with your reaction - he/she would rather provide other
explanations."
*   t_remind_not_deny_disagree:-remindT(Case,S1), not denyrespS(Case,S1),*
*   disagreeT(Case,S1).*
*   "If you are reminded something and it was not denied, do not keep disagreeing - just*
continue bringing your point across."
*   agree_understand_problem:-agreeS(Case,S1), understandprobT(Case,S1).*
*   "If you agreed with something and it is followed by your opponent having understood*
the problem - this is an inconsistent steps. To understand a problem, you opponent needs
yourself to express it in one way or another but not to agree on it."
*   cheat_agree:-cheatT(Case,S1), agreeS(Case,S1).*
*   "You are saying that you agreed with what you think your opponent were lying about.*
Confirm that this was the case."
*   repetitive_request:-featureS(_fs), findall(_m, (member(_m, _fs), _mfull=..[_m,Case,S3],*
call(_mfull)), _ms), len(_ms,_lms), _lms>1.
*   "As you indicate, yourself or your opponent have made repetitive request; make sure*
you intend to mention this."

Fig. 4.14 The clauses expressing criteria of the scenario implausibility to generate warnings for the complaint author/evaluator. The clause satisfaction initiates an associated textual advice. Clauses are shown as they are implemented in Prolog (variables have the form '_'). The last clause uses meta-programming to verify whether there is a double occurrence of a mental action in a scenario

are forms of interactions between human agents. Elements of the language that expresses these interactions are referred to as locutions, speech acts (Bach and Harnish 1979), utterances, or *communicative actions* (we are going to keep using the last term).

The foundation of the current theory of *speech acts* was developed by (Austin 1962) where he explores the performative utterances, aiming to prove that when people speak, they are doing more than simply conveying information—they act. A speech act is essentially a theory that asserts the claim that *in saying something, we perform something*. It is an action that is performed by means of language. An example from the domain of customer complaints would be a performative act of a judge during a hearing when s/he says "I now pronounce that the complaint is solved." Due to Austin's designation of speech acts, sentences like this adopt a notion of action. The judge's sentence is not a report of the action; it *is* the action indeed.

However, every sentence does not take on the same linguistic action. Austin distinguishes between three types of linguistic acts: the act *of* saying something, what one *does* in saying it, and what one does *by* saying it. He labels them *Locutionary*, *Illocutionary*, and *Perlocutionary*, respectively (Farrell 2006). A locutionary act is simply saying something about the world, e.g. a declarative sentence such as "The product does not work." This sentence is not posing a question, promising, or commanding anything. It simply states something about the world, containing purely propositional content. This type of act is the most basic, and does not require much more explanation.

The illocutionary act includes promising, questioning, admitting, hypothesizing, etc. The locutionary act was simply the act of saying something, while the illocutionary act is performed *in* saying something. For example, "A company promises to support the product after it is sold" asserts more than simply stating a sentence about the world. It includes an *assertion* that is performative in nature. Illocutionary acts are very prominent in language, and are frequently in use in complaint scenarios.

The third type of linguistic acts is *perlocutionary* ones. These are non-conventional sentences that cause a natural condition or state in a person. These acts de-emphasize the actual intentions, and focus on the effects on the hearer. Acts of frightening or convincing depend on the response of another person. If a perlocutionary act is successful, then it seems safe to say that an illocutionary acts has successfully taken place.

Austin's speech act theory has been fairly influential since its inception. There have been certain improvements and clarifications made to speech acts that are worth noting; in particular, (Searle 1979) development upon Austin's insistence such acts cannot perform two different ways. Searle shows that illocutionary acts can act in two different ways.

Let us consider the following situation of a quarrel between two people, Peter and Nick. By describing a situation of strong dissatisfaction with Nick's behavior (locutionary component) in a writing style of Peter that is designed to have the force of a warning (illocutionary component), Peter may actually frighten Nick and make him give in to his requests (perlocutionary component). We can analyze whether Nick presents his communicative actions of herself and those of his opponent consistently in terms of these components, which we are going to do by means of machine learning.

Approximating scenarios of multiagent interactions, we follow along the lines of communicative actions' division into *constatives* and *performatives*.

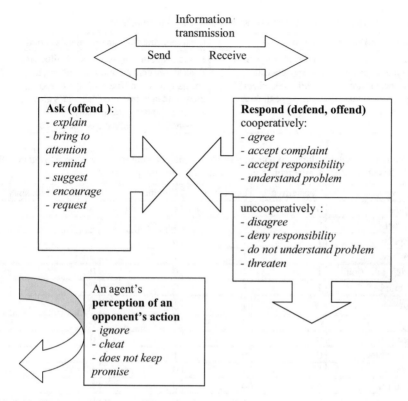

Fig. 4.15 The classes of communicative actions of conflicting human agents

- Constatives describe or report some state of affairs such that it is possible to assess whether they are false or true.
- Performatives, on the other hand, are *fortunate* or *unfortunate*, *sincere* or *insincere*, *realistic* or *unrealistic*, and, finally valid or invalid, which is the focus of the current study. Performatives address the attitude of an the agent performing the linguistic act, including his thoughts, feelings, and intentions.

It turns out that it is much more efficient to automatically analyze the group of performatives than that of constatives, because the former is domain-independent; in case of complaints there is always a lack of information to judge on constatives (Fig. 4.15).

To choose communicative actions to adequately represent an inter-human conflict, we have selected the most frequently used ones from our structured database of complaints (Table 4.2, Galitsky and Peterson 2005).

A number of *computational* approaches have attempted to discover and categorize how the agents' attitudes and communicative actions are related to each other in the case of computational simulation of human agents (Searle 1979). As we have mentioned above, applying machine learning to the attitudes and communicative

Table 4.2 The set of communicative actions from a typical complaint

Customer describes his own action	Customer describes an opponent's action
Agree, explain, suggest, bring company's attention, remind, allow, try, request, understand, inform, confirm, ask, check, ignore, convince, disagree, appeal, deny, threaten	Agree, explain, suggest, remind, allow, try, request, understand, inform, confirm, ask, check, ignore, convince, disagree, appeal, deny, threaten, bring to customer's attention, accept complaint, accept/deny responsibilities, encourage, cheat

Table 4.3 Selected attributes of communicative actions, adapting speech act theory to our domain. The attributes for *allow* are highlighted (mentioned in the example below)

Speech Acts	Constatives	Directives	Commissives	Acknowledgements
Agree	0	0	1	0
Accept	0	0	1	1
Explain	1	1	0	0
Suggest	0	1	1	0
Bring_attention	1	1	0	0
Remind	1	1	0	0
allow	1	1	1	0
Try	0	0	1	0
Request	0	1	0	0
Understand	0	0	1	1
Inform	1	1	0	1
Confirm	1	0	0	1
Ask	0	1	0	0
Check	1	0	0	1
Ignore	1	0	0	1
Convince	0	1	1	0
Disagree	1	0	1	0
Appeal	0	1	0	1
Deny	1	1	0	0
Threaten	0	1	1	0

actions, we are primarily concerned with how these approaches can provide a unified and robust framework for finding a similarity between the communicative actions. The theory of speech acts seems to be one of the most promising approaches to categorizing communicative actions in terms of their roles. Following (Bach and Harnish 1979), we consider four categories of illocutionary communicative actions with major representatives *stating, requesting, promising and apologizing*. Each speech act is related to a single category only in the framework of the speech act theory. For our purpose, each speech act is extracted from text automatically, or is selected from a list by a user as a word, may belong to multiple categories (Table 4.3).

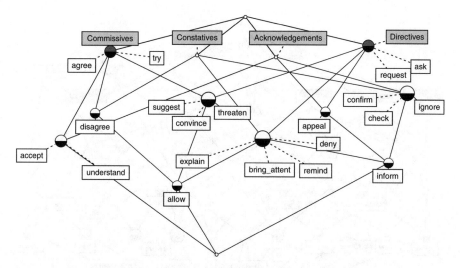

Fig. 4.16 The concept lattice for communicative actions adapting speech act theory to our domain. Each communicative action does not have a unique set of attributes: calculation of similarity might be inadequate

Now we can calculate the similarity between communicative actions as a set (an overlap) of speech act categories they belong to. To estimate how fruitful the speech act-theoretical approach is for calculating the similarities between communicative actions, we build a concept lattice (Ganter and Wille 1999) for communicative actions as objects and speech act categories as their features (*Constatives, Directives, Commissives*, and *Acknowledgements*). It the concept lattice, each node is assigned a set of features and a set of objects. For each node, all features assigned to nodes, assessable when navigating the lattice upwards, are satisfied by the objects assigned to this node. In Fig. 4.16, we show either features or objects for each node. For example, let us consider the node assigned with the object *allow.* Navigating the edges up, we access the *disagree* and then *Commissives* and *Constatives* node, triple *suggest-convince-threaten* node and then *Commissives* and *Directives,* and four-tuple *explain-bring_attention-remind-deny* and then *Directives.* Hence the lattice is showing that the object *allow* satisfies three out of four *features Commissives, Directives, and Constative* (as we have specified in the Table 4.3, grayed row).

As the reader can see, this direct Speech Act – theoretical approach is inadequate for uniform coverage of communicative actions in conflict scenarios. Some communicative actions (e.g. agree, try) are described by the selected features more accurately, whereas *suggest-convince-threaten* and tuple *explain-bring_attention-remind-deny* cannot be distinguished under this categorization at all. Hence four features of the Speech Act theory are insufficient to differentiate between twenty communicative actions which have been evaluated to be a minimal set to express an inter-human conflict (Galitsky et al. 2008). Hence more attributes are needed to

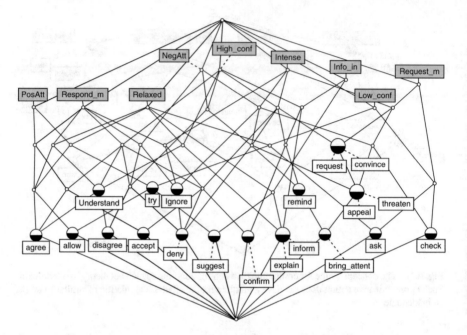

Fig. 4.17 The resultant concept lattice for communicative actions with adjusted definitions. Each communicative action has a unique set of attributes

be taken into account to find an adequate means to compute similarities between communicative actions.

We proceed to the solution which turned out to be the most robust and plausible (Fig. 4.17). To extend the speech act–based means of expressing similarity between communicative actions, we introduce five attributes each of which reflects a particular semantic parameter for communicative activity (Table 4.4):

- *Positive/negative attitude* expresses whether a communicative action is a cooperative (friendly, helpful) move (1), uncooperative (unfriendly, unhelpful) move (−1), neither or both (hard to tell, 0).
- *Request/respond mode* specifies whether a communicative action is expected to be followed by a reaction (1), constitutes a response (follows) a previous request, neither or both (hard to tell, 0).
- *Info supply/no info supply* tells if a communicative action brings in an additional data about the conflict (1), does not bring any information (−1), 0; does not occur here.
- *High/low confidence* specifies the confidence of the preceding mental state so that a particular communicative action is chosen, high knowledge/confidence (1), lack of knowledge/confidence (−1), neither or both is possible (0).
- *Intense/relaxed mode* says about the potential emotional load: high (1), low (−1), neutral (0) emotional loads are possible.

Table 4.4 Augmented attributes of communicative actions

Communicative action	Attributes				
	Positive/negative attitude	Request/respond mode	Info supply/ no info supply	High/low confidence	Intense/relaxed mode
Agree	1	−1	−1	1	−1
Accept	1	−1	−1	1	1
Explain	0	−1	1	1	−1
Suggest	1	0	1	−1	−1
Bring_attention	1	1	1	1	1
Remind	−1	0	1	1	1
Allow	1	−1	−1	−1	−1
Try	1	0	−1	−1	−1
Request	0	1	−1	1	1
Understand	0	−1	−1	1	−1
Inform	0	0	1	1	−1
Confirm	0	−1	1	1	1
Ask	0	1	−1	−1	−1
Check	−1	1	−1	−1	1
Ignore	−1	−1	−1	−1	1
Convince	0	1	1	1	−1
Disagree	−1	−1	−1	1	−1
Appeal	−1	1	1	1	1
Deny	−1	−1	−1	1	1
Threaten	−1	1	−1	1	1

Note that out of the set of meanings for each communicative action, we merge its subset into a single meaning. This merge is performed, taking into account relations between the meanings of the given communicative actions and those of the other ones (Galitsky 2006).

Formal concept analysis (FCA, Ganter and Wille 1999) was used to characterize the set of communicative actions in the context of our framework. In FCA, a (formal) context consists of a set of objects G, a set of attributes M, and an indication of which objects have which attributes. A *concept* is a pair containing both a natural property cluster and its corresponding natural object cluster. A "natural" object cluster is the set of all objects that share a common subset of properties, and a "natural" property cluster is the set of all properties shared by one of the natural object clusters. Given a set of objects G and a set of attributes M, a concept is defined to be a pair (G_i, M_i) such that

1. $G_i \subseteq G$;
2. $M_i \subseteq M$;
3. every object in G_i has every attribute in M_i;
4. for every object in G that is not in G_i, there is an attribute in M_i that the object does not have;
5. for every attribute in M that is not in M_i, there is an object in G_i that does not have that attribute.

Given a concept (G_i, M_i), the set G_i is called the *extent* of the concept, and the set M_i is called the *intent*. Concepts can be partially ordered by inclusion: if (G_i, M_i) and (G_j, M_j) are concepts, a partial order $\leq$ can be defined, where $(G_i, M_i) \leq (G_j, M_j)$ whenever $G_i \subseteq G_j$. Equivalently, $(G_i, M_i) \leq (G_j, M_j)$ whenever $M_j \subseteq M_i$. In general, attributes may allow multiple values (many-valued attributes), characterizing many-valued contexts. By applying so-called conceptual scaling, many-valued contexts can be transformed to one-valued scaled contexts from which concepts can be computed. The family of these concepts obeys the mathematical axioms defining a lattice, and is called a concept lattice or Galois lattice.

So-called *line diagrams* are used in order to succinctly represent information about intents and extents of formal context in a concept lattice. Nodes are circles that can be labeled with (a) both attributes and objects; (b) attributes; (c) objects or (d) none. In order to consider some distinguished labels, some nodes appear as circles which are half-filled in their lower part (labelled with objects only), and nodes which are half-filled in their upper part (labelled with attributes only). Nodes which are empty circles have no particular labels. In order to provide a formal characterization of the communicative actions in S_{freq} in terms of their attributes a concept lattice was obtained. Nominal scaling was applied on the first and second attributes (the third, fourth and fifth attributes were already two-valued). As a result of this scaling, we obtained nine two-valued attributes associated with different possible values of the original five attributes: PosAtt (1), NegAtt (-1), Request (1), Respond (-1), InfoIn (1), High_Conf (1), Low_Conf (-1), Intense (1), Relaxed (-1). It must be remarked that some particular two-valued attributes, derived from the original attributes, are not considered for building the resulting concept lattice shown in Fig. 4.17, as they do not contribute strongly in distinguishing communicative actions from each other. The resulting scaled context had nine two-valued attributes, resulting in the concept lattice.

The ConExp software (Yevtushenko 2005) was used to construct and visualize the concept lattice of communicative actions and their associated nine two-valued attributes. Some selected nodes are provided with descriptions of the corresponding "intents" and "extents" subscribed to show how certain communicative actions are semantically related to each other. The concept lattice illustrates the semantics of communicative actions, and shows how to cover different meanings in the knowledge domain of customer–company interaction in complaint scenarios. The concept lattice illustrates the semantics of communicative actions; it shows how the choice of attribute-based expressions covers the totality of possible meanings in the knowledge domain of interaction between human agents.

After scaling the many-valued context of communicative actions, descriptions of communicative action are given by 9-tuples of attributes, ordered in the usual way. Thus, vertex labels of generalizations of scenario graphs are given by intents of the scaled context of communicative actions.

Before we proceed to the formal model of scenarios in terms of graphs, we define a conflict scenario as a sequence of communicative actions, each of which is a *reaction* to the previous communicative actions of opponents. This reaction is constrained by *interaction protocols* by means of enumeration of *valid* scenarios

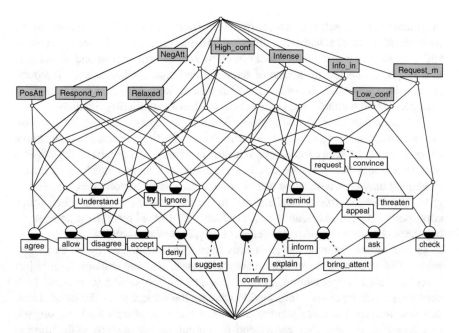

Fig. 4.18 The resultant concept lattice for communicative actions with adjusted definitions. Each communicative action has a unique set of attributes

where this protocol is assumed to be correct. Multiagent conflict is a scenario where agents have inconsistent intentions (about states):

want(AgentFor, State), want(AgentAgainst, not State).

The scenario is defined as a sequence of communicative actions. Usually, if the sequence of communicative actions of customer support is "adequate", a complaint does not arise. A conflict can be defined as a *logical inconsistency*. Our definition of complaint scenario includes inconsistencies in both mental and physical spaces.

The actions which agents select are physical and mental. We consider the special class of mental actions used for communications, and refer to them as communicative actions (Searle 1979). To visually represent the communicative actions agents use, we rely on concept lattices. We form attributes of communicative actions according to our model and draw the concept lattice (Fig. 4.18, see Galitsky and de la Rosa 2011 for more details).

4.3.6 Defining Scenario as Graphs

In order to provide a computational approach to represent complaints, we will define the notion of complaint scenario, a graph-based formalization for representing customer–company dialogues. In such scenarios we will distinguish a number of communicative actions, which from empirical evidence have proven to be representative for characterizing different possible interactions between customer and company in a complaint scenario. Such actions will correspond to vertices in a graph, connected by means of temporal and causal relationships. Temporal relationships formalize the order in which actions were advanced in a complaint dialogue, whereas attack relationships help to identify conflicting situations.

To form a data structure for machine learning, we approximate an inter-human interaction scenario as a sequence of communicative actions, ordered in time, with a causal relation between certain communicative actions (more precisely, the subjects of these actions). Scenarios are simplified to allow for effective matching by means of graphs: only communicative actions remain as a most important component to reflect the dialogue structure and express similarities between scenarios. Each vertex corresponds to a communicative action, which is performed by either proponent, or opponent. An arc (oriented edge) denotes a sequence of two actions.

In our model communicative actions have two parameters: agent name and subject (information transmitted, a cause addressed, a reason explained, an object described, etc.). Representing scenarios as graphs, we take into account both parameters. Arc types bear information whether the subject stays the same. Thick arcs link vertices that correspond to communicative actions with the same subject; thin arcs link vertices that correspond to communicative actions with different subject. The curve arcs denote a causal link between the arguments of mental actions.

Let us consider an example of a scenario and its graph (Figs. 4.19 and 4.20). The causal link here is [ask] (the service is not as advertised) [disagree] – failures in a service contract (and, therefore, the service is not as advertised) [disagree] – failures in a service contract (and, therefore, the service is not as advertised), and also [requested] – (to send to my home) [reminded] them to mail it (requested a thing and then reminded about it).

One of the most important tasks in assisting negotiations and resolving inter-human conflicts is the validity assessment. A scenario (in particular, a complaint) is valid if it is plausible, internally consistent, and also consistent with available domain-specific knowledge. In case of inter-human conflicts or negotiations, such domain-specific knowledge is frequently unavailable. In this book, we demonstrate that a wide class of scenarios of various natures can be assigned to class of valid

---

I asked why the service was not as advertised——
    They *explained* that I did not understand the advertised features properly
I *disagreed* and *confirmed* the particular failures in a service contract
    They *agreed* with my points and *suggested* compensation
I *accepted* it and *requested* to send it to my home address together with explanations on how it happened.
    They *promised* to send it to me.
In a month time I *reminded* them to mail it to me
After two months I *asked* what happened with my compensation...

Fig. 4.19 A sample complaint scenario

Fig. 4.20 A graph
representation for scenario

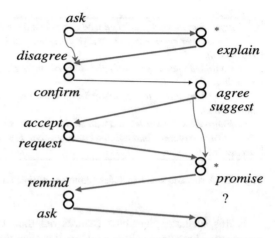

or invalid based on communicative actions and relationships between their subjects
only. The accuracy of such classification is sufficient for deployment in decision-
support systems, where final judgment is. To provide a framework for learning
communicative actions, we need to select their attributes.

Note that first two sentences (and the respective subgraph comprising two
vertices) are about the current transaction, three sentences after (and the respective
subgraph comprising three vertices) address the *unfair charge,* and the last sentence
is probably related to both issues above. Hence the vertices of two respective
subgraphs are linked with thick arcs (*explain-accept*) and (*remind-deny-disagree*).

In formal conflict scenarios extracted from text there can be multiple communicative actions per step, for example *I disagreed ... and suggested....* The former
communicative action describes how an agent receives a message (*accept, agree,
reject,* etc.) from an opponent, and the latter one describes the attitude of this agent
initiating a request (*suggest, explain,* etc.), or reaction to the opponent's action.
Sometimes, either of the above actions is omitted in textual description of conflicts.
Frequently, a communicative action, which is assumed but not mentioned explicitly,
can be deduced. In this chapter for the sake of simplicity we will consider single
action per step, performing the comparative analysis of scenarios.

There is a commonsense causal link *between being charged an unfair fee*
and *intention to have this amount of money back* which is expressed by the arc
between *remind* and *disagree.* Semantically, arcs with causal labels between vertices
for communicative actions express the causal links between the arguments of
communicative actions rather than between the communicative actions themselves.

How would one handle commonsense reasoning patterns in our domain? We need
specific commonsense knowledge to link such statements as *unfair fee* with *deposit
back.* An ontology which would give us sufficient knowledge is not available and it
would be extremely hard and expensive to build for a variety of complaint domains.
Therefore, our data structure for machine learning just includes causal links (and
not background knowledge).

> *I **explained** that my check bounced (I wrote it after I made a deposit).*
>
>   *A customer service representative **accepted** that it usually takes some time to process the deposit.*
>
>   *I **reminded** that I was unfairly charged an overdraft fee a month ago in a similar situation.*
>
>   *They **denied** that it was unfair because the overdraft fee was disclosed in my account information.*
>
>   *I **disagreed** with their fee and wanted this fee deposited back to my account.*
>
>   *They **explained** that nothing can be done at this point and that I need to look into the account rules closer.*

Fig. 4.21 A scenario which includes communicative actions of a proponent and an opponent

Is this scenario plausible? It turns out that it is not. First of all, having the background knowledge about banking, it is clear that the customer wrongly assumed that the funds become available immediately after a deposit is made. However, it is not really viable to store this information in a generic complaint management system; therefore, we further research into the legitimacy of the observed sequence of communicative actions. "Being in an attack mode (*reminding*) after a previous attack (*explaining*) was *accepted*" does not look like a cooperative mood. Moreover, keep disagreeing concerning the subject which has just being *denied* (speaking more precisely, a commonsense implication of this subject) is not an adequate negotiation strategy. On the other hand, if a similar scenario (in terms of the structure of communicative actions) has been assigned by a domain expert as *invalid*, we would want the machine learning system to relate the scenario Fig. 4.21 to the same class even if there are no explicit reasons.

Hence our analysis of the domain of customer complaints shows that to relate a scenario to a class without domain-specific knowledge, one needs to analyze a sequence of communicative actions and certain relations between their subjects. Otherwise, one would have to code all relevant domain knowledge which is well-known to be an extremely hard problem and non-feasible for a practical application.

We proceed with the description of our scenario dataset used for classifier training. This dataset contains two sets of complaint scenarios: showing a good attitude of a complainant (consistent plot with proper argumentation, a *valid complaint*) on the left, and a bad attitude of a complainant (inconsistent plot with certain flaws, implausible or irrational scenarios, an *invalid complaint*) on the right (Fig. 4.22).

Each scenario includes two to six interaction *steps*, each consisting of communicative actions with the alternating first attribute {*request – respond – additional request or other follow up*}. A step comprises one or more consequent actions with the same subject. Within a step, vertices for communicative actions with common argument are linked with *thick* arcs.

For example, *suggest* from scenario V2 (Fig. 4.22) is linked by a thin arc to communicative action *ignore*, whose argument is not logically linked to the argument of *suggest* (the subject of suggestion). The first step of V2 includes *ignore-deny-ignore-threaten*; these communicative actions have the same subject (it is not

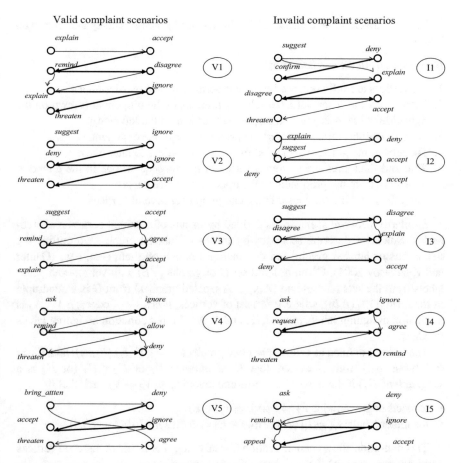

Fig. 4.22 A fragment of the training set of scenarios

specified in the graph of conflict scenario). The vertices of these communicative actions with the same argument are linked by the *thick* arcs. For example, it could be ***ignored*** *refund because of a wrong mailing address,* ***deny*** *the reason that the refund has been ignored* [*because of a wrong mailing address*], ***ignore*** *the denial* [*... concerning a wrong mailing address*], *and* ***threatening*** *for that ignorant behavior* [*... concerning a wrong mailing address*]. We have *wrong mailing address* as the common subject *S* of communicative actions *ignore-deny-ignore-threaten* which we approximate as

ignore(A1, S) & deny(A2,S) & ignore(A1,S) & threaten(A2, S), keeping in mind the scenario graph. In such approximation we write *deny(A2, S)* for the fact that *A2 denied the reason that the refund has been ignored because of S.* Indeed, *ignore(A1, S) & deny(A2,S) & ignore(A1,S) & threaten(A2, S).* Without a scenario graph, the best representation of the above in our language would be

ignore(A1, S) & deny(A2, ignore(A1, S)) & ignore(A1, deny(A2, ignore(A1, S))) & threaten(A2, ignore(A1, deny(A2, ignore(A1, S)))).

Let us enumerate the constraints for the scenario graph (Galitsky and Perterson 2005):

Definition 20 In the scenario graph:

1. All vertices are fully ordered by the temporal sequence (earlier-later);
2. Each vertex has a special label relating it either to the proponent (drawn on the right side in Fig. 4.20) or to the opponent (drawn on the left side);
3. Vertices denote actions either of the proponent or of the opponent;
4. The arcs of the graph are oriented from earlier vertices to later ones;
5. Thin and thick arcs point from a vertex to the subsequent one in the temporal sequence (from the proponent to the opponent or vice versa);
6. Curly arcs, staying for causal links, can jump over several vertices.

Similarity between scenarios is defined by means of maximal common subscenarios. Since we describe scenarios by means of labeled graphs, we outline the definitions of labeled graphs and domination relation on them (see, e.g., (Ganter and Kuznetsov 2001). Given ordered set G of graphs (V,E) with vertex- and edge-labels from the sets $(\Lambda_\varsigma, \preceq$ and $(\Lambda_E, \preceq)$. A labeled graph Γ from G is a quadruple of the form $((V,l),(E,b))$, where V is a set of vertices, E is a set of edges, $l: V \hat{} \Lambda_\varsigma$ is a function assigning labels to vertices, and $b: E \hat{} \Lambda_E$ is a function assigning labels to edges.

The order is defined as follows: For two graphs $\Gamma_1 := ((V_1,l_1),(E_1,b_1))$ and $\Gamma_2 := ((V_2,l_2),(E_2,b_2))$ from G we say that Γ_1 *dominates* Γ_2 or $\Gamma_2 \leq \Gamma_1$ (or Γ_2 is a *subgraph* of Γ_1) if there exists a one-to-one mapping $\varphi: V_2 \to V_1$ such that it

- respects edges: $(v,w) \in E_2 \Rightarrow (\varphi(v), \varphi(w)) \in E_1$,
- fits under labels: $l_2(v \preceq l_1(\varphi(v)), (v,w) \in E_2 \Rightarrow b_2(v,w) \preceq b_1(\varphi(v), \varphi(w))$.

This definition allows generalization ("weakening") of labels of matched vertices when passing from the "larger" graph G_1 to "smaller" graph G_2.

Now, generalization Z of a pair of scenario graphs X and Y (or their similarity), denoted by $X \hat{} Y = Z$, is the set of all inclusion-maximal common subgraphs of X and Y, each of them satisfying the following additional conditions:

- To be matched, two vertices from graphs X and Y must denote communicative actions of the same agent;
- Each common subgraph from Z contains at least one thick arc.

If the conditions above cannot be met then the common subgraph does not exist. This definition is easily extended to finding generalizations of several graphs (e.g., see Ganter and Kuznetsov 2001; Kuznetsov 1999). The subsumption order μ on pairs of graph sets X and Y is naturally defined as $X \mu Y := X *Y = X$.

Computing relation $\Gamma_2 \leq \Gamma_1$ for arbitrary graphs Γ_2 and Γ_1 is an NP-complete problem (since it is a generalization of the subgraph isomorphism problem from (Garey and Johnson 1979)). Finding $X * Y = Z$ for arbitrary X, Y, and Z is generally an NP-hard problem. In (Ganter and Kuznetsov 2001) a method based on so-called projections was proposed, which allows one to establish a trade-off between accuracy of representation by labeled graphs and complexity of computations with them. In particular, for a fixed size of projections, the worst-case time complexity of computing operation $*$ and testing relation $\leq$ becomes constant.

4.3.7   Machine Learning of Conflict Scenarios

The following conditions hold when a scenario graph U is assigned to a class (we consider positive classification, i.e., to valid complaints, the classification to invalid complaints is made similarly, Fig. 4.23).

Similarity Condition 21.

1. U is similar to (has a nonempty common scenario subgraph of) a positive example R+. It is possible that the same graph has also a nonempty common scenario subgraph with a negative example R−. This is means that the graph is similar to both positive and negative examples.
2. For any negative example R⁻, if U is similar to R⁻ (i.e., U $*$ R⁻ $\neq \varnothing$) then U $*$ R⁻ μ U $*$ R⁺. This condition introduces the measure of similarity and says that to be assigned to a class, the similarity between the unknown graph U and the closest (in terms of μ) scenario from the positive class should be higher than the similarity between U and each negative example (i.e., representative of the class of invalid complaints).

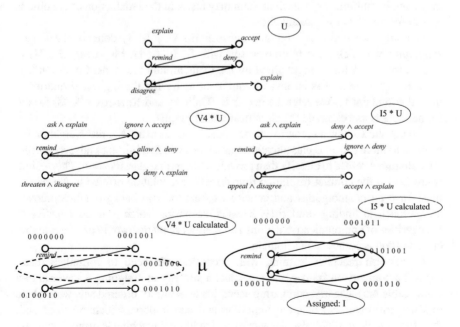

Fig. 4.23 A scenario with unknown label and the procedure of its classification

This condition introduces the measure of similarity and says that to be assigned to a class, the similarity between the unknown graph U and the closest scenario from the positive class should be higher than the similarity between U and each negative example (i.e., representative of the class of invalid complaints).

Condition 2 implies that there is a positive example R^+ such that for no R^- one has $U_* R^+ \mu R^-$, i.e., there is no counterexample to this generalization of positive examples.

Let us now proceed to the example of a particular U in Fig. 4.23 on the top. The task is to determine whether U belongs to the class of valid complaints (on the left of Fig. 4.4) or to the classes of invalid complaints (on the right); these classes are mutually exclusive.

We observe that V_4 is the graph of the highest similarity with U among all graphs from the set $\{V_1, \ldots V_5\}$ and find the common sub-scenario $U_* V_4$. Its only thick arc is derived from the thick arc between vertices with labels *remind* and *deny* of U and the thick arc between vertices with labels *remind* and *allow* of V_4. The first vertex of this thick arc of $U_* V_4$ is *remind* $\wedge$ *remind* = *remind*, the second is *allow* $\wedge$ *deny* = <0 0 0 1 0 0 0> ($U_* V_4$ is calculated at the left bottom). Other arcs of $U_* V_4$ are as follows: that from the vertex with the label *remind* to the vertex with the label <0 0 0 1 0 0 0>; the arc from the vertex with the label <0 0 0 1 0 0 1 > to the vertex with the label *remind*; the arc from the vertex with the label <0 0 0 1 0 0 0> the vertex with the label <0 1 0 0 0 1 0>. These arcs are thin, unless both respective arcs of $U_* V_4$ are thick (the latter is not the case here). Naturally, common subscenario may contain multiple steps, each of them may result in the satisfaction of conditions 1) – 2) for the class assignment above.

Similarly, we build the common subscenario $U_* I_5$; I_5 delivers the largest subgraph (two thick arcs) in comparison with I_1, I_2, I_3, I_4. Moreover, $U_* V_4 \mu U_* I_5$, this inclusion is highlighted by the ovals around the steps. Condition 2 is satisfied. Therefore, U is an invalid complaint as having the highest similarity to invalid complaint I_5. We refer the reader to (Galitsky and Kuznetsov 2008) for the further details and examples of classifications of graphs.

Having shown how a scenario can be related to class using Nearest Neighbor, we proceed to more cautious classification framework which minimizes false negatives: it would rather refuse to classify than provide a borderline classification. This feature is crucial for the conflict resolution domain where a solution offered to the parties must have an unambiguous and concise explanation and background. Moreover, an approach to finding similarities between scenarios which is more sensitive to peculiarities of communicative actions and conflict scenarios would deliver a higher classification accuracy in our domain.

To perform machine learning with scenarios, we need to formalize them, suggest a comparison framework and select a strategy of assigning a scenario to a class (Table 4.5). Clearly, comparing scenarios as arbitrary ordered sets would lead to a uniform treatment of more important and less important scenario steps and, therefore, would compromise the accuracy. Traditional machine learning technique (including Inductive Logic Programming) seems inapplicable due to a peculiar data structure of scenarios, especially of complaint scenarios.

Table 4.5 Evaluation of the adequacy of scenario representation language

Domain/dataset	Number of scenarios	Percentage of scenarios which were successfully represented as graphs by experts	Percentage of scenarios which were (at least partially) reconstructed from the graph	Percentage of scenarios which were properly represented and reconstructed	Percentage of properly related to a class (being adequately represented), 2 classes
Complaints-Bank 1 (Galitsky 2006)	20	85	75	65	72
Complaints-Bank 2	20	80	75	60	75
Complaints-Bank 3	20	95	85	75	78
Conflict between communities of agents	2	50	50	50	No eval
Emotional interactions (revealed communicative actions plus emotions)	12	75	67	58	60

4.3.8   Linked Sub-Scenarios

One of the most important information that a scenario comprises is its linked sub-scenario. A sequence of mental states is referred as to *linked* if the meta-variables of each mental meta-predicate of this sequence are instantiated by the same formula W. A basic example here is the typical unit of an arbitrary discourse, *I asked about a feature of object and she responded, specifying this feature for the object.* In this case W = *Feature(Object)*, where predicate *Feature* is uninstantiated at the time of asking but instantiated at the time of answering:

$$ask(i, she, Feature(Object)) \rightarrow answer(she, i, Feature(Object)),$$

'→' denotes the sequence of actions.

Let us now consider a more complex example of a linked sub-scenario, including mental states and physical actions and states:

> *I deposited my child support check and they sent it back to me saying that they could not deposit a business check into a personal account. It clearly states on the front it is child support from Brazoria County and on the back that it is payable to me.*

This fragment is represented as the background info part:

> *deposit(i, check(child_support)), send(bankOfAmerica, i, check(child_support)),*
> followed by the scenario itself:
> *inform(bankOfAmerica, i, not deposit(me, check(child_support)),*
> *believe(i, accept(Bank, check(child_support))).*

In this complaint sub-scenario, the mental predicates above (including physical predicate *deposit* which plays here the role of initial mental predicate) have the term *check(child_support)* as the value of metavariable W. Therefore, the scenario above is a linked sub-scenario of the complaint which is based on the conflict of bank's and customer's beliefs concerning a deposit of checks (issued by a particular institution). Given a particular linked sub-scenario, finding a similar sub-scenario in another complaint would mean that these two complaints are originated by a belief conflict of the same structure. At the same time, the semantics of linking meta-variable (*check(child_support)*) in our example identifies a particular physical parameter and is too specific to judge on the conflict. Moreover, the physical parameter above is independent on the plot of the scenario and may be combined (and serve as an argument of a mental action) with an arbitrary scenario. This discussion provided an additional justification of our mental action-based formal model of a scenario.

Let us continue with the example above; the complainant writes:

> *This is the second time in the last 3 months this bank has done this. The first time I went in they had to pay me $150 in fees because of the error. Then I get an insufficient funds from an automatic transfer that says the $2000 transfer couldn't happen. Well the auto transfer is for $20 and now the account is negative 1400 and some change. I hate these people. When I went in the first time they did this, the manager said "Oh well stupid error" and thought I didn't hear her. I will be removing all funds from this incompetent bank and trying some place else!*

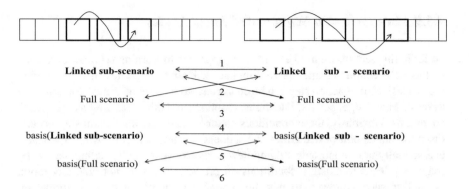

Fig. 4.24 The order of the search for common mental actions and emotions for a pair of scenarios (on the *left* and on the *right*)

As the reader observes, in this sample conflict the plot does not carry on with the same physical predicate. Above is a rather chaotic and emotional enumeration of previous events which do not form a linked sub-scenario that is well-suited for complaint identification (matching with a similar sub-scenario).

Overall scenario above is a representative for the class of complaints *Customer believes company did not follow its rules*. For the purposes of this study, the classes of complaints are drawn based on the mental attitudes of complainants and their opponents; linked sub-scenarios form the criterion of belonging to the class. Note that a linked sub-scenario in our example does not have to occur in the beginning of the whole scenario: its background may precede the essential part (linked sub-scenario).

Hence, to find a similarity between two scenarios, we need to find their common linked sub-scenario via the search for a match on predicate-by-predicate basis (Fig. 4.24). If it is checked to be impossible, a linked sub-scenario of one complaint is matched against the whole scenario of another one. If such the attempt fails, the whole scenarios are tried to be matched against each other. If two scenarios do not have common sequence of (linked) predicates, we perform their comparison as the ordered sets of mental actions.

As the reader may feel at this point, the problem of finding a similarity for two scenarios is not adequately reducible to the task of finding an intersection of the set of mental predicates for each scenario, even if we consider additional scenario-specific constraints above. Looking for intersections between the sets, which are the sets of formulas (not arbitrary elements), we take advantage of the operation of *term anti-unification* (Sect. 7.4.2, Reynolds 1970). In case of unary predicates anti-unification turns into a set-theoretic intersection.

Given a pair of scenarios, anti-unification yields a third scenario that comprises the common features (mental actions) of input scenarios. We intend our algorithm for search of similarity (Fig. 4.24) to reveal as many common features as possible.

4.3.9 Scenario as a Sequence of Local Logics

So far in this section we used an inductive approach to learning behavior of agents. In this sub-section we attempt to simulate deductive properties of a developing scenario. Each interaction step can be characterized by a set of mental conditions in terms of knowledge, beliefs, intentions, emotions and others, as well as "physical" conditions. Obviously, these conditions change when new interaction step occurs. From the standpoint of deduction, the sequence of interaction steps for a scenario is essentially non-monotonic: adding new steps (conventionally, adding new facts) frequently leads to existing conditions on previous states do not hold any more. We select such approach to non-monotonicity as local logics as a formalism to represent development of scenarios where new interaction steps of agents occur.

For the purpose of concept learning we were concerned with the structure of communicative action, however for the deductive system we need some sort of completeness for pre- and post-conditions of communicative actions. These can be obtained as prepositions being extracted from text, or deduced from domain specific rules like "early withdrawal $=>$ penalty", or from mental world-specific rules such as "loss of money $=>$ negative emotion". In this section we treat propositions irrespectively of their source.

In the formalism to be presented, *situations* are associated with mental states. Multiple situations *like though of being cheated on by an opponent, being misinformed, the plan to counter-attack being discovered* are associated with the state *change communication topic and formulate a new request* (This state can be followed with communicative action *remind* followed by *request*, for example). *Propositions* are interpreted as conditions on current mental states.

Definition 22 A *Boolean classification* (a Boolean logic without the relation |- for sets of propositions (Barwise 1975; Barwise and Perry 1983)) A $=< S, \Sigma, |=,$ &, $\neg >$ consists of a non-empty set S of situations, a set Σ propositions, a binary relation "true in" $| = $ on S x Σ, conjunction & and negation $\neg$. Boolean classification satisfies the following conditions for conjunction and negation: s $| = p_1$ & p_2 iff s $| = p_1$ and s $| = p_2$,

$$s \ |= \neg p \text{ iff } s \ |\neq p.$$

Boolean classification adopts the basic Gentzen sequent calculus approach to logic, and Γ |- Δ means that the conjunction of the propositions in Γ entails the disjunction of the propositions in Δ as a non-logical component of a formal system, combined with any kind of logical component. A pair of sets of propositions $< \Gamma, \Delta >$ is called a *sequent*. For example,

<{"this book is great"^"he enjoyed this book" & "this book covers math"^"he referred to this book preparing for math test" & "I recommend this book for beginners"^"Will suit a beginner reader well"},

{good_for_students $\vee$ good_for_mathematicians $\vee \neg$ suitable for biologists} is a sequent for book reading recommendation. This kind of sequents can be obtained by information extraction from text, where those sentence generalization expressions are selected from text which gave non-trivial results (generalization score is above threshold).

A Boolean *local* logic L = <A, |-, N > consists of a Boolean classification and binary relation |- of inferability for a pair of sets of propositions, and a set of *normal* situations N $\subseteq$ S. Normal situations satisfy the following conditions:

Entailment: The relation |- satisfies all usual Gentzen rules for classical propositional logic, including identity a |- a, weakening Γ |- $\Delta \Rightarrow \Gamma$, Γ' |- Δ, Δ', and global cut

Γ, Σ_0 |- Δ, Σ_1 for each partition < Σ_0, Σ_1 >of some set $\Sigma' \Rightarrow \Gamma$|- Δ. Also *normal* situations are those situations s such that:

for any Γ|- Δ and s | = p for all p$\in\Gamma$ =>s | = q for some q$\in\Delta$. By default, situations are normal. The use of normal situations in a local logic L imitates assumptions which are implicit background knowledge within L.

A local logic is *sound* if its every situation is normal. L is *complete* if

- for all sets of propositions Γ, Δ, Γ |- Δ,

- then there is a normal situation s such that s | = p for every p$\in\Gamma$ and s | = $\neg$q for every q $\in\Delta$.

It is possible to introduce a partial order on a pair of logics L_1 and L_2 on a fixed classification A: $L_1 < L_2$ iff:

- For all sets Γ, Δ of propositions, Γ |-$_{L1}$ $\Delta \Rightarrow \Gamma$ |-$_{L2}$ Δ, and
- Every situation which is normal in L_2 is normal L_1.

Given this formalism, we state that individual information extraction occurs relatively to an implicit local logic. If either natural language expression or targeted extraction (constraints or normal situations) changes, then there is a potential that normal situations or constraints change respectively as well. This is how local logics implement non-monotonicity.

We now take advantage of the theorem introduced in (Barwise & Seligman 1997).

The local logics on a given classification form a complete lattice under ordering <.

Observation 23 Hence a given behavior scenario developing in time forms a complete lattice. At each point in time, current scenario can be valid, invalid or undetermined; validity assessment does not correlate with order on a sequence of developing scenarios directly.

4.4   Some Applications of Formalized ToM

4.4.1   *Learning Conflicts Between Communities of Agents*

It is worth explaining to CwA that communities of agents can be characterized by
"collective" communication actions in a similar way to individual agents. Hence
using the developed machinery, it is possible to represent the development of a
conflict between communities of agents, so that the whole community is represented
by a single agent, all the way towards a national-level and international conflict.
The problem of conflict resolution in this is of an enormous importance and has a
substantial educational value.

To demonstrate an example of a graph representation for a conflict involving
three groups of agents, we consider an analysis (Fang et al. 1993) of a nasty
groundwater contamination conflict. Elmira, a Canadian town draws its municipal
water from an underground aquifer. Ontario Ministry of the Environment (MoE)
discovered that the aquifer was contaminated by a carcinogen. Suspicion fell on
the Elmira pesticide products plant of Uniroyal Chemical Ltd. (Uniroyal), which
had a history of environmental problems. MoE issued a Control Order under the
Environmental Protection Act of Ontario, requiring that Uniroyal implement a
long-term collection and treatment system, and carry out any necessary cleanup
under Ministry supervision. Uniroyal immediately exercised its right to appeal.
Meanwhile, various interest groups formed and attempted to influence the process
through lobbying and other means. Of particular note was the Local Government
that took common positions in the dispute and, encouraged by the Ministry, hired
independent consultants. MoE's objective was to carry out its mandate as efficiently
as possible; Uniroyal wanted the Control Order modified or rescinded; Local
Government wanted to protect its citizens and its industrial base.

We highlight the communicative actions used by the main groups of agents as
well as the options under the control of each decision maker. MoE controls the
option to modify the Control Order to make it more acceptable to Uniroyal (called
Modify in Table 4.6). Uniroyal can lengthen the appeal process.

(Delay), accept the current Control Order (Accept), or abandon its Elmira
operations (Abandon). Finally, Local Government can insist that the original
Control Order be applied (Insist).

Moving from the status quo (state 1) via the transitional non-cooperative
equilibrium (state 5) to the final cooperative equilibrium (state 8) in the Elmira
groundwater contamination dispute.

We now outline the original approach of the authors in treatment conflict as a
sequence of states with selections of options in cooperative and non-cooperative
equilibriums. Each of the nine feasible states is a possible scenario of this simple
model, and is represented by a column of Y's and N's. A Y indicates that Yes, the
option opposite the Y is selected by the decision maker controlling it, while an N
means No, the option is not taken. For example, state 8, the far right column in

Table 4.6 A conflict between private and governmental entities

Decision Makers and Options	Status Quo		Noncooperative Equilibrium		Cooperative Equilibrium
MoE					
1. Modify	N		N	→	Y
Uniroyal					
2. Delay	Y		Y	→	N
3. Accept	N		N	→	Y
4. Abandon	N		N		N
Local Givernment					
5. Insist	N	→	Y		Y
State Number	1		5		8

Table 4.6, is the scenario where MoE modifies the Control Order (selects option 1) and Uniroyal accepts this modification (chooses option 3), while Local Government continues to support the original Control Order (selecting option 5).

We proceed to the problem of relating a conflict between communities of human agents to a class of *violent* outcome and *non-violent* outcome. If a conflict at a given development stage is similar to a number of conflicts which have been peacefully resolved, then one can expect the same outcome. In this case an interference of national or international communities is probably not required. However, if this conflict is similar to the ones which have led to violence of any sort, an urgent action may be required.

Obviously, because of a very reduced and sparse dataset of conflicts between human communities, statistical approach would not be as helpful; rule based methods providing adequate explanations for decisions are required. We believe that a communicative actions-oriented knowledge representation machinery is adequate in this domain; Nearest neighbor machine learning may need to be extended into a more cautious one which would less likely deliver false negative.

We provide a brief example of an (abbreviated) textual description of a national conflict and its graph-based representation (Fig. 4.25). An expert is expected to build a graph representation manually using some kind of user interface.

4.4.2   Emotional Profile

We call *emotional profile* a formal representation of a sequence of emotional states through a textual discourse. Emotional profile is extracted from textual description of a conflict, where the e-mail author describes his/her interaction with other individuals. Emotional profile consists of a sequence of emotional states of interacting agents, where communicative actions are attached to these emotional states.

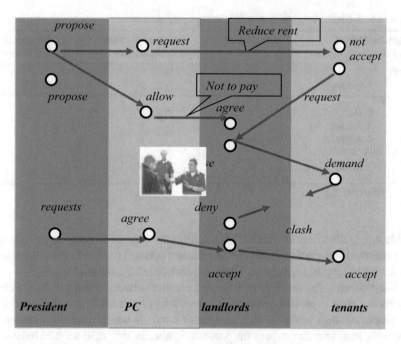

Fig. 4.25 Conflict representation between communities of human agents

Intensity of linguistic expressions for emotions has been the subject of extensive psychological studies (Kent and Nicholls 1977; Rouhana and Bar-Tal 1998); we base our categorization of emotions and qualitative expression for emotion intensity in these studies. We apply computational treatment to our observations in the domain of customer complaints (Galitsky 2004) that emotions are *amplified* by communicative actions. For example the expression *I was upset because of him* is considered to express a weaker intensity of emotion than the expression *He ignored my request and I got upset* with communicative actions *request-upset*. In our formal representation of the latter case the communicative action *ignore* is substituted into the emotion *upset* as the second parameter: *upset(i, ignore(he, request(i,_)))*. Emotional profile of a textual scenario includes one or more expressions in predicates for emotions, communicative actions and mental states for each sentence from this scenario mentioning emotional state. Moreover, we compute the intensity of emotion for each such sentence.

Intensity of an emotion for a sentence depends on the following factors:

1. The category of emotion (e.g. satisfaction (value = 0), *warning, distress, threat* (value = 1)), formed following the relevant psychological studies (Mehrabian 1995, Oatley and Jenkins 1996; Liu and Maes 2004);
2. Attachment of communicative action which amplifies the intensity of emotion by providing explicit explanation of its cause;
3. Occurrence of multiple emotions per sentence.

We have derived a numerical expression to calculate an emotional intensity for each sentence taking into account the above factors (we will discuss it informally in this chapter). Hence building an emotional profile as expression in predicates leads to a quantitative expression for how the total intensity of emotions evolves through the scenario. We call this numerical sequence an *intensity profile*.

To access the emotion level of the whole scenario, we track the evolution of the intensity of emotions. If it goes up and then goes down, one may conclude that a conflict occurred, and then has been resolved. A monotonous increase of emotion intensity would happen in case of an unresolved conflict (dispute). Conversely, a decrease in intensity means that involved parties are coming to an agreement. An oscillating intensity profile indicates more complex pattern of activity, and in most cases it reveals a strong emotional distress.

It has been confirmed by multiple studies (Kaplan 1981; Hecht 2003) that a terrorist attacker has experienced a substantial emotional distress at some points before committing a terrorist attack. Particularly, individuals who have run into certain problems in their life such as broken relationship, family and marriage troubles, employment difficulties, mental and physical illnesses, are approached by agents of terrorist network with proposal for participation in an attack. Therefore, if an individual from a category with a higher likelihood to belong to a terrorist network is discovered to be in an emotional distress, some preventive measures can be taken, including a meeting with a social worker, psychotherapeutic counseling, etc. Therefore, if an individual with such distinguishing patterns can be detected on the basis of email texts, some preventive measures can be taken within a broad spectrum (from offering to provide psychotherapeutic counseling to deviating police intelligence to follow him/her closer because of the potential danger he/she represents). Hence, an early recognition of such patterns of emotional distress is crucial as it provides the earliest warning of potential future terrorist activity.

What kind of data is available to judge on a current emotional state of an individual? One of the easiest ways is to follow a phone conversation and detect emotional states from the pitch of voice. However, the most robust and detailed analysis of emotional distress can be conducted given *textual data*. In this section, we introduce the methodology of *extraction of emotional profile* from text (e-mails) to provide an early notification of potential involvement of individuals from certain categories in terrorist activity.

In this section, we introduce the idea of building emotional profile of an email message to characterize the emotional distress of the author. Emotional profile is a way to combine meanings of individual words in sentences and then to merge expressions for emotions in these sentences for deriving a high-level characteristic of emotional load of a textual message. It turns out that explicit expressions for emotions are amplified by the words which are not explicit indications of emotions but characterize interaction between involved agents (their communicative actions, Searle 1979).

In the rest of this section, we present a number of examples for emotional profiles, analyze their features and comment on the issues of how to extract emotional profile from text. Then we propose a machine learning framework, which relates emotional profiles to the classes "No emotional distress" and "emotional distress exists" and evaluate it using the dataset of textual customer complaints.

4.4.3   Analyzing an Email from a Would-Be Terrorist Attacker

As an example, we present a fragment of correspondence between a would-be British suicide bomber (Fig. 4.26) and his relatives, who have been charged in connection to failing to notify authorities of a potential terrorist attack. We believe if a system, like described in the current paper, were available and could be applied to the email below, an emotional distress would be detected and a terrorist attack attempt could have been prevented.

We show expressions for emotions in bold and associated expressions for communicative actions or mental states in bold italic. As the reader observes, emotional

Selected text	negative positive ➤
...We are **happy** that you are focused in your studies. ...We all have to be *firm* and *focused* with reality as time is slipping away, and there is really *no time* to be **weak** and **emotional**... ...It does not *matter* of **consequences** to us in this life because we do *not* **fear** or *allow* to be **weak** ... ...The trouble is when our minds are a little **idle** and wander to **negative** *thoughts*, which is an old trick of Satan... Do not *attach yourself* to anything so much that your **suffering** is ongoing... We were *told to rejoice* not to be in a **depression** as we have the best of news for all our loved ones which will come to pass very quickly. You should not be **sad** but determined in your aims as we have a **tremendous** burden and duty on our heads in these times... Try to see life in this world as a job with variety of duties without emotions except to your Lord. In your spare time make ... rather than **worrying**. I wonder what **punishment** ... **ignorant** ... this **scares** me. ... is **happy** that you are in a **happy** *frame of mind*... Do not **worry** about ...kids. ...You married a real good woman she is very **happy** with you... Our **worry** is for religion...Everything else is emotional struggle. ...you will be specially **blessed** and **successful**... ...stay focused and determined...	

Fig. 4.26 Example of a email message where a detection of emotional distress could prevent a would-be terrorist attack. On the left: selected fragments where emotions are shown in bold and expressions which amplify them – in italic bold. On the right: emotion intensity profile, negative to positive from left to right

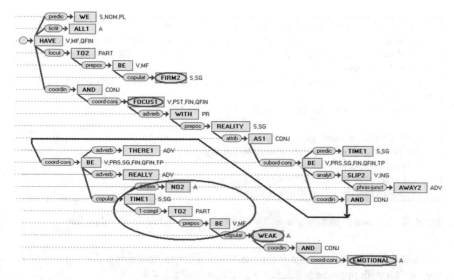

Fig. 4.27 A parse tree for the second sentence in Fig. 4.26

profile in this email is very peculiar. Primarily, there are very strong oscillations of the emotional intensity. These oscillations are medium at the beginning of message, stay negative at the middle portion of it and become very volatile towards the end of the message.

There are multiple forms of expressions whose meanings can be classified as communicative actions or mental states; this example is a good illustration for how expressions indicating emotions are amplified. Also, one can see that a dependent occurrence of emotions amplifies their individual intensity (someone is **happy** that you are **happy**).

A parsing tree for the second sentence in Fig 4.26 is shown in Fig. 4.27. Indications of emotions are shown in small ovals, we extract the words with explicit meanings for emotion (*firm, week, emotional*) and the one which has a meaning of emotion because of the particular way it occurs in the sentence (*focus* in a passive voice). Emotions *week, emotional* are amplified by the expression *no time to be* (shown by a larger oval) with the meaning *I encourage you to be,* which is an imperative communication state. Natural language algorithms of extracting emotions from text is beyond the scope of this book.

4.4.4 Reasoning with Emotional Profiles

We now proceed to the example where extracted emotions and communicative actions are formalized (Fig. 4.28). Each sentence is represented individually; emotions are predicates over agents, and communicative actions range over domain-specific parameters

I was surprised and requested so that they check my account.

It was disgusting that they ignored my request because no transaction has been agreed.

I did not confirm that I wanted to withdraw funds from my account because I was frustrated with them.

Being upset I explained that the balance was wrong for some reasons beyond their understanding.

Please do not deny responsibilities for what you have done to me.

not request(i, check(they)) & surprise(i),
ignore(they,request(i,agree(transaction)))&disgusting(i),
not confirm(i, not want(i,withdraw)) & frustrate(i),
explain(i, understand(they, wrong(balance))) & upset(i),
imperative(not deny(they, do(they, me))).

Fig. 4.28 A message describing interaction with opponents and its emotional profile

Indeed, a typical message with emotional distress contains a description of an interaction with opponents (Galitsky and Tumarkina 2004).

Advanced treatment of text is required to build and analyze an emotional profile. A keyword-based analysis for emotional entities by itself does not provide a sufficient evidence to conclude that an e-mail is aggressive, contains signs of distress, or a threat to someone. It is important to distinguish, for example *"I am afraid to say…"* and *"I am afraid of something"* (see Galitsky 2003 for more examples). Hence, detailed syntactic analysis, followed by full-scale *semantic* and *pragmatic* steps are required to obtain an adequate content for emotional profile. As to the building of emotional profile itself, reasoning is required to handle various patterns of relations between communicative actions and emotions.

Because of high logical complexity of natural language information extraction, the accuracy of construction of emotional profiles is rather limited. Therefore, additional logical means are required to find a consistent subset of extracted emotions and communicative actions. We select the defeasible logic programming (Garcia and Simari 2004) as an adequate reasoning means to handle unreliable knowledge extracted from text. This rule-based approach supports rules with exceptions. Analysis of emotional profiles allows judging on complaint validity, argumentation, level of frustration, and aggressiveness of its author. In this proposal, our focus is an accurate characterization of the last two parameters.

Emotions and communicative actions are extracted in the form of logic program, which is considered as defeasible one when one piece of evidence concerning emotional intensity is inconsistent with another piece of evidence. Such inconsistencies arise when certain syntactic features of text are ignored due to their complexity. For example, discrepancies with proper determinations of co-references between sentences may lead to the following problems while building an emotional profile

1. *His manners and other stuff pleased me* (positive emotion in connection with a person's mental (and possessions?)).
2. *I was fed up with his things* (strong negative emotion in connection to some object (material or behavioral ?) of (the same or different ?) person).

3. *I was appalled by his request to help him move his stuff* (even stronger negative emotion in connection to with (this or different ?) object of the same person above (which appears to be a material object ?))

Hence there are inconsistencies between the first and the second, and between the second and the third sentences. In accordance to the traditional logical artificial intelligence, nonmonotonic reasoning needs to come into play to compensate for the limitations of syntactic analysis. Such reasoning is expected to deliver a maximal consistent set of expressions for emotions (speaking more precisely, consistent parameters of these emotions). For our example, initially we obtain the expressions for emotions with the following options for arguments:

please([manner(he);things(he)],i), sad([things(he);behavior(he);

things(he1);behavior(he1)], i), shock(request(he, [action(things(he); actions(he)]),i).

After the implausible interpretations are defeated, we obtain the following:

please(manner(he), i), sad(things(he), i), shock(request(he, action(things)),i).

4.4.4.1 How Well Can a Conflict Be Represented via Communicative Actions?

In this section we use the Hocker-Wilmot Conflict Assessment Guide (Wehr 1979) to observe which characteristics of an inter-human conflicts can be described by our model, and which characteristics are not covered by it. We intentionally use the treatment of conflict used by sociologists to abstract away from our particular formalization.

The guide (Wehr 1979) is composed of a series of questions designed to focus on the components of conflict; it can be used to bring specific aspects of a conflict into focus and serve as a check on gaps in information about a conflict. We reduce this series of questions for brevity and provide our brief answers in bold.

1. Nature of the Conflict

    1. What are the "triggering events" that brought this conflict into mutual awareness? **Specific sequence of communicative actions and emotions like got denied – got upset – share with public**
    2. What is the historical context of this conflict in terms of (1) the ongoing relationship between the parties? **Some communicative actions (CAs) and References in subjects** and (2) other, external events within which this conflict is embedded? **References in subjects.**
    3. Conflict elements:

        1. How is the struggle being expressed by each party? **Fully by CAs**
        2. What are the perceived incompatible goals? **Fully by multiple subjects**
        3. What are the perceived scarce rewards? Rewards are mentioned explicitly in **subjects**

4. In what ways are the parties interdependent? **Semantic of CAs implies interdependence**.
5. How are they interfering with one another? **Semantic of CAs implies interference.**
6. How are they cooperating to keep the conflict in motion? **Semantic of CAs implies cooperations.**

4. Has the conflict vacillated between productive and destructive phases? **Indicated by CA sequences**

2. Styles of Conflict

   1. What individual styles did each party use? **Only as far as attitudes**
   2. How did the individual styles change during the course of the conflict? **Sometimes, mostly not.**
   3. How did the parties perceive the other's style? **Sometimes, mostly not.**
   4. In what way did a party's style reinforce the choices the other party made as the conflict progressed? **This is exactly what is learned in terms of CAs.**
   5. Were the style choices primarily symmetrical or complementary? **We learned this in terms of CAs.**
   6. From an external perspective, what were the advantages and disadvantages of each style within this particular conflict?
   7. Can the overall system be characterized as having a predominant style? What do the participants say about the relationship as a whole? **Style is reflected as an overall scenario structure.**
   8. From an external perspective, where would this conflict system be placed in terms of cohesion and adaptability?
   9. Would any of the other system descriptions aptly summarize the system dynamics?

3. Power

   1. What attitudes about their own and the other's power does each party have? Do they talk openly about power, or is it not discussed? Power is expressed as an attribute of CA
   2. What do the parties see as their own and the other's dependencies on one another? As an external observer, can you classify some dependencies that they do not list? **These dependencies are expressed in semantics of verbs for CAs, but we do not treat that explicitly.**
   3. What power currencies do the parties see themselves and the other possessing? **Beyond our model.**
   4. In what ways do the parties disagree on the balance of power between them? Do they underestimate their own or the other's influence? **Very superficial treatment: semantics of verbs sometimes indicate relationships between powers.**
   5. What impact does each party's assessment of power have on subsequent choices in the conflict?

6. What evidence of destructive "power balancing" occurs?
7. In what ways do observers of the conflict agree and disagree with the parties' assessments of their power?
8. What are some unused sources of power that are present?

4. Goals

1. How do the parties clarify their goals? Do they phrase them in individualistic or system terms? **This is expressed in NL and we differentiate: 'I want' vs 'This is how we do it . . .'.**
2. What does each party think the other's goals are? Are they similar or dissimilar to the perceptions of self-goals? **Expressed by the sequence of CAs, like "if you** *warn* **me that** ... **I** *deny* **[this or other subject]".**
3. How have the goals been altered from the beginning of the conflict to the present? In what ways are the prospective, transactive, and retrospective goals similar or dissimilar? **This is sometimes, but not always represented via CAs, for example where an agent transition from an inquiry to feeling of revenge.**

5. Tactics

1. Do the participants appear to strategize about their conflict choices or remain spontaneous? **It is usually hard to extract from textual description of a conflict.**
2. How does each party view the other's strategizing? **Some CAs like** *confirm* **provide indication on how opponents' strategies are anticipated.**

6. Assessment

1. What rules of repetitive patterns characterize this conflict? **Clearly indicated by the sequence of CAs**
2. Can quantitative instruments be used to give information about elements of the conflict? **Not in the proposed model**

4.4.5   Evaluation of Adequateness of Representation

To demonstrate that the proposed representation language of labeled graphs is adequate to represent scenarios of interactions between human agents in various domains, we performed the evaluation of coding to graph/decoding from graph and evaluate distortion of communicative action-related information. We conducted the evaluation with respect to the criteria on how the suggested model based on communicative actions can represent real-world scenarios including complaints, conflict between communities of agents and emotional interactions.

Complainants had a task to read a textual complaint and draw a graph so that another team member (a company representative) could comprehend it (and briefly sketch the plot as a text). A third team member (judge) then compared the original complaint and the one written by the company representative as perceived from the form. The result of this comparison was the judgment on whether the scenario structure has been dramatically distorted in respect to the validity of a given complaint.

It must be noted that less than 15 % of complaints were hard to capture by means of communicative actions. We also observed that about a third of complaints lost important details and could not be adequately restored (although they might still be properly related to a class). Nevertheless, one can see that the proposed representation mechanism is adequate for representing so complex and ambiguous structures as textual complaints in most cases.

Note that in our approach the role of defeat relationships and causal links between the subjects of communicative actions is to represent common features of scenarios, and not to determine the validity of claims being communicated. Communicative actions of one scenario are matched against those of another scenario, and attack relationships between arguments are matched against those of another scenario, irrespectively of the validity of these arguments.

Conducting the evaluation of adequateness in other domains, we split the members of evaluation team into reporters, assessors and judges. Reporters represented scenarios as graphs, and assessors decoded the perceived structure of communicative actions back into text. Finally, the judges compared the original description (be it text or other media in the case of wireless interaction) with the respective originals.

For the banks, one can track deviation of one dataset versus another, which is 10–15 % of the third set versus the first two sets. This is due to the lower variability of scenarios, which makes it easier to represent and reconstruct it (classification accuracy is comparable). Recognition for banking complaints is almost as accurate as coding via graph (representation), but not the reconstruction of the structure of interactions between complainants and their opponents.

Although it is possible to demonstrate the adequacy of representation language, it is rather hard to obtain data for conflicts between communities of agents, so with only one case presented in Fig. 4.29 one succeeded in understanding the discourse of the conflict from the graph. Coding emotional profiles via graphs similar to Fig. 4.25 was not as expressive as in the case of complaints, and classification accuracy is closer to the scenario reconstruction than to the scenario representation accuracy. Indeed, the proposed language via communicative actions captures peculiarity of emotional profiles in a lesser degree than the structure of complaint scenarios. We were unable to evaluate the security assessment scenarios in real world; however we obtained sufficient data to track the accuracy for wireless interactions. In terms of representation it is as good as complaint scenarios, but the reconstruction (which is the most important operation) accuracy is lower than for complaints, and the accuracy of classification lies in between representation and reconstruction. In such domain as emotional interaction there is much higher loss of information then in the other domains, however proper classification (with providing background on *why* a given scenario is related to a class) gives a little bit better results.

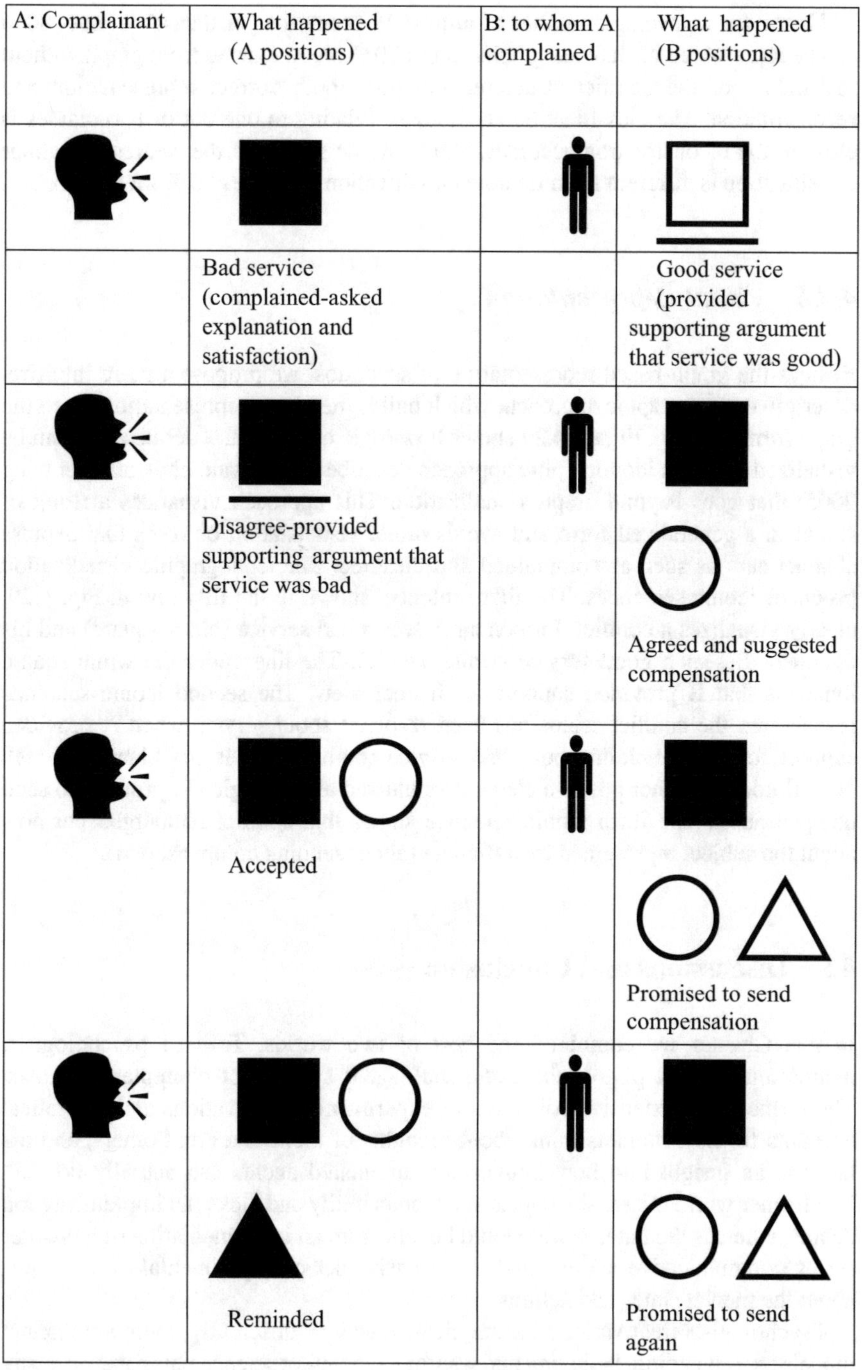

A: Complainant	What happened (A positions)	B: to whom A complained	What happened (B positions)
	Bad service (complained-asked explanation and satisfaction)		Good service (provided supporting argument that service was good)
	Disagree-provided supporting argument that service was bad		Agreed and suggested compensation
	Accepted		Promised to send compensation
	Reminded		Promised to send again

Fig. 4.29 Iconic visualization of the logic of conflict deliberation

Hence for an average number of almost 19 scenarios per dataset, almost 80 % can be represented via labeled graphs, about 70 % reconstructed from graph without major loss of the conflict structure, and 60 % both correct representation and reconstruction. The classification accuracy of relating to one out of two classes is close to the reconstruction accuracy. Note that the setting of the Nearest Neighbor classification is different from random classification that gives 50 % for two classes.

4.4.6   Visual Representation

Besides the graph-based representation of scenarios, we propose a more intuitive, descriptive iconographic approach, which builds the visual representation given the graph formalization. Figure 4.29 shows how logic of complaint deliberation can be visualized using an iconographic approach described in (Kovalerchuk and Schwing 2005) that goes beyond graph visualization. This approach visualizes a result of action in a generalized form and avoids direct visualization of verbs that express abstract actions such as complained and disagree. The iconographic visualization produces iconic sentences. The first sentence, shown in the first row in Fig. 4.29, clearly visualizes a conflict. Proponent A sees a bad service (black square) and his opponent B sees a good service (white square). The line under the white square indicates that B provided support for his/her view. The second iconic sentence reveals that the conflict seems has been resolved about service when A provided support for his/her claim about bad service (both A and B see black squares). Now B added another positive element visualized as a triangle – a promise to send compensation. The forth iconic sentence shows that conflict reemerged but now about the subject represented by a triangle (about sending compensation).

4.5   Discussions and Conclusion

In this Chapter we combined the best of two worlds, ToM of psychologists, neuroscientists and philosophers and multiagent systems of computer scientists. The former is an extensive collection of experimental observations and theoretical accounts for how humans think about thoughts of themselves and others, and the latter is an insight into how human and automated agents can actually do that. The former world misses the consistency, plausibility and lacks the implementation details, whereas the latter world would benefit from an implementation of a broader set of communicative actions and an extensive set of experimental observations about the mental states and actions.

Psychologists treat various communicative actions differently; there are distinct models for pretending, believing and wanting. Computer science puts forward a way to systematically treat mental states and actions within a unified framework. All communicative actions are given multiple definitions in the same format, for each meaning. As a result, a better structured and compact representation of mental world than the original ToM is obtained, suitable for both teaching CwA and designing intelligent agents for operating in the mental world. Formalizing ToM, the major finding is that the mental entities do not just randomly coexist in the mental world, but instead form a basis of *knowledge-belief-intention*, so that most of them can be defined in this basis, including emotions.

To formally represent the theoretical note of theory-theory, we used a meta-theoretic approach. Then communicative actions can be defined as metapredicates, and it becomes convenient to cover a multitude of meanings by such definitions. Hence basic and derived metapredicates become units of a linguistic model of the mental world. Both logical and linguistic models are suitable to be taught to CwA as we will demonstrate in Chap. 8.

In this Chapter we have discussed the applications of modal logic for reasoning about mental world. Clearly, a lot of observations about the multiagent behavior can be deduced from the axioms; however the set of theorems does not constitute a basis to enumerate a set of consecutive mental states. We conclude that for the generic implementation of reasoning simulation is required, which is implemented as en exhaustive search in the space of possible behaviors. It has been observed in this study that the simulation for realistic mental states for a few agents is not computationally intensive. Simulation is the second way of interpretation for the Theory-of-Mind, along with theory-theory one.

The theory, models and architectures of intelligent agents and ToM are based BDI approach. Although this functions well for single agents it has been long recognized that this approach falls short for multiagent systems. It lacks appropriate social aspects to make natural interaction possible. The original concept for intelligent agents was based on a (simple) idea of how people reason about actions. (Dignum et al. 2014) proposed to go back to the foundation of BDI and to acknowledge that people are in the core social beings. People don't function as rational agents with the addition of some "sociality" modules to make them aware of other people. Rather people are social at the base and this sociality pervades all our reasoning, motivation, and any other aspect of our behavior. The authors proposed a new set of core cognitive elements to replace the BDI approach and discuss the paradigm of a social landscape. They also aim at a radical change in the way the community creates social agents and believe that the new approach incorporates previous work, such as BDI. Their claim is that deliberation about actions and BDI are certainly a part of how agents cope with a dynamic world, but are not the core part of social agents that are part of a social world interacting with other agents and humans in a natural way.

Having formalized individual communicative actions, we then proposed a computational model on how to represent interactions such as conflicts between humans via a structure of their communicative actions. We then introduced a machine learning approach suitable to tackle such structures to relate a formalized conflict scenario to a class. It has been developed and evaluated in one domain (customer complaints), and then used as a knowledge representation means in other domains of distinct natures. The number and structure of classes depend on a domain, but the criteria expressed by sequences of communicative actions have been shown to be relevant for expressing commonalities between scenarios.

The representation language is that of labeled directed acyclic graphs with generalization operator on them. For machine learning, the scenarios are represented as a sequence of communicative actions attached to agents; these actions are grouped by subjects. Scenario discourse is represented by subject change and brings in additional structure to the scenario, together with causal links between these subjects of communicative actions. Argumentation defeat relationships between the subjects of communicative actions (as a specific case of causal link) are coded in the graph and used by machine learning as well.

We explored the role of communicative actions in representing various kinds of conflicts in multiagent systems and discovered that proper formalization of communicative actions is essential to judge on conflicts. Having conducted the comparative evaluation of classification accuracies in multiple domains, we came to conclusion that a graph-based communicative action-focused approach is one of the most adequate for automated learning how to classify conflicts and predict their outcomes.

Based on speech act theory, we designed the set of attributes for communicative actions and showed how the procedure of relating a complaint to a class can be implemented as Nearest Neighbor learning machinery. The approach to learn scenarios of inter-human interactions (encoded as sequences of communicative actions) is believed to be original on one hand and universal on the other hand. We believe that rather few computational approach has been applied to such problem as understanding customer complaints, and the other domains where mining for communicative actions seem to be useful have not been tackled computationally either.

Overall, there has been a strong interest to computational issues of mental attitudes over the last few decades. A series of studies have addressed reasoning about emotional and mental states, building emotion-enabled automated agents, emotion recognition from text, facial image and speech. Emotions are considered as an important component of intelligence and its models which involve the mental world. The universal formal model of emotion is one of the most difficult problems on the way to build an automated agent that demonstrates the behavior, perceived by humans as emotional one (El-Nasr and Skubic 1998; Sloman 1999). In this book we formalized emotions in a way suitable for teaching CwA and verified our formalization in a number of applied domains where emotions play a specific role. We believe the current paper is one of the first addressing the problem of using the sequence of emotional states to improve the accuracy of extraction of information about multiagent conflict.

Extracting and parameterizing human attitudes from text has found a variety of applications, (including behavior modeling and demographic profiling) and a number of computational techniques have been deployed. (Liu and Maes 2004) implement a generic framework for processing a corpus of personal texts and estimating the affect of the text at the sentence and concept level. Concepts, topics, and episodes are extracted from text and associated with their respective affective valence scores; each < concept, affective valence score > pair constitutes a single exposure of an attitude. The analysis of each personal text yields many attitude exposures, which accumulate in an affective memory system. The affective memory system has a reflexive component, in which repeated attitude exposures are required to form a stable attitude, a method that follows the classical conditioning in psychology.

We believe the current book is one of the first attempts targeting machine learning in the domain with such complex structure as inter-human interactions described in natural language. Our approach extends the expressiveness of representation language for agents' attitudes, using twenty communicative actions linked by a concept lattice. It can be applied to an arbitrary domain including inter-human conflicts, obviously characterized in natural language.

The evaluation of the model shows that it is an adequate technique to handle complex objects (both in terms of knowledge representation and reasoning). This includes communicative actions of multiagent interactions. The Nearest Neighbors approach was found suitable to relate an inter-human conflict scenario to a class. Evaluation using the dataset of formalized real-world complaints showed a satisfactory performance. The proposed method for formal representation of conflict scenarios allows their classification as well as teaching to CwA.

References

Alexander G, Raja A, Durfee E, Musliner D (2007) Design paradigms for meta-control in multi-agent systems In: Raja A, Cox MT (eds) Proceedings of the first international workshop on metareasoning in agent-based systems, AAMAS-07, pp 92–103

Austin JL (1962) How to do things with words. Oxford University Press, Oxford

Bach K, Harnish R (1979) Linguistic communication and speech acts. MIT Press, Cambridge, MA

Baron-Cohen S (2000) Theory of mind and autism: a fifteen year review. In: Baron-Cohen S, Tagar-Flusberg H, Cohen DJ (eds) Understanding other minds, vol A. Oxford University Press, Oxford, pp 3–20

Barwise J (1975) Admissible sets and structures. Springer, Berlin

Barwise J, Perry J (1983) Situations and attitudes. MIT Press, Cambridge, MA/London

Barwise KJ, Seligman J (1997) Information flow: the logic of distributed systems. Cambridge University Press, Cambridge

Boella G, Hulstijn V, van der Torre L (2004) Persuasion strategies in dialogue. In: Grasso F, Reed C (eds) In: Proceedings of the ECAI workshop on Computational Models of Natural Argument (CMNA'04), Valencia

Bratman ME (1987) Intention, plans and practical reason. Harvard University Press, Cambridge, MA

Breazeal C (1998) A motivational system for regulating human-robot interactions. In: Proceedings of the fifteenth national conference on AI (AAAI-98)

Carley K (1997) Extracting team mental models. J Organ Behav 18:533–538

Chang C-W, Chin-Tsai L, Lian-Qing W (2009) Mining the text information to optimizing the customer relationship management. Expert Syst Appl 36(2 Part 1):1433–1443

Chesnevar CI, Simari G, Alsinet T, Godo L (2004) A logic programming framework for possibilistic argumentation with vague knowledge. In: Proceedings of the international conference in Uncertainty in Artificial Intelligence (UAI 2004), Banff, Canada, pp 76–84

Cox MT, Raja A (2007) Metareasoning: a manifesto. AAAI-Workshop

Cox MT, Ram A (1999) Introspective multistrategy learning: on the construction of learning strategies. Artif Intell 112:1–55

Criscuolo G, Giunchiglia F, Serafini L (2002) A foundation for Metareasoning Part II: the model theory. J Log Comput 12(1):167–208

Dignum F, Hofstede GJ, Prada R (2014) From autistic to social agents. In: Proceedings of the 2014 IC on autonomous agents and multi-agent systems. pp 1161–1164

d'Inverno M, Kinny D, Luck M, Wooldridge M (1998) A formal specification of dMARS. In: Singh, Rao and Wooldridge (eds) Intelligent Agents IV: proceedings of the 4th International workshop on agent theories, architectures and languages, LNAI 1365, pp 155–176

Dunbar RIM, Launay J, Curry O (2015) The complexity of jokes is limited by cognitive constraints on mentalizing. Hum Nat:1–11

El-Nasr MS, Skubic M (1998) A fuzzy emotional agent for decision- making in a mobile robot. In: Proceedings of WCCI'98, Anchorage, AK, USA

Fagin R, Halpern JY, Moses Y, Vardi MY (1996) Reasoning about knowledge. MIT Press, Cambridge, MA/London

Fang L, Hipel KW, Kilgour DM (1993) Interactive decision making: the graph model for conflict resolution. Wiley, New York

Farrel J (2006) Philosophy of Language. www.farrell.blogs.com/Writings/Speech-Acts.pdf

Galitsky B (2002) On the training of mental reasoning: searching the works of literature. FLAIRS – 02, Pensacola Beach

Galitsky B (2003) Natural language question answering system: technique of semantic headers. Advanced Knowledge International, Adelaide

Galitsky B (2004) A library of behaviors: implementing commonsense reasoning about mental world. 8th international conference on knowledge-based intelligent information system. LNAI 3215, pp 307–313

Galitsky B (2005) Implementing commonsense reasoning via semantic skeletons for answering complex questions. In: FLAIRS – 05, May 15–17, Clearwater Bearch, FL

Galitsky B (2006) Reasoning about mental attitudes of complaining customers. Knowl-Based Syst Elsevier 19(7):592–615

Galitsky B (2015) Team formation by children with Autism. Foundations of autonomy and its (Cyber) threats: from individuals to interdependence: papers from the 2015 AAAI spring symposium

Galitsky B, de la Rosa JL (2011) Concept-based learning of human behavior for customer relationship management. Special issue on information engineering applications based on lattices. Inform Sci 181(10) pp 2016–2035

Galitsky BA, Kuznetsov SO (2008) Learning communicative actions of conflicting human agents. J Exp Theor Artif Intell 20(4):277–317

Galitsky B, Kuznetsov SO, Kovalerchuk B (2008) Argumentation vs meta-argumentation for the assessment of multi-agent conflict. In: 2008 AAAI workshop on meta-reasoning. AAAI tech report. http://www.aaai.org/Library/Workshops/2008/ws08-07-011.php

Galitsky B, Pampapathi R (2005) Can many agents answer questions better than one? First Monday 10(1). http://firstmonday.org/ojs/index.php/fm/article/view/1204/1124

Galitsky B, Peterson D (2005) On the peculiarities of default reasoning of children with Autism. In: FLAIRS – 05, May 15–17, Clearwater Bearch, FL

Galitsky B, Tumarkina I (2004) Justification of customer complaints using mental actions and emotional states. FLAIRS – 04, Miami

Galitsky B, González MP, Chesñevar CI (2009) A novel approach for classifying customer complaints through graphs similarities in argumentative dialogues. Decis Support Syst 46(3):717–729

Ganter B, Kuznetsov S (2001) 'Pattern structures and their projections'. In: Stumme G, Delugach H (ed) Proceedings of the 9th International Conference on Conceptual Structures, ICCS'01. lecture notes in artificial intelligence, 2120, pp 129–142

Ganter B, Wille R (1999) Formal concept analysis: mathematical foundations. Springer, Berlin

Garcia A, Simari G (2004) Defeasible logic programming: an argumentative approach. Theory Pract Logic Program 4:95–138

Garey MR, Johnson DS (1979) Computers and intractability: a guide to the theory of NP-completeness. Freeman, San Francisco

Hecht R (2003) Deadly history, terrorism, and political violence 15:35–47. Suicide terrorism, Bibliography, 2004. Available from: www.maxwell.af.mil/au/aul/bibs/terrsuic/suite.htm

Johnson MW, McBurney P, Parsons S (2005) A mathematical model of dialog. Electron Notes Theor Comput Sci 141(5):33–48

Kaplan A (1981) The psychodynamics of terrorism. In: Alexander Y, Gleason J (eds) Behavioral and quantitative perspectives on terrorism. Pergamon Press, New York

Kent I, Nicholls W (1977) The psychodynamics of terrorism. Ment Health Soc 4(1 Suppl 2):1–8

Kipper K, Korhonen A, Ryant N, Palmer M (2008) A large-scale classification of English verbs. Lang Resour Eval J 42:21–40

Kovalerchuk B, Schwing J (eds) (2005) Visual and spatial analysis: advances in data mining reasoning and problem solving. Springer, Berlin

Kuznetsov SO (1999) Learning of simple conceptual graphs from positive and negative examples. In: Zytkow J, Rauch J (eds) Proceedings of 3rd conference on principles of data mining and knowledge discovery (PKDD 1999). Lecture notes in artificial intelligence, vol 1704. Springer, pp 384–392

Levesque HJ, Reiter R, Lesperance Y, Lin F, Scherl RB (1997) GOLOG: A logic programming language for dynamic domains. J Log Program 31:59–84

Liu H, Maes P (2004) What would they think? A computational model of attitudes. In: Proceedings of the ACM international conference on Intelligent User Interfaces (IUI 2004). Madeira, Funchal, Portugal

McCarthy J (1979) Ascribing mental qualities to machines. In: Ringle M (ed) Philosophical perspectives in artificial intelligence. Humanities Press, Atlantic Highlands

McCarthy J (1995) Making robots conscious of their mental states. In: Proceedings of the machine intelligence conference 15

Mehrabian A (1971) Nonverbal betrayal of feeling. J Exp Res Pers 5:64–73

Mehrabian A (1995) Framework for a comprehensive description and measurement of emotional states. Genet Soc Gen Psychol Monogr 121:339–361

Muller HJ, Dieng R (eds) (2000) Computational conflicts: conflict modeling for distributed intelligent systems. Springer, New York

Nodine M, Unruh A (2000) Constructing robust conversation policies in dynamic agent communities. In: Dignum F, Creaves M (eds) Issues in agent communication. Springer, Berlin

Oatley K, Jenkins J (1996) Understanding emotions. Blackwell, Oxford

Pilowsky T, Yirmiya N, Arbelle S, Mozes T (2000) Theory of mind abilities of children with schizophrenia, children with autism, and normally developing children. Schizophr Res 42(2):145–155

Rahwan I, Ramchurn SD, Jennings NR, McBurney P, Parsons S, Sonenberg L (2003) Argumentation-based negotiation. Knowl Eng Rev 18(4):343–375

Ram A, Moorman K (eds) (1999) Understanding language understanding: computational models of reading. The MIT Press, Cambridge, MA

Rao AS, Georgeff, MP (1995) BDI-agents: from theory to practice. In: Proceedings of the first International Conference on Multiagent Systems (ICMAS' 1995)

Reynolds JC (1970) Transformational systems and the algebraic structure of atomic formulas. Mach Intell 5:135–151. Edinburgh University Press, USA

Riesbeck CK, Schank RC, Goldman NM, Rieger CJ (1975) Inference and paraphrase by computer. J ACM 22(3):309–328

Rouhana NN, Bar-Tal D (1998) Psychological dynamics of intractable ethno national conflicts: the Israeli-Palestinian case. Am Psychol 53:761–770

Schank R (1969) A conceptual dependency parser for natural language. In: Proceedings of the 1969 conference on computational linguistics, Sweden, pp 1–3

Scheutz M (2001) Agents with or without emotions, FLAIRS-01, Pensacola Beach, pp 89–93

Searle J (1979) Expression and meaning studies in the theory of speech acts. Cambridge University
    Press, Cambridge/New York
Shanahan M (1997) Solving the frame problem. MIT Press, Cambridge, MA
Shardanand U, Maes P (1995) Social information filtering: algorithms for automating 'word
    of mouth'. In: Proceedings of the conference human factors in computing systems CHI'95,
    pp 210–127
Shoham Y (1993) Agent oriented programming. Artif Intell 60(1):51–92
Sloman A (1999) Damasio, Descartes, alarms and meta-management. 1998 IEEE international
    conference on systems, man, and cybernetics, 1998
Sloman A (2000) Architecture-based conceptions of mind. In: Proceedings of the 11th international
    congress of logic, methodology and philosophy of science, Dordrecht, Kluwer, p 397
Wehr P (1979) Conflict regulation. Westview Press, Boulder
Wooldridge M (2000) Reasoning about rational agents. The MIT Press, Cambridge, MA
Yevtushenko SA (2005) ConExp software. http://www.sf.net/projects/conexp?

Chapter 5
Theory of Mind Engine

Having presented intuitive ToM and formalized it in previous two Chapters, we now build a ToM engine that is supposed to reproduce reasoning and behavior associated with ToM-capable humans in some approximated form. We will enable this engine to be ToM-competent: it should be capable of correctly answering questions in ToM scenarios. To obtain correct answers, ToM engine needs to properly infer the mental states (who *knows* what, who *wants* what) that include these answers. How can we assure that the ToM engine completes all such exercises and question properly?

We require the ToM engine to derive a *complete* sequence of mental states, given a ToM task (which we refer to as *initial mental state*). We then expect such completeness to reproduce rationality and intelligence in reasoning in the mental world. This feature of completeness can be achieved not only because of the limited number of entities describing the manifold of activities in the mental world, but also because these entities can be defined in a basis of just three mental actions, *knowledge, belief* and *intention*.

Once ToM engine is designed, we will evaluate it with a number of various scenarios in mental world. We refer to the ToM engine as a *natural language multiagent mental simulator*, NL_MAMS.

Kaiser and Shiffrar (2009) write that PwA tend to view other people and objects alike. It is as if they view the world through a lens devoid of emotion. People and objects appear to hold the same level of significance. In this chapter we design the lens through which everything exists in the mental, emotional world only.

5.1 The Task of NL_MAMS

The NL_MAMS inputs formal or natural language descriptions of initial mental states of interacting agents. It outputs deterministic scenarios of plausible, rational behaviors of these agents in the mental world. The NL_MAMS is capable of

© Springer International Publishing Switzerland 2016 177
B. Galitsky, *Computational Autism*, Human–Computer Interaction Series,
DOI 10.1007/978-3-319-39972-0_5

analyzing and predicting the consequences of mental and physical actions of actions (Galitsky 2002, 2013). The output of the NL_MAMS is the sequence of mental formulas expressing the states that are the results of the committed actions (behaviors) chosen by these agents.

Obviously, we cannot reproduce the richness and variability of the real mental sub-world of the real world by our ToM engine. To properly frame the capabilities of the ToM simulator, we specify the *available library of behaviors* for each agent to choose. To reproduce certain scenarios and certain ToM tasks, we define a minimal set of behaviors providing successful solutions to these tasks. The scope of the ToM engine (the totality of generated scenarios) is determined by a library of behaviors loaded into the system. This library contains definitions of mental entities such as deceive, so that an NL_MAMS agent can chose it if its preconditions can be satisfied at a given state and this action leads to most desired or least undesired reachable states.

The NL_MAMS can be viewed from the multiple perspectives:

A *planner* in the mental world. Given a current state and constraints in the form of implausible or irrational agents' actions, build a plan of actions to satisfy these constraints.

A *simulator* of the mental world. Given the set of constraints for allowed actions give, simulate an activity of an agent searching for a best action. An agent first searches through all possible actions of his opponents according to his knowledge about their beliefs, and then searches through his own options having found those of opponents.

A *game player in the mental world*. The simulator settings could be reduced to the game-theoretic ones if the mutual beliefs of agents are complete or absent, and intentions are uniform (a trivial case of multiagent scenario, Rosenschein and Zlotkin 1994).

A *prediction engine* in the mental world. Given previous initial mental states and their outcomes, or sequences of mental states, the system learns from them and predicts the outcome for an unknown initial mental state. This engine can also be viewed as a machine learning or induction one.

A *reasoning engine* about the mental world. An axiomatic system for a given ToM session includes the initial mental states and behavioral library of definitions of mental entities as axioms. Theorems include deduced mental actions and mental states which form a sequence. If mental state s_1 is inferred relying on action a_1 that is in turn inferred relying on state s_0, then s_0, a_1 and s_1 are ordered in time correspondingly.

Since the NL_MAMS possesses definitions of mental entities, it is capable of representing natural language expressions that include mental entities as mental formulas. Words for physical states and actions are merged and form parameters of these entities. Therefore we assign to the NL_MAMS the capability of *understanding* natural language messages from its user and other agents. The NL_MAMS extracts the expressions, which mention explicitly or assume implicitly mental states and actions of involved agents.

Modeling of multiagent interaction takes into account possible *ambiguity* of messages that is inherent in a natural language dialog. For each mental entity extracted from text, such as *inform*, the NL_MAMS forms a disjunction of mental formulas for each meaning of this entity

inform1(A,B,S) ∪ *inform2(A,B,S)* ∪ *inform3(A,B,S)* according to multiple clauses for *inform*.

The NL_MAMS imitates the multiagent behaviors that are caused by possible misunderstanding of one agent by another because of the ambiguity of mental entities. Under the search of optimal action or reaction, the set of meanings for received entities is (exhaustively) analyzed with respect to avoiding the least wanted state (assuming this state may be achieved as a result of a particular understanding of a message). In this book we will not touch upon the natural language component of the NL_MAMS and refer the reader to (Galitsky 2003) for the description of message understanding issues in mental domains and sample applications of question answering.

5.2   Simulating Reasoning About Mental States

Over the last three decades, intelligent software systems have been assisting humans in a wide range of their activities including information seeking, shopping, education, negotiation, etc. However, a major bottleneck for penetration of such system into these domains is understanding human factors involved in respective activities. A personalized software system must be capable of modeling mental attitudes of users including their intentions, knowledge, and beliefs. Moreover, software systems need to be competent to handle various behavior forms of users' proponents and opponents, associated with systems' functionality, such as *pretending, lying, offending*, and *forgiving*.

In this chapter we build a generic simulation environment for reasoning about mental attitudes. We intend this environment to be integrated as a component with a behavior-prediction software in a particular domain where understanding mental attitudes of users and/or prediction of their mental states is required (Winograd and Flores 1986; Shoham 1993; Wooldridge 2000). In particular, it is important in the domains of internet auction, where understanding intentions of sellers and buyers is a key. A combination of the reactive and the deliberate approaches to multiagent architecture is used in this study to approximate the decision making of conflicting human agents communicating using rather extensive vocabulary of speech acts.

Intelligent software and web services are expected to be taking into consideration multiple static human factors including age, gender, education, location, social background, etc. (Yu et al. 2003; Li et al. 2003). In this Chapter we focus on dynamic human factors such as beliefs and intentions of human agents which are fairly important for a system to keep track of while assisting a user. Moreover, in addition to such mental attitudes as knowledge, belief, desire, and intention, we treat more complex mental states and actions such as *pretending, cheating, offending, forgiving, explaining* etc. Our simulation framework is independent of the user interface or the way mental attitudes are obtained from a user; they may be extracted from text (Galitsky 2003) or specified via a form explicitly (Galitsky 2006).

Reasoning about mental attributes and behavior patterns is an important component of human intellectual activity. Quite a few formalisms have been suggested to reproduce the peculiarities of human reasoning in the way of logical calculi. In these calculi the laws of "mental world" are encoded via axioms, and derived theorems are expected to describe the states and actions of agents in the mental world. It has been comprehended a few decades ago that staying within the bounds of classical logic, it is hard to represent the certain phenomenology of human reasoning. Non-classical logics have enabled artificial intelligence to model reasoning of agents in time and space, in the conditions of uncertainty and inconsistency, and reasoning about the behaviors of each other. Particularly, the modal logics are quite successful means to represent the notion of knowledge, belief and intention in connection to the other ("physical") properties of the real world (Fagin et al. 1996). However, nowadays there is still a lack of complex real-world examples, based on a software implementation of non-classical calculi.

In recent years an attention to formal modeling of various forms of human reasoning and mental behavior has strongly risen, particularly in connection with software applications in business and educational domains. A series of phenomena in human reasoning have been represented in such computational approaches as reasoning about action (Shanahan 1997), knowledge, space and time, nonmonotonic and counterfactual reasoning, etc. as well as in user modeling. Nevertheless, a generic computational framework for reasoning about mental states which is suitable for software applications is yet to be developed (Walton and Krabbe 1995; d'Inverno et al. 1998; Olivia et al. 1999; Tamma et al. 2005).

Our intention is to construct a framework to simulate human reasoning in the mental word in as detailed way as possible (compare with Shoham 1993; Sloman 2000). Building the practical systems which model the mental world (Galitsky 2003), we have been evaluating whether a pure axiomatic reasoning delivers sufficiently rich number of theorems to adequately describe the mental states of agents. We tend to believe that a simulation-based (procedural, reactive) approach rather than a deductive reasoning-based one is suitable to express the laws of mental world and to apply them to produce as realistic scenarios as possible for practical applications. The main goal of the desired system is *obtaining a set of consecutive mental states,* which are expected to *follow the initial mental state* that is given. We look for a solution to this problem which is as close to the natural behavior (from the experts' viewpoint) as possible.

We have already verified that the simulation approach is applicable in a variety of domain of various natures (Galitsky 2003). In this Chapter we present in details the implementation and evaluation of NL_MAMS, analyze how the library of behaviors affects the functionality of the simulator, and outline its application domains and integration with other reasoning and machine learning components.

To proceed from the partial cases of multiagent systems, where the reasoning-based approach proved successful, towards the generic implementation, we will attempt to address the following issues:

- Rather weak subset of commonsense laws of mental world is expressible via assertions between modalities;
- Too few theorems are deducible from the axioms for modalities as laws of mental world to describe its phenomena in detail;
- Attempts to build sound and complete (in logical sense) formalizations of mental world are associated with the drop of the expressiveness of resultant language: only a subset of observed mental states can be reproduced;
- Representing mental entities as independent modalities moves the modal logic-based approach away from the natural language, which is capable of merging the multiple cohesive meanings in a single lexical unit for mental entity;
- Implementation of reasoning as a first-order theorem proving is inefficient; also, it seems to be hard to directly take advantage of the practical limitation on the complexity of mental formulas.
- First-order logic (particularly, modal and lambda calculi) is oriented to handle certain phenomena of natural language such as quantification and especially language syntax-semantic connections (e.g. Montague grammars). At the same time, it is harder to adjust these calculi (furthermore, their model theories) to the peculiarities of ambiguity in mental natural language expressions, processing derived mental states and actions.

Analyzing these limitations, one may come to conclusions that the mental world is quite different from physical world in terms of how the reasoning is organized. Since 1980s, a number of control architectures for practical reasoning agents have been proposed; however, most of them have been deployed only in limited artificial environments, and very few have been accepted for the field-tested applications.

To mention the current applications of reasoning about knowledge which are based on modal logic, these are communication protocols and reliability, multiagent scheduling and temporal constraint satisfaction.

Hence the following developments to be presented in this chapter need to occur:

1. Using simulation of decision-making rather than representing it as a pure deduction (see e.g. Bousquet et al. 2004);
2. Describing the multiagent interaction, ascend from the level of atomic actions of agents to the level of behaviors;
3. Limiting the complexity of mental formulas;
4. Following closer the natural language in describing the mental world, using a wide range of entities (this has been explored with respect to acceptance by a multiagent community by Lara and Alfonseca (2000));
5. Taking advantage of approximation machinery. We express an arbitrary mental entity through the basis *knowledge-belief-intention* (*informing, deceiving, pretending, reconciling* etc., Galitsky 2006);

6. Using a hybrid reasoning system *combining* simulation of decision-making with the set of typical behaviors specified as axioms
7. Increasing the *expressiveness* of representation language by means of using an extensive set of formalized mental entities beyond *belief* and *desire*.

5.3   Implementation of Simulation

Decision-making of agents in our settings is primarily concerned with choice of actions to achieve desired states. Generally speaking, agents have immediate and long-term goals of mental and physical states, and sometimes explicit intentions of actions.

5.3.1   Choosing the Best Action Considering Yourself Only

Let us first consider an action selection algorithm in a trivial case, where an agent does not consider possible actions of others. Of particular importance to our interests are systems that allow agents to learn about and model their *own* teammates and then use that knowledge to improve collaboration. Kaminka and Frenkel (2005) presents a technique that allows one agent (a coach) to predict the future behavior of other agents (its own team and the opponent team) in order to coordinate activities by observing those agents and building a model of their behavior. Observations are translated into a time series of recognized atomic behaviors, and these into subsequences that characterize a team (although not necessarily a single agent). Kaminka and Tambe (2000) investigated just how much monitoring of another agent is sufficient for an agent to be an effective teammate.

To choose the best action, each agent considers each action it can currently perform (Fig. 5.1). Firstly, each agent selects a set of actions it can legally perform at the current step (physically available for the agents, acceptable in terms of the norms, etc.). Such an action may be explicitly wanted or not; also, this action may belong to a sequence of actions in accordance with a form of behavior that has been chosen at a previous step or is about to be chosen. In the former case, the agent may resume the chosen behavior form or abort it.

Having a set of actions that are legal to be currently performed, the agent applies a preference relation. This relation is defined on states and actions and sets the following order (1 is preferred over 2–5, 2 is preferred over 3–5, etc.):

1. Explicitly preferred (wanted) action
2. The action that leads to a desired state that is not current.
3. Action that eliminates an unwanted state that is current.
4. Action that does not lead to an unwanted state that is not current.
5. Action that does not eliminate a wanted state that is current.

Initial mental state

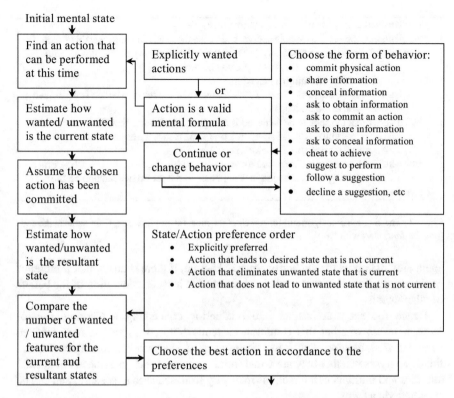

Fig. 5.1 The chart for the choice of action, involving own agent capabilities and world knowledge (simplified case)

In our representation language the sequence of preference conditions is as follows:

```
want(A, ChosenAction),
want(A, State), not State, assume(ChosenAction), State,
want(A, not State), State, assume(ChosenAction), not State,
not ( want( not State), not State, assume(ChosenAction),
State ),
not ( want( State), State, assume(ChosenAction), not State
) .
```

Agent's actions to select from can be atomic or compound. A compound action which includes a mutually-dependent typical sequence of actions is called a *behavior* (Sect. 4.3). A compound action of a given agent may include actions of other agents and various intermediate states, some of which the agent may want to avoid. The agent decides either to perform the action delivering the least unwanted state or action of another agent, or to do nothing. If there are multiple possible actions which do not lead, in the agent's belief, to unwanted consequences, this

```
chooseAction(Agent,ChosenActions):-
% generates the set of available actions and chose those leading to acceptable states
findall( PossibleAction, ( % finds all objects satisfying conditions below
     availableAction(Agent, PossibleAction),
          % choosing (forming) a behavior
     assume(PossibleAction), % assume that the selected action is performed
     acceptableState(Agent),
% To verify that the state to be achieved is acceptable (not worse than the current state)
     clean_assume(PossibleAction), % cleans the assumptions
   ), AccumulatedPossibleActions),
  chooseBestActions(AccumulatedPossibleActions,        ChosenAc-
tions). % choosing the best action in accordance to the preference relation on the set of
accessible states
```

Fig. 5.2 The single-agent algorithm for search of the most favorable action. Comments to the code (*courier font*) start with '%'

agent either chooses the explicitly preferred action, if there is an explicit preference predicate, or the action whose choice involves the least consideration of the beliefs of other agents.

Hence the agent A has an initial intention concerning a *ChosenAction* or *State*, assesses whether this condition currently holds, then selects the preferred *ChosenAction*, assumes that it has been executed, deduces the consequences, and finally analyses whether they are preferential. The preference, parameters of agents' attitudes and multiagent interactions may vary from scenario to scenario and can be specified via a form.

Before an action can be assumed, NL_MAMS needs to check that a potential action is a valid mental formula (Sect. 4.2). A valid mental formula is neither an axiom (such as *an agent knows what it knows*) nor implausible formula (such as literally viewing *someone else's mental state*).

A resultant state comprises one or more explicitly wanted or unwanted states; the agent performs the comparative analysis of preferences on a state-by-state basis. Figure 5.2 presents an algorithm for the search of the most favorable action as a simple logic program for the case of a single agent.

Hence in the simplified model without simulating decision-making of others, the agent performs the exhaustive search through all currently legal actions for all possible consequences. For each such action, the agent assumes he has executed it and estimates the consequences.

5.3.2   Choosing the Best Action Taking into Account Action Selection Analysis of Others

We start with the premise that humans use themselves as an approximate, initial model of their teammates and opponents. Therefore, we based the simulation of the teammate's decision making on the robot's own knowledge of the situation and its decision process. To predict the teammate's choice of actions in a collaborative strategy, we modeled the human as following the self-centered strategy. The result of the simulation is made available to the base model by inserting the result into the "imaginal" buffer of possible opponents' actions. The availability of the results of the mental simulation facilitates the agent's completion of its own decision making. The effect is that the robotic agent yields to what it believes is the human's choice. While this simple model of teamwork allows us to demonstrate the concept and the implementation of the simulation of the teammate, we proceed to the simulation mode which uses the collaborative strategy recursively.

The high-level algorithm for the choice of a most favorable action (Fig. 5.3), taking into account decision-making of the opponents, is presented below as a logic program (Fig. 5.4). Note that in addition to Fig. 5.2 we have the predicate *assumeOtherAgents(Agent, OthersActions)* which is preceded by the predicate.

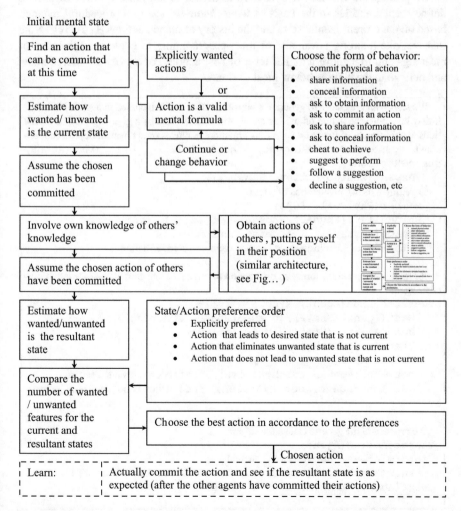

Fig. 5.3 The chart for the choice of action involving simulation of the choice of action by other agents. The model of learning within our framework is depicted on the bottom by dotted lines

involveKnowledgeOfOthers(Agent): the agent's perspective of knowledge and intentions of its opponents needs to be invoked before this agent simulates the choice of the most favorable actions by each of these opponents.

5.3.3 The Library of Available Behaviors

We have discovered that the totality of mental entities can be expressed in the basis *want- know-believe* (Galitsky 2003). The clauses for pre-conditions of behaviors (as aggregated mental actions) we define in this section indeed contain these predicates. The head of each clause is the predicate generateAction(Agent, GeneratedAction, History) which returns the second argument.

We present the clauses for behaviors in details to introduce a flavor of how to define mental entities in the basis of *want- know-believe* in a procedural manner, based on the current mental state and the history of mental actions History. Note that we take a strong advantage of meta-programming to express a wider set of meanings and to achieve a higher level of abstraction. For brevity we merge know and believe in the clauses below most of times.

We start with the clause to generate a physical action that is included in agent's intention. It may be a potential action of another agent, which is selected by a given agent. The clause finds a subformula of intention so that its argument is ranges over physical objects (not actions). generateAction(Agent,   ActionFull,   _):-   want(Agent, StateORAction),
    expand(StateORAction, SOAs) !],
% getting a list of all subterms of a term
  member(PhysFull, SOAs),
  PhysFull=..[PhysAct,WhoWhat, Object|_], % a phys action
  argrep(PhysFull, 1, Agent, ActionFull).
% substitution of itself instead of another agent into selected action

%The following clause forms an own action for an agent that causes desired state of another agent
generateAction(Agent, MyAction, _):-
    want(Agent, State),(clause(State, MyAction);
    know(Agent, (State:- MyAction))),
    State=..[_,OthAg|_],OthAg\=Agent,
    MyAction=..[_, Agent|_],
    not want(Agent, not MyAction), % it is not an unwanted action
    not know(Agent, not MyAction). % this action is not known as impossible

We proceed to the generic clause for *inform*
generateAction(Agent,
  inform(Agent, Addressee, Smth),_):-
    know(Agent,want(Addressee, know(Addressee, Smth)));
  want(Agent, know(Addressee, Smth)).

If an agent is being informed, it should possibly add a belief (reaction to being in-formed)

```
generateAction(Agent, assert(believe(Agent, Smth)),
    History):- % has been informed at a previous step
  prevStep(inform(AgentInform, Agent, Fact), History),
  not believe(Agent, not Smth),
  not know(Agent, not Smth),
  not believe(Agent, not trust(Agent, Smth)).
```

The following clause specifies how an agent forms mistrust when it discovers that it is being informed a lie

```
generateAction(Agent,
  believe(Agent, not trust(Agent, Smth)), History):-
  prevStep(inform(AgentInform, Agent, Fact),
   History),
  %checking if it's a previous action
  member( FactOp , LastHistory),opposite(Fact, FactOp).
```

The clause clarifying when to ask with intention to gain knowledge and possibly believe that someone knows looks like

```
generateAction(Agent, ask(Agent, InformAgent, Smth),
_):-
  [!((want(Agent, know(Agent, Smth)), believe(Agent,
  know(InformAgent, Smth)),
  nonvar(Smth) ); ( want(Agent, know(Agent, Smth)),
  nonvar(Smth) )),
  ifthen(var(InformAgent), (allAgents(Ags),
  member(InformAgent, Ags))) !].
```

The clause introduces the conditions for when to answer: history includes asking, an agent answers if it knows and/or wants addressee to know; believe/know options are con-sidered

```
generateAction(Agent, ActionFull, History):-
  prevStep(ask(AgentAsk, Agent, Smth), LastHistory), (
  (believe(Agent, Smth),
  want(Agent, know(AskAgent, Smth)),
  ActionFull= answer(Agent, AgentAsk,
    believe(Agent,Smth)) );
  (believe(Agent, not Smth),
  want(Agent, know(AskAgent, Smth)),
  ActionFull= answer(Agent, AgentAsk, believe(Agent,
  not Smth)) );
  ( (know(Agent, SmthRelevant);
  believe(Agent, SmthRelevant)),
  expand(SmthRelevant, SmthRE), member(Smth, SmthRE),
```

```
   ActionFull= answer(Agent, AgentAsk, SmthRelevant) )).
```

We proceed to the clause for generation of a suggestion. If an agent wants someone's action and does not have a belief that this agent does not want to perform that action then that action is suggested.

```
generateAction(Agent,
    suggest(Agent, OtherAg, OtherAgAction), History):-
  want(Agent, OtherAgAction),
  OtherAgAction=..[Action, OtherAg|_],
  not believe(Agent,
    not want(OtherAg,   OtherAgAction)),
  not member(Action, [know, believe, want] ),
  Agent\=OtherAg, allAgents(Ags), member(OtherAg, Ags).
```

If an agent is being suggested something, the following clause specify the conditions to follow these suggestions

```
generateAction(Agent, Smth, History):-
  prevStep(suggest(AgentAsk, Agent, Smth),History),
  ( (Smth=..[Action, Agent|_]);
  ( (Smth=(not NSmth)), NSmth=..[Action, Agent|_])),
  Agent\=AgentAsk.
```

The following clause is applicable to the agent which is going to try not to share information to / to conceal from/ to suggest not to not inform another agent

```
generateAction(Agent, ActionFull, _) :-
  want(Agent, not OtherAgAction),
    OtherAgAction=..[_, OtherAg|_],
  (believe(Agent, believe(ThirdAgent,
    OtherAgActionCondition));
  know(ThirdAgent, OtherAgActionCondition)),
  Agent\=OtherAg, Agent\=ThirdAgent,
    ThirdAgent \= OtherAg,
  ifthen((know(Agent, (
  OtherAgAction:-
    believe(OtherAg,OtherAgActionCondition)));
    clause(OtherAgAction,
    believe(OtherAg, OtherAgActionCondition));
    ),
  ActionFull=suggest(Agent, ThirdAgent,
  not inform(ThirdAgent, OtherAg,
                    OtherAgActionCondition))),
  ifthen(( know(Agent, (OtherAgAction:-
    believe(OtherAg, not OtherAgActionCondition)));
```

```
  clause(OtherAgAction,   believe(OtherAg,   not   OtherAgAction-
Condition));
  believe(Agent, (OtherAgAction:-
        believe(OtherAg, not OtherAgActionCondition)))
     ),
  ActionFull=suggest(Agent, ThirdAgent,
  inform(ThirdAgent, OtherAg,
                        not OtherAgActionCondition))).
```

We proceed to the clause for intentional cheating/informing to make someone perform desired action

```
generateAction(Agent, ActionFull, _):-
  want(Agent, OtherAgAction),
  OtherAgAction=..[_, OtherAg|_],
  (know(Agent, (OtherAgAction:-
      believe(OtherAg, OtherAgActionCondition)));
  clause(OtherAgAction,
  know(OtherAg, OtherAgActionCondition));
  know(Agent, (OtherAgAction:-
              know(OtherAg, OtherAgActionCondition)))),
  Agent\=OtherAg,
  ifthenelse( ( know(Agent,
                   not want(OtherAg, OtherAgAction));
  believe(Agent, not OtherAgActionCondition) ),
  (ActionFull=..
  [cheat, Agent, OtherAg, OtherAgActionCondition];
  ActionFull=..[inform, Agent, OtherAg, OtherAgActionCondi-
tion])).
```

The diagram Fig. 5.5 depicts relations between mental actions. *Suggesting* is a partial case of *asking*, *asking* and *suggesting* may have a goal to *initiate_action*. *Cheating* is a partial case of *informing* with untruthful information, which may or may not have a goal of initiating an opponent's action. Both *informing* and *cheating* may form *responding*, all these mental actions may serve the purpose of *initiate_action*. Committing *a physical action* may also be *following advice*.

As to the causal links, usually *asking* and sometimes *informing* causes *responding*, *suggesting* may cause *following* it (*follow_advice*), cheating and initiation of action may cause *committing of this* (*physical*) *action*.

5.4 Evaluation of NL_MAMS

In this section we assess the performance of the NL_MAMS with respect to a number of characteristics to make a judgment about its educational value for CwA.

A practical commonsense reasoning system such as NL_MAMS can be characterized in terms of the following parameters:

```
chooseAction(Agent,ChosenActions, History):-
% generates the set of available actions and chose those leading to acceptable states
findall( PossibleAction, ( % finds all objects satisfying conditions below
availableAction(Agent, PossibleAction, History),
         % choosing (forming) a behavior
assume(PossibleAction), % assume that the selected action is performed
involveKnowledgeOfOthers(Agent),
                 %substitutes own knowledge by own knowledge of others' knowledge
  assumeOtherAgents(Agent, OthersActions),
  % Similar assumption concerning others'actions. They are obtained based on the
  % acceptable states of the others from the viewpoint of the given agent.
  % Here the agent thinks for its opponents what would they do to achieve their goals
  acceptableState(Agent),
% To verify that the state to be achieved is acceptable (not worse than the current state)
    clean_assume(PossibleAction), % cleans the assumptions
  ), AccumulatedPossibleActions),
chooseBestActions(AccumulatedPossibleActions,        ChosenAc-
tions). % choosing the best action in accordance to the preference relation on the set of
accessible states
```

Fig. 5.4 The predicate *availableAction* (From Fig. 5.2) will be the focus of our considerations of behavior forms in the following section

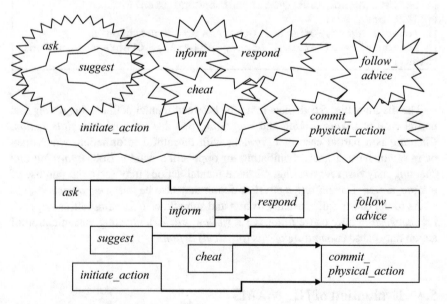

Fig. 5.5 The relations between the behaviors

1. *Correctness.* To evaluate the correctness of the NL_MAMS, we compare the scenarios built by NL_MAMS with those built by human experts. The adequacy of a reasoning system like NL_MAMS to the real mental world can be evaluated by means of a representation of a set of scenarios of multiagent interaction (focused on mental attitudes) collected from a variety of domains.
2. The *coverage* of possible behaviors. To evaluate the *coverage* of real-world scenarios, we collect the dataset from various domains. For this dataset, we verify that NL_MAMS's reasoning can link the initial mental state, mentioned in a scenario from this dataset, with the final mental state from that scenario. The link is implemented via the library of behaviors; and our evaluation of coverage is indeed an estimate of how the encoded set of behaviors covers the totality of real-world scenarios with respect to the resultant mental states.
3. Scenario *complexity.* To evaluate the highest *complexity* of scenarios the NL_MAMS can handle we vary the *number* of behaviors of various agents combined in a single scenario. Maximum complexity is the number of behaviors such that the correctness of obtained scenarios dramatically falls when this number is incremented. In other words, if a scenario complexity exceeds this number, there is a significant deviation of scenarios generated by the NL_MAMS from those natural for human experts, given the same initial mental states.
4. The *expressiveness* of representation language. Evaluating the expressiveness of representation language, we are concerned with the information lost when scenario representation is converted from the natural to the formal language. Importance of the lost information is estimated taken into account the caused deviation of resultant mental states. The information is usually lost because the number of meanings of mental entities explicitly represented as behaviors is obviously lower than respective number of meanings in a natural language description of a scenario of inter-human interactions. Evaluation of the expressiveness of representation language is tightly connected with natural language information extraction focused on mental entities presented in Galitsky and Kuznetsov (2008). We will not conduct the evaluation of expressiveness in this book, but mention that the NL_MAMS's vocabulary includes the generic template for physical actions and rather extensive set of lexical units and synonyms for the common-usage mental attributes.

For the purpose of estimating the parameters (1)–(3) above we form two following datasets of textual scenarios to be represented by the NL_MAMS:

(a) The scenarios that were suggested to illustrate certain peculiarities of reasoning about mental world (frame problems, defaults, circumscription, argumentation, belief updates, reasoning about knowledge, time and space, reasoning in legal, educational, medical domains, etc.). Seventy-two such scenarios have been collected over the duration of NL_MAMS project (over 7 years). There are no special criteria for inclusion to this dataset except that the mental states and actions should be explicitly mentioned.
(b) The uniform set of multiagent conflict scenarios (textual complaints) obtained and subject to manual formal representation from the public complaint database

(e.g. PlanetFeedback.com). Complaints describe interaction between a complainant and company representatives; these conflicting scenarios are mostly occurring in a mental space. Fifty-eight banking complaints has been obtained and converted into formal representation (Galitsky and Kuznetsov 2008) to serve as the evaluation dataset. Complaint selection was random in terms of content: all banking complaints submitted within a month that describe at least 4 steps of interactions (pairs of communicative actions) between the involved parties.

The role of the dataset (a) which is fairly diverse is to compare the performance of NL_MAMS with other systems in mental as well as non-mental reasoning. Also, most of the scenarios from this dataset are accompanied with their formal representations. This dataset is used as a basis to estimate the correctness and coverage by behaviors, since existing formal representations allows unambiguous comparison of the original and NL_MAMS-based representations.

We use the dataset (b) of customer complaints to estimate the coverage with higher accuracy than the former dataset and to estimate scenario complexity, since a high number of scenarios for each complexity are available. Since we used a superset of the dataset (b) to evaluate our scenario learning framework for communicative actions only (Chap. 3), we also use it for correctness evaluation based on a specific class of plausible and implausible scenarios. NL_MAMS is expected to build plausible (valid) scenarios only, and not build implausible (invalid) scenarios.

Although NL_MAMS is a prediction system, we evaluate a plausibility of results rather than a prediction accuracy: the real mental world is too rich and diverse to be predictable in terms of the proposed model. Although the precision can be satisfactory, the recall of NL_MAMS is really low. We expect the NL_MAMS to yield at least a single plausible scenario of multiagent interaction; we do not target yielding the totality of possible resultant mental states.

5.4.1 Evaluation of Correctness

We used the dataset (a) above formed by compiling examples found in the logical AI literature to evaluate the correctness. For each formalized scenario, NL_MAMS was fed with the initial mental state (explicitly mentioned in these scenarios). We verified whether the NL_MAMS can yield the sequence of further mental states from this scenario. If a given scenario required adding a new form of behavior, the respective clause for this behavior was added.

The results of the correctness evaluation are shown in the Table 5.1. The first column presents an origin of a scenario, and the second column contains a number of scenarios for each group. The third column shows the number of scenarios of each origin, where it is necessary to add a clause for a new behavior or alter an existing clause, given the behavior library before this evaluation. The fourth column enumerates some of the behaviors for each group of scenarios that have to be

Table 5.1 Evaluation of correctness

Origin of a scenario: reasoning domain	Number of scenarios	Number of scenarios where new behavior has to be added	Required additional forms of behavior (selected examples)	Number of scenarios where the correct representation was achieved
Modal logic, BDI model (e.g. Wooldridge 2000)	15	6	Changing mind, giving up, advising other to give up	11
Reasoning about action (e.g Reiter 1993)	16	12	Change action parameters	13
Default reasoning (e.g. Gabbay 1999)	18	6	Changing mind	12
Argumentation (e.g. Weigand and de Moor 2004)	13	4	Defeating previous statement, breaking a loop in actions, threaten	9
Other multiagent models (negotiation, auction, coalition formation, assistance) (e.g. Olivia et al. 1999)	10	3	Agree, disagree, confirm, deny	9
Total	72	31 (43 %)		54 (75 %)

added to reproduce them. We observed that the scenarios requiring a modification of the behavior library constitutes 43 % of the total number of scenarios. Finally, the fifth column presents the number of scenarios for each group that allowed correct representation (with or without a modification). We observed that 75 % of the total number of scenarios was subject to correct representations. In other 25 % of cases, either the underlying reasoning was too complex, or initial mental states were lacking the information necessary to correctly derive consecutive mental states.

In addition to the above evaluation we observed that in most cases the agents' behavior that is generated by the NL_MAMS is perceived by its users and assessors as a sequence of natural and expected choices. If it is not the case, the NL_MAMS backs its scenario up by providing the motivation and the protocol of exhaustive search through the lists of available actions at each step. A user might disagree with the selected form of behavior, but she will at least understand the motivations. Furthermore, handling manifold of meanings caused by the necessity to represent NL input increases system flexibility and makes it closer to the real world in imitation of human reasoning and human behavior.

5.4.2   Evaluation of Coverage

As a result of the evaluation of correctness, the behavior library has been extended (trained) to accommodate atypical behaviors from the dataset (a). Evaluating the

Table 5.2 Evaluation of the behavioral coverage of scenarios

Form of behavior	Training, 72 scenarios from logical AI literature		Test, 58 complaint scenarios	
	# of scenarios	% of scenarios	# of scenarios	% of scenarios
Perform own physical action	70	97	57	98
Achieving desired state of another agent	21	28	29	50
Informing	14	19	23	40
Updating belief while being informed	5	7	17	29
Forming mistrust	7	9	32	55
Asking to gain knowledge	29	39	19	33
Answering	18	24	14	24
Generating suggestion	26	35	21	36
Following suggestion	14	19	18	31
Avoiding sharing/suggesting not to inform	12	16	13	22
Cheating to achieve an action	17	23	5	9
New forms of behavior	–	–	**14**	**19**

Note that a particular behavior form may occur in a scenario more than once. The bottom row depicts the number of cases that require a modification of the behavior library

coverage, we assess how frequent an occurrence of each behavior form is in the complaint dataset (b) which did not participate in the training of the behavior forms. In this section we conduct the evaluation of the accumulated behavior library and overall system performance.

We observed that the trained behaviors adequately cover the test domain (Table 5.2). All clauses for behaviors that were obtained in the domain of randomly accumulated scenarios were employed in forming the sequence of consecutive mental states in the test domain. Conversely, to explain a rational multiagent behavior of proponents and opponents in complaint scenarios in 81 % of cases, it is sufficient to use accumulated clauses for behaviors. The remaining 19 % of complaint scenarios the NL_MAMS failed to reproduce, relying on the accumulated library of behaviors and its simulation machinery. Each scenario contains on average 3.2 forms of behavior in the training dataset and 4.3 forms of behavior in the test dataset.

Clearly, formal descriptions of the behavior of complainants and their opponents in more detail would benefit from additional complaint-specific behavior patterns. However, we revealed that increasing the complexity of the formal descriptions of textual scenarios does not make them more consistent, because the majority of intermediate mental states are not explicitly mentioned. Hence we come to the conclusion that the formed library of behaviors is sufficient to provide an adequate (most consistent) description of multiagent interactions between a complainant and his opponents. And since customer complaints domain is a source of fairly complex examples of conflicts in mental world, we can expect the NL_MAMS to satisfactorily perform in other, simpler domains.

Note that our evaluation is by no means intended to predict the behavior of scenario agents; instead, we try to include all necessary information in the initial mental state so that the scenario is generated as a respective sequence. The problem of prediction the consecutive mental states under a lack of information is posed differently (Galitsky 2006) and requires machine learning and reasoning about actions (Galitsky et al. 2009) components in addition to NL_MAMS (Sect. 7.4).

5.4.3   Evaluation of Complexity

The complexity of scenarios the NL_MAMS can handle significantly exceeds that of the textual information on mental attributes of human and automatic agents comprehensible by a user. We observe that the NL_MAMS's performance is much higher than the humans' performance in spite of the fact that reasoning about mental states is natural and frequent task for a human user. To characterize the computational tractability of the suggested approach, we take into account that at each step NL_MAMS considers about 30 available behavior forms for each agent.

In the process of multiagent communication and while behavior decision-making, the NL_MAMS analyses the formulas of complexity (the number of nested mental predicates) below four (Sect. 4.2). For the totality of all well-written mental formulas the system recognizes whether a formula is an axiom, meaningful or meaningless expression (Galitsky and Kuznetsov 2008). For an arbitrary set of such formulas as an initial condition for NL_MAMS, it either finds a contradiction or synthesizes the scenario of multiagent behavior.

We used the dataset (b) of formalized complaints and its extension by longer scenarios to estimate how the correctness of representations depends on scenario complexity, measured as a number of behavior forms. We observed that the maximum complexity of the scenarios NL_MAMS can handle reliably is 4 behavior forms. Exceeding this number, the correctness of generated scenarios falls to as low as 52 % for 5 behavior forms and to just 34 % for 6 behavior forms. The results show that when a scenario contains 5–6 behaviors, the NL_MAMS is frequently unable to represent its last one-two mental states towards the end. Instead, it significantly deviates from what an expert would think of a natural behavior of participating agents (Table 5.3).

To analyze how nested expressions for mental states and actions are represented by the NL_MAMS, we assessed the correctness of scenarios representation grouping scenarios by the *maximum number of nested mental actions or states in a scenario* (Table 5.4). One can see an abrupt drop in the correctness of scenario representation when the complexity of nested expressions exceeds four.

Table 5.3 Estimating the maximum complexity of scenarios for NL_MAMS: number of behavior forms

Number of behavior forms per scenario	Correctness of scenario representation, %
2	85
3	80
4	75
5	50
6	35

Table 5.4 Estimating the maximum complexity of scenarios for NL_MAMS: number of behavior forms

Maximum number of nested mental actions or states in a scenario	Correctness of scenario representation, %
1	85
2	75
3	80
4	60
5	30
6	25

As to the expressiveness of NL_MAMS's representation language, one can estimate its sensitivity to a deviation of meanings of mental entities presenting initial conditions. We formulate the sensitivity statement for the NL_MAMS as follows:

Sensitivity Hypothesis For any two mental formulas μ and μ' for respective entities specifying initial mental states, there exist two initial mental states of s and s' yielding different scenarios. $\mu \in s$ and $\mu' \in s'$ are such that the simulator forms distinct multiagent scenarios $s \to s_1, \ldots, s_n$ and $s' \to s_1', \ldots, s_k'$. Therefore, NL_MAMS is capable of taking into account the difference between any two mental formulas (or two distinct mental entities) while building a sequence of mental states.

The conclusion of our assessment is that the NL_MAMS is suitable for assistance with rehabilitation of CwA reasoning.

5.5   Accompanying Reasoning Systems and Application Domains

The main conjecture of the evaluation section above is that NL_MAMS is good at exactly what it is expected to do: yielding a plausible sequence of mental states given the initial one. However, to take into account additional information about the agents, previous experience and cases involving these agents, their particular circumstances, features of the physical environment, etc., it is important to involve other reasoning components. Integrating the NL_MAMS simulation with other reasoning methodologies including deductive, inductive and abductive is necessary for processing mental attitudes together with domain-specific knowledge (compare with Stein and Barnden 1995).

Table 5.5 enumerates the accompanying reasoning components and presents the sample chunks of knowledge from the domain of customer complaints. These components have been implemented in the system for conflict resolution (Sect. 4.3), which heavily relies on mental states and communicative actions of involved parties (Galitsky et al. 2009). The complaint domain is use to demonstrate the upper bound of the complexity of the mental world as a subject of reasoning. For autistic rehabilitation, a hybrid reasoning system is required to support a broader set of scenarios with a substantial diversity of physical states and actions.

To demonstrate the universality of our approach to reasoning about mental attitudes, we enumerate the other problem domains where NL_MAMS has been deployed or used for simulation or knowledge representation:

- Solving constraint satisfaction problem in the environment of conflicting human and automatic agents (scheduling for the broadcasting industry);
- Training of negotiation and other decision-making skills; querying the works of literature using mental states of their characters (Galitsky 2004);
- Automatic synthesis of scenarios (e.g. for Internet advertisements);
- Analysis and classification of the characters of fairy tales;
- Modeling mental states of investors for market predictions;
- Extracting mental states of participating agents from text; understanding customers' complaints;
- Extraction of the mental behavior patterns from the wireless-based location services data;
- Simulating the relationships between economic agents.

5.6   HCI Issues of Autistic Training

The user interface of NL_MAMS allows the user to input description of scenarios via plain English. The form (Fig. 5.6) shows an example in which a user specified a scenario (the Sally Anne story from (Baron-Cohen et al. 1985) in English. This user then pressed the button [Load (translate into formal expressions)].

The result of pressing this button is the mental formulas seen in the combo box. The combo box allows users to highlight parses they like and to edit those that need refinement – in the case of inaccuracies in formal representations. Although a beginning user would not be able to notice such inaccuracies, we know from prior experience that CwA who spent significant time with NL_MAMS are able to refine them. In fact, we have found that experienced users are able to skip the English to formal logic translation step and enter their scenario descriptions directly in formal logic notation.

Table 5.5 Accompanying reasoning systems. We use the Prolog variables *Cust* and *Comp* for "customer" and "company" respectively

Component name	Component role	Sample encoded knowledge for the component

Behavior simulation: reasoning about mental states and actions, NL_MAMS	To provide a simulation environment for agents' choice of future mental actions, given the current mental state of interacting agents. The unit includes the library of behaviors available for agents. It yields the consecutive mental states given the initial one, simulating the decision-making process of agents	*forgive(Cust, Comp, WrongAdvice):-*
		  advice(Comp, Cust, WrongAdvice), *be-*
		lieve(Cust, know(Comp,
		  not (howToFix(Happen):- WrongAdvice))),
		  explain(Comp, *Cust,* *believe(Comp,*
		(howToFix(Happen):- *WrongAdvice)* *))).*
		trust(Cust, Comp).

Classical deductive clauses	To define entities, to specify links between them which always hold	*followAdviceNoResult :- ask(Cust, Comp, what(Happen)),*
		  suggest(Comp, Cust, satisfaction(Cust)) :-
		    howToFix(Happen)),
		  do(Cust, howToFix(Happen)), not satisfaction(Cust).

Defeasible rules	To specify when some entities may support serve as arguments for a given entity	*justified_complaint* *-<* *lieCS,* *con-* *sistent_discourse.* *~ justified_complaint-< consistent_discourse, ~* *loss(Cust).*

Default rules	To specify when an entity (prerequisite) *always* serves as the condition for the given entity of interest (consequent) if an additional assumption takes place (justification). If justification is not available (cannot be formulated, implicit), a default rule is interpreted as a respective defeasible one. Default rules may be conflicting, therefore implementation of operational semantics may be required	$\dfrac{lieCS:\ mention\_biz\_rule}{justified\_complaint}$ $\dfrac{justified\_complaint:\ lieCS}{cust\_compensation}$ $\dfrac{not\ requested(cust\_compensation):\ lieCS}{cust\_compensation}$
Reasoning about action: plan building rules so that the assistant agent can advise on future actions	To specify what the future (physical) action of an agents will be, given the pre-conditions of possible actions and their effects, taking into account the current development (of interaction between agents). Our implementation of reasoning about action allows online acquisition of action pre-conditions (Galitsky 2006)	$poss(do(Cust,\ fixProd(WayToFix))$:- suggest(Comp, Cust, Satisfaction :- howToFix(Happen)), lost_trust(Cust, CustServ). holds(disinformed, do(E, S)):- $E = explainWronglyCS.$
Machine learning: matching the cases *Jasmine*	To predict the future interaction of involved agents and to determine their parameters given the previously accumulated cases (represented as sequences of communicative actions). Matching a current formalized complaint with the dataset of complaints with assigned status.	*askt(Cust, P1). explain(Comp, P1). disagree(Cust,P1). confirm(Cust, P1), agree(Comp,P2), suggest(Comp, P2), accept(Cust, P2), request(Cust, P2), promise(Comp, P2), remind(Cust, P2), ask(Cust, P2).* Note two subjects of communicative actions: *P1* and *P2*.

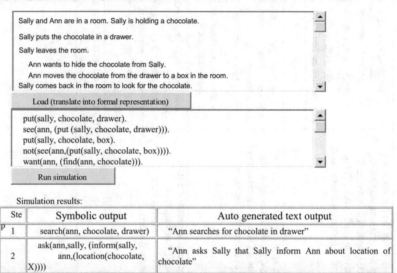

Training of Mental Reasoning using NL_MAMS

This educational tool develops general analytical skills, your capability to grasp a complex situation quickly, creative decision making and situational memory. For the scenario below, try to understand it and predict what each agent would do. Then, running the simulator, please compare its solution with your own. You may also want to modify the initial mental states of involved agents and observe how their resultant behaviour changes.

Specify the agents' and simulator parameters

> Sally and Ann are in a room. Sally is holding a chocolate.
>
> Sally puts the chocolate in a drawer.
>
> Sally leaves the room.
>
>   Ann wants to hide the chocolate from Sally.
>   Ann moves the chocolate from the drawer to a box in the room.
> Sally comes back in the room to look for the chocolate.

Load (translate into formal representation)

    put(sally, chocolate, drawer).
    see(ann, (put (sally, chocolate, drawer))).
    put(sally, chocolate, box).
    not(see(ann,(put(sally, chocolate, box)))).
    want(ann, (find(ann, chocolate))).

Run simulation

Simulation results:

Ste p	Symbolic output	Auto generated text output
1	search(ann, chocolate, drawer)	"Ann searches for chocolate in drawer"
2	ask(ann,sally, (inform(sally, ann,(location(chocolate, X))))	"Ann asks Sally that Sally inform Ann about location of chocolate"

Fig. 5.6 The NL_MAMS user interface for rehabilitation of autistic reasoning (advanced scenario). This exercise is one of the easiest for autistic trainees; it introduces the simplest connection of "not seeing → not knowing"

Once the user feels ready, he or she can press the [Run Simulation] button. This will cause the simulation to run. The results of running the simulation are the candidate answer to the question "What will happen next?" The results of running the simulation can be seen in the bottom of Fig. 5.7. There the user can see that in this case a two-step plan was generated. Most frequently, 3–5 steps are generated, and sometimes up to 8–10 steps. Each step is depicted in via its formal logic notation and via an automatically generated English rendering of that step.

In Table 5.6 we show the rules from our theory of mind library that fired in the process of running the simulation. Note that the rules may fire recursively. Some fired based on the initial states and others fired on intermediate results.

In our example we use a first-order Sallie-Ann test scenario, which is focused on the axiom "not seeing leads to not knowing". To be able to approach the application of this axiom, a number of general knowledge-related axioms should be applied, including a particular case of *searching* (with a specific pre-condition for our scenario), as well as generic axiom for an *informing* behavior. Notice a meta-predicate *epistemic_trans* which links uninstantiated expression *Query* with

There are three friends: Mike (m), Nick(n) and Peter(p). They got together tonight to have fun but their favorite toy is missing...

The friends take information from each other rather seriously, although they sometimes may want to tell a lie each other. The information concerning their mental states includes the permanent attitudes of the friends, as well as their particular moods for tonight.

Nick's mental state	Peter's mental state	Mike's mental state
Nick believes that Mike wants Peter to get the toy, and Nick wants Mike to get it. And also Nick would get if no one else does, but would not like to.	Peter does not want to get the toy himself and believes that Mike would not get it anyway. Also, Peter believes that Mike believes that Nick wants Mike to get it. Peter wants Mike to know that Peter would not get the toy himself. However, Peter would get the toy if he knows (someone tells him) that Nick wants him (Peter) to get it.	Mike wants either Nick or Peter to get the toy. Mike knows that Nick does not want Peter to get it. Mike would get the toy if Peter believes (is said) that Nick wants himself (Mike) to get it.

Form the statement using list boxes below

[Nick ▼] [want ▼] [inform ▼] [Peter ▼] [toy is bad ▼] [None ▼]

[None ▼] [Nick ▼] [None ▼] [None ▼]   or input in natural language

Nick wants Peter to inform Nick if the toy is bad.

[What will the children do?]   Read the scenario (generated sequence of mental states) below:

Nick's future actions	Peter's future actions	Mike's future actions
inform(n,p,want(m,get(p,toy)))	*inform(p,m,not get(p,toy))*	*cheat(m,p,want(n,get(p,toy)))*
cheat(n,p,want(m,get(p,toy)))	*nothing*	*inform(m,n,not get(m,toy))*
inform(n,p,get(m,toy))	*nothing*	*cheat(m,n,get(m,toy))*
ask(n,m,not get(m,toy))	*nothing*	*inform(m,p,not want(n,get(p,toy)))*
ask(n,m,get(m,toy))	***get(p, toy)***	*answer(m,n,not get(m,toy))*

Fig. 5.7 The NL_MAMS user interface for rehabilitation of autistic reasoning (advanced mode). This exercise is fairly complicates for autistic trainees; it can be challenging for adults to suggest an appropriate conflict resolution strategy

its instantiated version *QueryProposition* (this instantiation occurs when the body of the respective clause is called).

The user can select the subset of formulas specifying the initial mental state to monitor how the resultant scenario is changed. The system visualizes the semantic relationships between mental entities, a single physical entity and the agents involved. The parameters of NL_MAMS are specified using the form Fig. 5.8.

5.7   Other ToM-Related Systems

In the last two decades, interest in the formal modeling of various forms of human reasoning and in simulation of mental behavior has risen strongly. A series of phenomena in human reasoning have been reflected in such approaches as reasoning about actions and knowledge, nonmonotonic reasoning, etc. Modal logic-based

Table 5.6 English glosses and symbolic representation for behaviors

English gloss	Symbolic representation
IF an *Agent* wants to know in what Place some Object is and if he/she believes that Object is in that Place THEN he/she will search Place for Object.	*search(Agent, Object, Place) :- (* *want(Agent, know(Agent,* *location(Object,Place)) ,* *believe(Agent, location(Object,Place))*
IF *Agent1* sees *Agent2* put *Object* in *Place* THEN *Agent1* believes that the location of *Object* is *Place*.	*believe(Agent1, location(Object,Place)) :- see(Agent1,* *put(Agent2, Object, Place))*
Agent1 asks *Agent2* about *Query* IF *Agent1* want to know answer to this *query* and believes that *Agent2* knows *QueryProposition*.	*ask(Agent1, Agent2, Query) :-* *wants(Agent1, know(Agent1, QueryProposition)),* *not(know(Agent1, QueryProposition),* *believe(Agent1,* *knows(Agent2, QueryProposition)),* *epistemic_trans(Query, QueryProposition).*
Partial case of the above, where query is a binary predicate *BinaryPredicate(Subject,Object))*	*asks(Agent1, Agent2,* *BinaryPredicate(Subject,Object)) :-* *wants(Agent1, know(Agent1,* *BinaryPredicate(Subject, UnknownObject)),* *not(know(Agent1,* *BinaryPredicate(Subject, Object)),* *believe(Agent1,* *knows(Agent2, BinaryPredicate(Subject,Object)),* *epistemic_trans(UnknownObject, UnknownObject).*
Metapredicate which operates with expressions, either substituting variables in them, or checking that one expression can be turned into another by substitution. Can be treated as Prolog unification test.	*epistemic_trans(Query, QueryProposition).*
Not seeing leads to not knowing	*not(know(Agent, Proposition)) :- not(see(Agent, Proposition))*

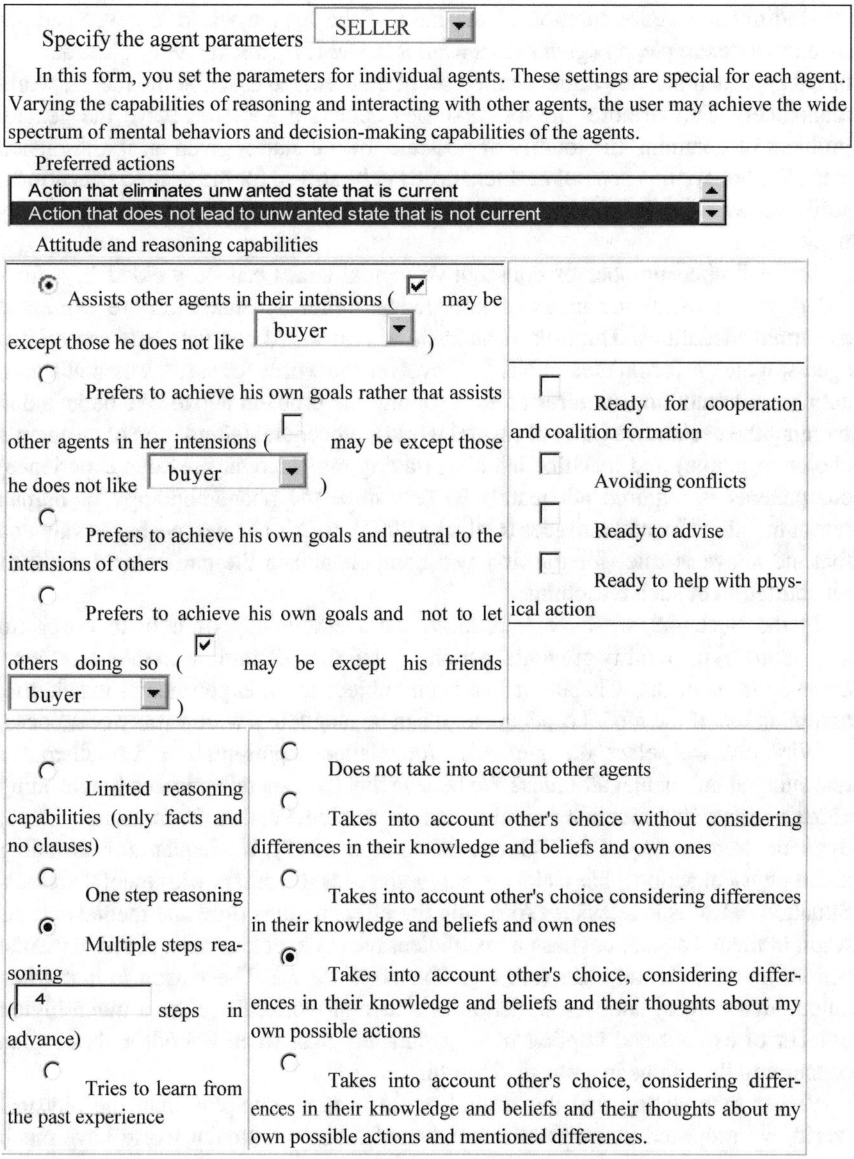

Specify the agent parameters | SELLER   ▼ |

In this form, you set the parameters for individual agents. These settings are special for each agent. Varying the capabilities of reasoning and interacting with other agents, the user may achieve the wide spectrum of mental behaviors and decision-making capabilities of the agents.

Preferred actions

| Action that eliminates unwanted state that is current | ▲ |
| Action that does not lead to unwanted state that is not current | ▼ |

Attitude and reasoning capabilities

(•)   Assists other agents in their intensions (☑ may be except those he does not like | buyer ▼ |)

( )   Prefers to achieve his own goals rather that assists other agents in her intensions (☐ may be except those he does not like | buyer ▼ |)

☐   Ready for cooperation and coalition formation

( )   Prefers to achieve his own goals and neutral to the intensions of others

☐   Avoiding conflicts

( )   Prefers to achieve his own goals and   not to let others doing so (☑ may be except his friends | buyer ▼ |)

☐   Ready to advise

☐   Ready to help with physical action

( )   Limited reasoning capabilities (only facts and no clauses)

( )   Does not take into account other agents

( )   Takes into account other's choice without considering differences in their knowledge and beliefs and own ones

( )   One step reasoning

( )   Takes into account other's choice considering differences in their knowledge and beliefs and own ones

(•)   Multiple steps reasoning (4   steps   in advance)

(•)   Takes into account other's choice, considering differences in their knowledge and beliefs and their thoughts about my own possible actions

( )   Tries to learn from the past experience

( )   Takes into account other's choice, considering differences in their knowledge and beliefs and their thoughts about my own possible actions and mentioned differences.

Fig. 5.8 Specifying the parameters of agents involved: attitude and reasoning capabilities. Varying these parameters, a rehabilitation specialist may adjust NL_MAMS to reproduce mental reasoning of a particular trainee

and situation calculus–based approaches have become the most popular in formal modeling of mental attitudes (McCarthy 1995; Fagin et al. 1996; Wooldridge 2000). However, these approaches had to be extended for the purpose of creation of an educational software that possesses such the capabilities.

Traditionally, representation of the laws of the mental world is developed via axioms (for example, *an agent knows what it knows* (Fagin et al. 1996)). The axiom–based approach delivers rather limited set of theorems to describe the mental world realistically. Furthermore, the axiom–based approach does not solve the general problem of obtaining the totality of possible mental states, given an initial mental state. We believe this general problem needs to be solved for the desired educational software: we want the children to be capable of reasoning starting from an arbitrary mental state.

Just a limited number of consecutive mental states can be yielded in a first-order system where meanings of knowledge, belief and intention are expressed as formal modalities. The task of analysis of real-world conflicts between human agents, which is formulated in NL and involves the words for various mental states, actions and emotions, requires at least solving the problem above. We believe that merging the declarative (laws of mental world), procedural (simulation of an agent's choice of action) and machine learning (taking into account previous experience) components is required adequately to reproduce the phenomenology of human reasoning about mental attitudes (Galitsky 2003). In this chapter, we have evaluated that the above is true (for the first two components) in the particular domain of rehabilitation of such reasoning.

In the Sect. 4.2 we have introduced the methodology of how to cover (to approximate) the totality of mental actions by building definitions in the basis *want-know-believe*. In this Chapter it has been subject to an experimental evaluation, assuming that if the model is adequate, it can be taught to a wide variety of trainees.

Why did we select the particular knowledge representation formalism for reasoning about mental attitudes? We believe that the general approach to reasoning about actions, the situation calculus and its implementation for reasoning about dynamic domains (e.g. GOLOG, (Levesque et al. 1997)) is adequate for reasoning about physical actions, but lacks the expressiveness to operate with mental actions. Situation calculus is relevant expressing the effect axioms (how the mental actions result in mental states) but has an insufficient means to determine a possible mental action, given a mental state (see e.g. Shanahan 1997)). The reason is that when an automatic agent chooses an action in a mental world, there are a much higher number of explicit and implicit input parameters than when a robot makes a plan concerning its actions in a physical world.

Rather than stating that the mental world is more complex than the physical world, we proposed that a smaller number of facts in a mental world have much more complex structure of causal links, and the very nature of these links is quite different from other reasoning domains. Indeed, our training methodology takes advantage of the compactness of entities of the mental world, focusing on the skill to build links between these entities.

We demonstrated that reasoning about mental world can be implemented via exhaustive search through the possible behaviors, evaluating achieved mental states. Generic representation of reasoning about mental world may be viewed as augmentation of logical axioms to perform reasoning about a particular domain (represented by means of applied axioms). Therefore we follow along the line of classical axiomatic method stating that the same set of logical axioms is sufficient to perform reasoning in an arbitrary domain. In this book we observed that the set of behaviors observed in one domain can be applied in an intact form to another domain with different physical axioms to produce adequate multiagent scenarios.

For an arbitrary set of mental formulas as an initial condition for NL_MAMS, it either finds a contradiction or synthesizes the scenario of multiagent behavior. NL_MAMS's vocabulary included the generic template for physical actions and rather extensive set of lexical units and synonyms for the common-usage mental entities. Also, it is worth mentioning that although each natural language has its own peculiarities of reasoning about mental attributes, replacing one natural language by another does not affect the suggested model for the mental world, as far as our experiments indicated.

In this book we have discussed the applications of modal logic for reasoning about mental world. Clearly, a lot of observations about the multiagent behavior can be deduced from the axioms; however the set of theorems does not constitute a basis to enumerate a set of consecutive mental states. We conclude that for the generic implementation of reasoning simulation is required, which is implemented as an exhaustive search in the space of possible behaviors. It has been observed in this study that the simulation for realistic mental states for a few agents is not computationally intensive.

Similar to the traditional settings of multiagent systems and the BDI model, both an initial mental state and the one to be predicted are specified in terms of *intentions, knowledge* and *beliefs*. However, the implementation of prediction is based on the defined behaviors as means to transit from one state to another. This is in contrast to the traditional approach where the pre-conditions of mental actions and mental states as effects of these actions are formulated in terms of a rather limited number of entities for mental states including *intentions, knowledge* and *beliefs*. Obviously, using a wider set of mental entities to express behaviors, leveraging the machinery of deriving these behaviors from the basis, delivers *much richer* set of mental states than the traditional approach. In other words, going beyond the basis dramatically increases the expressiveness of the representation language for mental actions, making the formal description of multiagent interaction scenarios adequate to apply to the real world.

Simulation-type approaches have been successfully applied to reasoning about mental attitudes: they follow the idea to eliminate layers of belief operator in order to simplify the reasoning and representation steps compared to what would be needed in modal logic-based reasoning about mental states. In our approach, reasoning by agent A about agent B's belief is carried out by standing in B's shoes and applying B's own reasoning process directly to B's supposed beliefs, much as if they were A's own beliefs, in order to conclude what B might believe. In other words, our "simulation" is conducting reasoning within an alleged belief space of B, where the reasoning process is similar to what A would herself use if B's beliefs had been in A's own belief space.

In terms of how a society of agents can be characterized in terms of their mental states, the proposed approach can be characterized as a low-level and detailed (without a loss of information). As examples of higher level description of multiagent societies which involve mental states it is worth mentioning (Buzing et al. 2005) who showed that the pressure to cooperate leads to the evolution of communication skills facilitating cooperation. At this lower level, logic-based simulation comes into play rather than numerical simulation; aggregation of agents to express their attitudes and attributes quantitatively does not seem to be a plausible solution. Another example of a higher level multiagent model would be a social dilemma of (Axelrod 1984), where decisions that seem to make perfect sense from each individual's point of view can aggregate into outcomes that are unfavorable for all (Galan and Izquierdo 2005). Cooperative norms treat multiagent interactions at a more general level than our study, where individual communicative actions are selected. The NL_MAMS predicts the behavior in much narrower sense and in much more concrete manner than, for example, than the systems implementing the Theory of Reasoned Action and Theory of Planned Behavior (Ajzen and Fishbein 1980).

Building the environment for a low-level simulation involving basic verbalized attitudes and behavior forms of agents, we do not enable them with ability to learn, provide argumentation, or other higher level forms of behavior (Chesñevar et al. 2000; Stone and Veloso 2000). This is for the sake of more accurate evaluation of how basic mental actions and states can yield the real-world forms of behavior. However, the proposed simulation framework and representation language, which are logic-based, can accommodate more complex forms of behavior at a higher level of generality.

There are two types of application domains of the NL_MAMS beyond the autistic rehabilitation. Primarily, these are domains where simulation of beliefs of human agents is required (e.g. analysis buyers' behavior at e-commerce site). Another important type of NL_MAMS is a HCI setting where prediction of possible mental states of software users is essential (e.g. educational domain) simulation of human agent is necessary. Mental attitudes of a human agent constitute one of the most important components of the human factors any software system is expected to be aware of, and especially a personalized assistant. However, design and architecture of NL_MAMS follow the pragmatic purpose of being a generic efficient component of a wide range of large-scale systems, in particular, customer relation management (CRM) ones. Therefore, we don't target to build a computational model of the human cognitive process, unlike, for example, ACT-R approach (Anderson 1993) developed and used by cognitive psychologists.

NL_MAMS targets both cooperation and conflict domains. For the former, general models of teamwork and collaboration within AI include: STEAM and TEAMCORE (Tambe 1997), SharedPlans (Grosz and Kraus 1996) and COLLA-GEN (Rich and Sidner 1996). For a broad overview of teamwork in multiagent systems the reader is recommended (Stone and Veloso 2000).

There is a series of multiagent systems where agents are designed to implement *emotions* (Breazeal 1998). Also, a number of formalisms have been developed that handle the notion of emotion quite adequately (see e.g. Oatley and Jenkins 1996; Parameswaran 2001; Scheutz 2001). However, the target of our model for mental world, that includes emotions of participating agents, is quite different. As we experimentally discovered, to stimulate the emotional development of autistic trainees, the interface of the rehabilitation system does not have to display the emotional behavior explicitly; instead, the canonical explanation of the strict rules for emotions is required. We have learned from our experimental studies that when children start better operate with basic entities of knowing and believing and then proceed to the derived entities like *deceiving* and *pretending* using NL_MAMS, the further step to more complex mental and emotional behavior frequently comes easier and quite naturally.

Simulating the cognitive processes of another agent requires maintaining multiple worlds where epistemic states of individual agents can be loaded. The problem spaces in Soar (Rosenbloom et al. 1993) and alternate worlds in Polyscheme (Cassimatis 2005) are good examples for such capabilities, but most cognitive systems do not have such a mechanism. Soar's problem spaces facilitate subgoaling and have been used to anticipate opponent's behavior in the game of Quake (Laird 2001). Polyscheme's worlds are a general construct and allow for instantiation and manipulation of hypothetical, counterfactual, and even stochastic simulations. The alternate worlds in Polyscheme have been used to model spatial perspective-taking and theory of mind (Bello and Cassimatis 2006). The concept of simulating the cognitive processes of another agent (Trafton et al. 2013) suggested that an important consideration in designing an architecture for integrated intelligence, is how well the system works with a person. When a system uses representations and processes similar to a person's, it will be able to collaborate with a person better than a computational system that does not. Furthermore, such a system will be more compatible with human expectations of reasonable behavior, and thus more accommodating to the human. Kennedy et al. (2008) showed how the integration of mental simulation of a teammate within an embodied computational cognitive model can improve performance of the robotic teammate.

5.7.1 Commonsense Psychology System

Psychologists need to explicitly spell out a conceptual system of commonsense psychology. Smedslund (1989) is arguing that some knowledge engineering needs to be done in order to identify the implicit commonsense theories that people have of mental states and processes. What is remarkable about Smedslund and his research is that he has done two things that set him apart from other theorists in this area. First, he has attempted to execute this knowledge engineering task himself on a reasonably large scale, authoring a library of the concepts, definitions, and axioms of commonsense psychology that he calls "Psychologic" (Smedslund 1989). Second, he has attempted to validate the contents of this library of commonsense psychological knowledge by studying the degree to which people within and across cultures are in agreement about the truth of this knowledge. Smedslund describes Psychologic as follows:

"Psychologic is a project of explicating the implicit conceptual system of psychology embedded in ordinary language, or in other words, the basic assumptions and distinctions underlying our ways of thinking and talking about psychological phenomena. Psychologic identifies 22 primitive terms whose meanings are taken to be self-evident, namely terms for psychological states (aware, feel, want, belief, understand, strength), for temporal relationships (when, after, before, now), for action (act, talk, can, try, ability, difficulty, exertion), normative values (right, wrong, good, bad), and a term for people (person). Psychologic elaborates these primitive terms through 43 definitions, which take the form illustrated by the following examples, where the notation "= df" is taken to mean "is by definition equal to".

Definition 1.2.3 "Intentional" = df "directed by a preference for achieving a goal."

Definition 1.2.8 "X is relevant for achieving a goal G" = df "taking into account increases the likelihood of achieving G."

Definition 3.3.15 "Two wants are compatible" = df "Acting according to one of the two wants can be combined with acting according to the other."

Using these definitions, Psychologic presents 56 axioms to describe the conceptual relationships that exist between these terms, as in the following examples:

Axiom 3.5.1 The strength of P's belief X is directly proportional to P's estimate of the likelihood that X is the case.

Axiom 4.1.1 P's feeling follows from P's awareness of the relationship between P's wants and P's beliefs.

Axiom 5.3.15 All understanding depends on relevant pre-understanding.

Although the language of Psychologic is intended to be expressed by these primitive terms only, definitions, and axioms, the contents of Psychologic as a conceptual system are really elaborated in the statements that can be seen as direct consequences of this conceptual system. These consequences are presented in the form of 108 theorems, listed with short proofs written in English, and an additional 135 corollaries that are viewed as direct consequences of the axioms and theorems. Examples of each are as follows:

Theorem 1.2.10 P takes into account what P takes to be relevant for the achievement of P's goal.

Theorem 3.3.17 If the wants W1 and W2, are compatible, then they combine in such a way that W1 & W2 > W1 and W1 & W2 > W2.

Corollary 3.5.2 If P's belief A is stronger than P's belief B, then P's estimate of the likelihood of A is higher than P's estimate of the likelihood of A.

Corollary 3.7.3 Every person reflectively believes in the possibility of his or her nonexistence.

Smedslund's project has received a substantial amount of criticism within his own field, with detractors tending to outnumber advocates. Given the fair amount of discussion and academic debate of Smedslund's research that exists within this corner of the field of psychology, it is remarkable that this research remains so isolated from the other fields across the cognitive sciences that have a direct interest in commonsense psychology.

Smedslund draws no connection between his work and ongoing research on Theory of Mind in philosophy, to research on the acquisition of Theory of Mind in developmental and social psychology, or to work in the formalization of common-sense knowledge within the field of AI. At the same time, Smedslund's project has not received attention within these other fields. One should confirm that Smedslund advanced the inter-disciplinary connections between logic and psychology, given the degree to which each of these academic fields is isolated from each other.

5.7.2   A Symbolic Production-Based System

To better understand how engineering ToM Systems work, in this section we describe ACT-R is a hybrid symbolic/sub-symbolic production-based system. Modules in ACT-R are intended to represent relatively specific cognitive faculties such as declarative (fact-based) and procedural (rule-based) memory, visual and auditory perception, vocalization, and time perception. Buffers in ACT-R make up the working memory of a cognitive model. Some modules fill their buffers in response to the changes in the environment and all modules fill their buffers in response to explicit procedural requests. Like many production systems, ACT-R continuously matches production conditions against the working memory (buffers), selects a single production to fire, and then executes specified buffer changes and module requests which eventually result in updates to relevant buffers.

The project (Kennedy et al. 2008) embodied ACT-R on a human-scale robotic platform suited to use in indoor environments. It carries the sensors and provides onboard computing support for the multimodal sensing, navigation, and output. With ACT-R/E, Trafton et al. (2013) have extended the ACT-R architecture with rudimentary spatial reasoning (spatial module), localization and navigation faculties ("moval" module), and modified the visual, aural, and vocal modules to use actual robot sensors as shown in the architectural diagram in Fig. 5.9.

ACT-R architecture facilitates running additional cognitive models simultaneously. An ACT-R model consists of declarative and procedural memory and an initial goal. The ability of ACT-R to spawn a new model from within a running model allows cognitive system developers to represent and manipulate a mental model of another agent. To allow the base cognitive model to continue running while the simulation occurs, two models can run synchronously at the production-level. The flexibility of fixing the declarative memory and productions of the simulated mental model to a subset of the original model's allows the system to consider hypothetical and counterfactual situations.

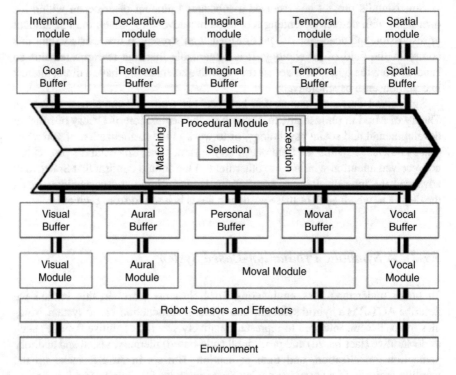

Fig. 5.9 ACT-R/E architecture (From Trafton et al. 2013)

5.8   Discussion and Conclusions

In this Chapter we constructed the engine which navigates through the mental world, operates with its language and makes decision on how the citizens of the mental world need to be tackled with. The functioning of this engine is an existential proof that a computational ToM exists and that it is sustainable, adaptable and intelligent as observed by external observers. ToM engine in the form of NL_MAMS is evaluated with respect to correctness, coverage and complexity, and can be integrated with other reasoning components and with machine learning, to perform both reasoning and cognitive tasks.

We demonstrated that reasoning about mental world can be implemented via exhaustive search through the possible actions and behaviors, evaluating achieved mental states. From the standpoint of axiomatic method, which combines pure (logical) axioms of inference with domain-specific (applied) axioms, generic representation of reasoning about mental world may be viewed as an augmentation of the former. Therefore we follow the classical axiomatic method stating that the same set of logical axioms is sufficient to perform reasoning in an arbitrary domain. In our case, the same axioms of the mental world (considered a pure, logical component) can be applied to an arbitrary physical world. In this chapter we have verified that the set of behaviors observed in one domain can be applied in an intact form to another domain with different physical axioms to produce adequate multiagent scenarios.

For an arbitrary set of mental formulas as an initial condition for NL_MAMS, it either finds a contradiction or synthesizes the scenario of multiagent behavior. NL_MAMS's vocabulary included the generic template for physical actions and rather extensive set of lexical units and synonyms for the common-usage mental entities. Also, it is worth mentioning that though each natural language has its own peculiarities of reasoning about mental attributes, replacing one natural language by another does not affect the suggested model for the mental world.

There are two aspects of NL_MAMS's contribution to the theory of mind training. Firstly, it introduces a new conceptual framework for treating mental entities in a way which the trainees are frequently ready to accommodate. The second aspect which seems to be more important for training practice is that NL_MAMS allows a much more persistent, consistent, and efficient approach because as a computer system, NL_MAMS can repeat exercises and vary them as many times as a trainee wishes. Moreover, a computer system is a more appealing interaction subject than a human peer in the case of autism.

It is worth mentioning that irrespectively of the capabilities of a particular child in mental reasoning and irrespectively of the NL_MAMS capabilities of delivering intuitive scenarios, the user interface of NL_MAMS kept the children attention quite tightly. Usually, it is rather hard to keep autistic trainees focused on any particular task; various means need to come into play to achieve such a focus, unless a relevant user interface is designed.

References

Ajzen I, Fishbein M (1980) Understanding attitudes and predicting social behavior. Prentice-Hall, Englewood Cliffs

Anderson J (1993) Rules of the mind. Lawrence Erlbaum Associates, Hillsdale

Axelrod R (1984) The evolution of cooperation. Basic Books, New York

Baron-Cohen S, Leslie AM, Frith U (1985) Does the autistic child have a "theory of mind"? Cognition 21:37–46

Bello P, Cassimatis N (2006) Developmental accounts of theory-of-mind acquisition: achieving clarity via computational cognitive modeling. In: Proceedings of the 28th annual conference of the Cognitive Science Society, pp 1014–1019

Bousquet O, Boucheron S, Lugosi G (2004) Introduction to statistical learning theory. Lect Notes in Artif Intell 3176:169–207

Breazeal C (1998) A motivational system for regulating human-robot interactions. In: Proceeding of the fifteenth national conference on AI (AAAI-98)

Buzing PC, Eiben AE, Schut MC (2005) Emerging communication and cooperation in evolving agent societies. J Artif Soc Soc Simul 8(1). http://jasss.soc.surrey.ac.uk/8/1/2.html

Cassimatis NL (2005) Integrating cognitive models based on different computational methods. Paper presented at the twenty-seventh annual conference of the Cognitive Science Society

Chesnevar C, Maguitman A, Loui R (2000) Logical models of argument. ACM Comput Surv 32(4):337–383 de Lara J, Alfonseca M (2000) Some strategies for the simulation of vocabulary agreement in multi-agent communities. J Artif Soc Soc Simul 3(4). http://www.soc.surrey.ac.uk/JASSS/3/4/2.html

d'Inverno M, Kinny D, Luck M, Wooldridge M (1998) A formal specification of dMARS, Intelligent Agents IV. In Singh, Rao, Wooldridge (eds) Proceedings of the 4th international workshop on agent theories, architectures and languages. LNAI 1365, pp 155–176

Fagin R, Halpern JY, Moses Y, Vardi MY (1996) Reasoning about knowledge. MIT Press, Cambridge, MA/London

Gabbay DM (1999) Action, time and default. In: Levesque HJ, Pirri F (eds) Logical foundations for cognitive agents. Springer, Berlin/Heidelberg/New York

Galan JM, Izquierdo LR (2005) Appearances can be deceiving: lessons learned re-implementing Axelrod's 'evolutionary approach to norms. J Artif Soc Soc Simul 8(3). http://jasss.soc.surrey.ac.uk/8/3/2.html

Galitsky B (2002) Extending the BDI model to accelerate the mental development of autistic patients. Second international conference on development & learning. Cambridge, MA

Galitsky B (2003) Natural language question answering system: technique of semantic headers. Advanced Knowledge Intl, Adelaide

Galitsky B (2004) A library of behaviors: implementing commonsense reasoning about mental world. KES 2004 LNAI 3215, pp 307–313

Galitsky B (2006) Reasoning about mental attitudes of complaining customers. Knowl-Based Syst Elsevier 19(7):592–615

Galitsky B (2013) A computational simulation tool for training autistic reasoning about mental attitudes. Knowl-Based Syst 50:25–43

Galitsky BA, Kuznetsov SO (2008) Learning communicative actions of conflicting human agents. J Exp Theor Artif Intell 20(4):277–317

Galitsky B, González MP, Chesñevar CI (2009) A novel approach for classifying customer complaints through graphs similarities in argumentative dialogues. Decis Support Syst 46(3):717–729

Grosz BJ, Kraus S (1996) Collaborative plans for complex group actions. AIJ 86:269–358

Kaiser MD, Shiffrar M (2009) The visual perception of motion by observers with autism spectrum disorders: a review and synthesis. Psychon Bull Rev 16:761–777

Kaminka GA, Frenkel I (2005) Flexible teamwork in behavior-based robots. In AAAI-05

Kaminka GA, Tambe M (2000) Robust multi-agent teams via socially-attentive monitoring. JAIR 12:105–147

Kennedy WG, Bugajska MD, Harrison AM, Trafton JG (2008) Like-me simulation as an effective and cognitively plausible basis for social robotics. Int J Soc Robot 1(2):181–194

Laird JE (2001) It knows what you're going to do: adding anticipation to a quakebot. In: Proceedings of the fifth international conference on autonomous agents. ACM, New York

Levesque HJ, Reiter R, Lesperance Y, Lin F, Scherl RB (1997) GOLOG: a logic programming language for dynamic domains. J Log Program 31:59–84

Li G, Hopgood AA, Weller MJ (2003) Shifting matrix management: a model for multi-agent cooperation. Eng Appl Artif Intell 16(3):191–201

McCarthy J (1995) Making robots conscious of their mental states. In: Proceedings of machine intelligence conference 15

Oatley K, Jenkins J (1996) Understanding emotions. Blackwell, Oxford

Olivia C, Chang CF, Enguix CF, Ghose AK (1999) Case-based BDI agents: an effective approach for intelligent search on the World Wide Web. Intelligent Agents in cyberspace. Papers from 1999 AAAI spring symposium

Parameswaran N (2001) Emotions in Intelligent Agents. FLAIRS-01, Pensacola Beach, pp 82–86

Reiter R (1993) Proving properties of states in the situational calculus. AI 64:337–351

Rich C, Sidner CL (1996) COLLAGEN: a collaboration manager for software interface agents. User Model User-Adap Inter 8(3–4):315–350

Rosenbloom PS, Laird JE, Newell A (1993) The SOAR papers. MIT Press, Cambridge, MA

Rosenschein J, Zlotkin G (1994) Rules of encounter: designing conventions for automated negotiation among computers. MIT Press, Cambridge, MA

Scheutz M (2001) Agents with or without emotions. FLAIRS-01, Pensacola Beach, pp 89–93

Shanahan M (1997) Solving the frame problem. MIT Press, Cambridge, MA

Shoham Y (1993) Agent oriented programming. Artif Intell 60(1):51–92

Sloman A (2000) Architecture-based conceptions of mind. In: Proceedings of the 11th international congress of logic, methodology and philosophy of science. Kluwer, Dordrecht, p 397

Smedslund J (1989) What is psychologic? Recent trends in theoretical psychology. In: Part of the series recent research in psychology, pp 453–457

Stein GC, Barnden JA (1995) Towards more flexible and common-sensical reasoning about beliefs. In 1995 AAAI spring symposium on representing mental states and mechanisms. AAAI Press, Menlo Park

Stone P, Veloso M (2000) Multiagent systems: a survey from a machine learning perspective. Auton Robot 8(3):345–383

Tambe M (1997) Agent architectures for flexible, practical teamwork. In: Proceedings of the national conference on artificial intelligence (AAAI). August, 1997

Tamma V, Phelps S, Dickinso I, Wooldridge M (2005) Ontologies for supporting negotiation in e-commerce. Eng Appl Artif Intell 18(2):223–236

Trafton GJ, Laura MH, Anthony MH, Franklin PT II, Sangeet SK, Alan CS (2013) ACT-R/E: an embodied cognitive architecture for human-robot interaction. J Hum-Robot Interact 2(1):30–55

Walton DN, Krabbe E (1995) Commitment in dialogue. Basic concepts of interpersonal reasoning. State University of New York Press, Albany

Weigand H, de Moor A (2004) Argumentation semantics of communicative action. In: Proceedings of the 9th international working conference on the Language-Action Perspective on communication modelling (LAP 2004), Rutgers University, NJ, USA

Winograd T, Flores F (1986) Understanding computers and cognition: a new foundation for design. Alex, Norwood

Wooldridge M (2000) Reasoning about rational agents. MIT Press, Cambridge, MA

Yu R, Iung B, Panetto H (2003) A multi-agents based E-maintenance system with case-based reasoning decision support. Eng Appl Artif Intell 16(4):321–333

Chapter 6
Reasoning Beyond the Mental World

Whereas for CwA reasoning about mental world is the key for they successful adaptation to the real world and development, other limitations of reasoning are needed to be addressed as well. We focus on various forms of reasoning and rationality and conclude which reasoning features need to be learned and in which form.

6.1 Mental vs Physical World

Mental-physical distinction is considered a fundamental cornerstone of ToM, and one that is not explicitly taught by parents or teachers. The test for this distinction involves the child listening to stories in which one character is having a mental experience (e.g., believing that the rain will start) whilst a second character is having a physical experience (e.g., getting wet from this rain). The experimenter then asks the subject to judge which operations the two characters can perform (e.g., which character can stroke the dog?). Whilst 3–4 year old normal children can easily make these judgments, thereby showing their good understanding of the differences between mental and physical entities and events, CwA have been found to be significantly impaired.

In the literature on autism, mental and physical worlds are usually considered from distinct standpoints in terms of children capability to reason about them. Baron-Cohen et al. (2001) define *folk psychology* as comprising both low-level social perception, and higher-level social intelligence.

Low-level here broadly refers to skills present in human infancy (Johnson 2000). These include being able to judge:

1. if something is a human agent, animal or neither (Premack 1990);
2. if another person is looking at you or not;

© Springer International Publishing Switzerland 2016 215
B. Galitsky, *Computational Autism*, Human–Computer Interaction Series,
DOI 10.1007/978-3-319-39972-0_6

3. if another individual is expressing a basic emotion (Ekman 1992), and if so, what type.
4. if engaging in shared attention, for example by following gaze or pointing gestures (Mundy and Crowson 1997; Tomasello 1988);
5. showing concern or basic empathy at another's distress, or responding appropriately to another's basic emotional;
6. being able to judge an agent's goal or basic intention (Premack 1990).

Higher-level here refers to skills present from early childhood and which continue to develop throughout the lifespan. These include the following:

1. Attribution of the bread spectrum of mental states to herself and others, including pretense, deception, belief (Leslie 1987);
2. being able to recognize and respond appropriately to complex emotions, not just basic ones (Harris et al. 1989);
3. being able to link such mind-reading to action, including language, and therefore to understand and produce pragmatically appropriate language (Tager-Flusberg 1989);
4. using mind-reading not only to make sense of others' behavior, but also to predict it, and even manipulate it;
5. having a sense of what is appropriate in different social contexts, based on what others will think of our own behavioral conduct;
6. having empathic understanding of another mind. This understanding includes the skills involved in normal reciprocal social relationships and in communication.

According to (Baron-Cohen et al. 2001), folk psychology domain is quite focused and narrowly defined with the focus of understanding the mental world and social causality between its inhabitants. At the same time, folk physics comprises both low-level perception of physical causality, and higher-level understanding of physical causality. Low-level here refers broadly to skills present in early human learning of th e physical world, such as the perception of physical causality (Leslie and Keeble 1987) and expectations concerning the positions, speeds and other properties of physical objects. Higher-level here refers to skills present from early childhood and which continue to develop throughout the lifespan, the entities related to mechanics (Karmiloff-Smith 1992). Similarly to folk psychology, folk physics is not expected to rely on a single cognitive process.

Both mental and physical domains:

1. are aspects of our causal cognition and are associated with causal links;
2. are acquired and/or developed in a universal way,
3. show little if any cultural variability,
4. have a specific but universal ontogenesis,
5. are adaptive,
6. may be open to neurological dissociation.

Baron-Cohen et al. (2001) employed the model that the human brain has evolved in at least two independent directions of cognition: folk psychology and folk physics. In the extreme case, severe autism may be characterized by a total lack of folk psychology (and thus "mindblindness"). Autism spectrum conditions come by degrees, so different points on the autistic spectrum may involve degrees of deficit in folk psychology (Baron-Cohen 1995). In CwA who have no accompanying mental disability (having intelligence in the normal range), the child's folk physics would develop not only normally, but even at a superior level. AS children were functioning significantly above their mental age in terms of folk physics, but significantly below their mental age in terms of folk psychology.

Impaired folk psychology, together with superior folk physics in AS might be partly the result of a genetic liability. This is because autism appears to be heritable (Gillberg 1991), and because there is every reason to expect that individuals with such a cognitive profile could have been selected for in hominid evolution. Good folk physics would have possess important advantages in using tools and hunting skills.

Different computer systems operate in physical and mental worlds, including multiagent systems. Control systems, device drivers and auto-pilots are examples of the former world, whereas search, recommendation, decision-support and customer care systems need to simulate and take into account user intent and mental worlds of their users (Galitsky et al. 2009).

6.1.1 Autistic Generalization

Although children with ASD can be guided to make a generalization from parts to whole, they have difficulty with inference making at the abstract level. Preschool CwA can categorize animate and inanimate objects based on surface features (Johnson and Rakison 2006). CwA tend to rely on explicit rules only to support inductive inferences such as an entity that have legs versus things that have wheels. These explicit rules lead them to make some inappropriate categorizations such as classifying a table as an animal. CwA are unable to perform a metareasoning task (Sect. 4.1.3) to decide when it requires the information on a prototype or some kind of abstract representation. For example, it is hard to CwA to formulate features of animate and inanimate objects that would distinguish these objects beyond surface appearances. CwA are delayed in the process of concept formation, performing more like infants than typically developing children of the same preschool age. However CwA sometimes rely on inductive reasoning to form categories, although they did not always attend to all the defining attributes. This suggests that CwA may rely on their ability to focus on details that are salient to them, ignoring other attributes that matter. Hence CwA may benefit from guided concept formation that calls attention to those attributes that distinguish one concept from another.

Abstract reasoning skills are particularly critical for reading comprehension, especially when reading narrative text. Reading expository text, such as a set of rules or directions, or descriptions of processes, requires less abstraction than reading narrative, where readers engage cognitive processes to infer character's traits, draw conclusions, and identify causal attributes. CwA typically prefer expository text, such as science texts. This may be because they find narrative text especially challenging because it required abstract and social reasoning patterns (Randi et al. 2010).

6.2   Reasoning, Cognitive Science and Rationality

Autistic individuals, along with machine intelligence systems, are considered less rational reasoners compared to control. In this section we treat in depth the issue of rationality and explore the directions rationality of CwA can be intervened.

Traditionally, rationality is taken to be a defining characteristic of human nature: "man is a rational animal," apparently capable of deliberate thought, planning, problem-solving, scientific theorizing and prediction, moral reasoning, and so forth. "Rational" means here a rational discourse where an agent wants to arrive at justified true belief. This definition of rationality is from an era oriented toward theory. A pragmatically oriented definition extends this concept of rationality to actions. "Rational agency" can be defined (MIT Encyclopedia of Cognitive Science) as a coherence requirement:

> agent must have a means-end competence to fit its actions or decisions, according to its beliefs or knowledge representations, to its desires or goal-structure.

Without such coherence there is no agent. The main condition here is *fit* that has a logical load. If an action is performed which is not part of a plan derived to achieve a given goal, there is no fit. In this sense checking the weather before getting online and logging on to the network is irrational, as well as first plugging out the power unit of a modem.

CwA are capable of making decisions, applying knowledge available to them and based on available beliefs, achieve their desires. For example, by bursting into tantrum and crying to make his mother give him some chips. His action of crying fits to the desire of getting chips, which would be hard to achieve otherwise.

At the same time, CwA are simplest such rational agents in terms of amount of knowledge and structure and depth of beliefs, due to their special cognitive skills.

Judged by these standards, reasoning of CCs, not just CwA in the laboratory is very poor and irrational (as shown by the seminal experiments of (Wason 1968) for logic and (Kahneman and Tversky 1972) for probability), and it has therefore been said that humans, both PwA and controls are actually not rational in the sense defined above. The objective is to make the reasoning of CwA as rational as possible.

Wason describes the students in his experiments showing irrationality of human thinking.

> The old ways of seeing things now look like absurd prejudices, but our highly intelligent student volunteers display analogous miniature prejudices when their premature conclu-

sions are challenged by the facts. As Kuhn has shown, old paradigms do not die in the face of a few counterexamples. In the same way, our volunteers do not often accommodate their thought to new observations, even those governed by logical necessity, in a deceptive problem situation. They will frequently deny the facts, or contradict themselves, rather than shift their frame of reference.

Stanovich (1999) discussion of rules governing reasoning introduces a distinction between normative, descriptive, and prescriptive rules. We give brief characterizations of the three kinds, followed by representative examples.

- *Normative rules*: reasoning as it should be, ideally. These rules should be taught to CwA in its original form

  - *Modus tollens*: $\neg q, p \to q / \neg p$
  - Bayes' theorem: $P(D \mid S) = P(S \mid D)P(D)/P(S)$.

- *Descriptive rules*: reasoning as it is actually practiced. These should be explained to CwA as being used by other people, so that CwA can better understand them. CwA are also encouraged to apply these rules if normative rules are not applicable.

  - Many people do not endorse *modus tollens* and believe that from $\neg q, p \to q$ nothing can be derived.
  - In doing probabilistic calculations people do not do normalization and assume $P(D \mid S) = P(S \mid D)$. For example, estimating a probability of a disease given a set of symptoms, specialists neglect the base rate, the one occurring among healthy people.

- *Prescriptive rules* result from taking into account our bounded rationality, i.e., computational limitations (due to the computational complexity of classical logic, and the even higher complexity of probability theory) and storage limitations (the impossibility of simultaneously representing all factors relevant to a computation, say, of a plan to achieve a given goal). Prescriptive rules should be taught to CwA for approximation of what can be derived in the real world.

  - The classically invalid principle $\neg q, p \wedge r \to q / \neg p \wedge \neg r$ is correct according to closed–world reasoning, which is computationally much less complex than classical propositional logic, and helps with memory issues when implemented in a computer.

In terms of these three kinds of rules, Stanovich distinguishes the following positions on the relationship between reasoning and rationality:

Human reasoning competence and performance is actually normatively correct. What appears to be incorrect reasoning can be explained by such maneuvers as different task construal, a different interpretation of logical terms, etc.

Actual human performance follows prescriptive rules, but the latter are in general (and necessarily) subnormal, because of the heavy computational demands of normatively correct reasoning. The performance of actual human reasoning still does not reach prescriptive standards, which are themselves subnormal; and this is a significant potential improvement area for rehabilitation of autistic reasoning.

In the life of CC, reasoning happens infrequently in everyday life, and mainly in schools. And for CC the true rationality is adaptiveness in taking quick decisions that are optimal given constraints of time and energy. On the contrary, we expect CwA who acquired reasoning skills and axioms as a result of training to reason intensively behaving in everyday life. Even though adaptation capabilities of CwA are rather limited, learned rules are supposed to compensate for it and still maintain acceptable behavior. Hence the role of learning and applying rules is higher for CwA compared with CC.

Interpretation of formal symbols is of high importance in reasoning. But even if interpretation is important, and interpretations may differ from person to person, people may reason in ways that are inconsistent with their chosen interpretation. From a methodological point of view this means that if one uses a particular interpretation to explain something, one must have evidence for the interpretation that is independent of this "something". Stanovich's scheme is predicated on the assumption that reasoning is about following rules from a fixed, given set, say classical logic, rules that should apply always and everywhere. For if there is no given set of rules which constitutes the norm, and the norm is instead relative to a "domain," then the domain may well include the cognitive constraints that gave rise to the notion of prescriptive rules, thus promoting the latter to the rank of norm.

Piaget's *logicism* (Piaget 1953) tells that the acquisition of formal-deductive operations is due to cognitive development. Piaget was the first to show that preschool children are not capable of applying classical predicate logic; they need to grow older to do that. This is in contradiction with Wason's selection task, a striking deviation from classical logical reasoning. Piaget's work can be considered as undermining the role of logic as an inference mechanism. A further criticism concerned the alleged slowness of logical inference mechanisms, especially when search is involved, for example when backtracking from a given goal. The production system of Newell and Simon only includes *modus ponens* rule, allowing fast forward inference process, but the other forms if inference are substantially slower.

A few decades back the production systems were used and explore the manipulation of mental representation. *Logicism* is one central characterizing of production system models which is followed in this book's rehabilitation strategy. As production systems involve, perception and action are added to production systems to approach active learning (Sect. 7.3). Modern production systems preserve Logicism and follow the *sense-think-act* cycle. At the same time, Piaget theory of cognitive development accepts the idea that Logicism is founded upon actions in the world. From both computational and experimental observations one can see that human cognition is based on *sense-think-act* and *sense-act* chains. The external world starts to play more important role in the cognition; some researchers argue that cognition is mediated by a set of cognitive agents (Minsky 2006). Then the process of thinking is not just application of logical rules but instead a combination of *sense-think-act* and *sense-act* chains which interact with the real world to solve problems (Wilson and Dupuis 2010).

If logical laws were like physical, empirical laws about psychological events, they would have to be approximate, preliminary and subject to refinement, like all laws in natural science. But logical laws are exact and unassailable, hence they cannot be empirical. Psychologism about logical laws also leads to skeptical relativism: as we observe in CwA, different people reason according to different logical laws, so that what is true for one person may not be true for another – truth, however, is absolute, not indexed to a person.

Stenning and van Lambalgen (2008) analyzed several tasks on which autistic people are known to fail, such as the false belief task and the box task, and find that these tasks have a common logical structure which is identical to that of the suppression task (McKenzie et al. 2011). This leads to a prediction for autistic people's behavior on the suppression task. Both adolescents with ASD and typically developing controls were presented with conditional reasoning problems using familiar content. The task relies on both valid and fallacious conditional inferences that would otherwise be suppressed if counterexample cases are brought to mind. Such suppression occurs when additional premises are presented, whose effect is to suggest such counterexample cases. In this study (Stenning and van Lambalgen 2008) predicted and observed that this suppression effect was substantially and significantly weaker for autistic participants than for CC. The authors conclude that CwA are less contextualized in their reasoning, a finding that can be linked to research on autism on a variety of other cognitive tasks.

6.3   Autistic Probabilistic and Counterfactual Reasoning

Probabilistic inference and conditioning calculates the conditional probabilities of dependence between states. If event A only correlated with event B dependent on event C, then C defeats A as a cause of B (Gopnik et al. 2001). Counterfactual and subtractive reasoning is focused on predicting mental states which are dependent on facts known to be false. Studies of typically developing children have shown strong associations between false belief and subtractive reasoning tasks (Harris et al. 1996; Peterson and Galitsky 2004).

Counterfactual version of the false belief task has been proposed by Riggs et al. (2000). This task was intended to show that difficulties in counterfactual reasoning cause unsuccessful performance in the false belief task. In each condition, a false belief state task and a corresponding physical state task in the same domain were constructed. For example, the following image of the Maxi task was constructed: a child, a mother-doll and an experimenter are in a kitchen. The child sees that there is a chocolate in the fridge. The mother-doll now bakes a chocolate cake, in the process of which the chocolate moves from fridge to cupboard. The experimenter now asks the child: *Where would the chocolate be if mother hadn't baked a cake?*

The structure of answers is highly correlated with that on the false belief task. Before the cut-off age of four, the child answers: 'in the cupboard'; afterwards, she answers 'in the fridge'. There is no ToM involved in answering correctly; instead one needs insight into the commonsense reasoning inertia of the world: states only change when they are affected by actions, explicit causes. It is unclear what causes the younger child to answer 'in the cupboard': a simple failure to apply inertial reasoning can bring the response 'it could be anywhere', due to the events that could have happened in this alternative world.

Answers such as this would be yielded by applying causal reasoning without closed world reasoning for occurrences of events. The answer 'in the cupboard' more likely reflects a failure to apply causal reasoning altogether, turning instead to a "default" response. In one out of three of (Riggs and Peterson 2000) experiments the false belief task was considerably more difficult for the children than the counterfactual task, since ToM reasoning is the hardest for CwA.

Peterson and Bowler (2000) demonstrated this issue by comparing CwA, CC and children with severe learning problems' performance on false belief tasks and counterfactual tasks. CC showed high correlation on these tasks, but a dissociation turned out to be obvious in both CwA and children with severe learning problems. For all children, the majority of those who failed the counterfactual task also failed the false belief task, due to the fact that the counterfactual reasoning domain is necessary for the false belief domain. Three-quarters of the typically developing children who completed the counterfactual task also pass the false belief task, but these ratios go down in the other groups: sixty % in children with learning difficulties, 44 % CwA. The authors suggest that one factor is the necessity to 'generate' Maxi's false belief, whereas in the counterfactual task the false statement is given. The authors also show the correlation of this feature with other supposed failures of the ability to generalize in autism (Sect. 6.4), such as the difficulty of spontaneous recall compared to cued recall. In the false belief task the CwA and CC have to see the relevance of Maxi's not observing the crucial event to perform the computation. In the counterfactual task all the ingredients are given, and only an inertial computation is necessary.

In terms of CwA education, our conclusion is that the axioms of inertia need to be taught for both mental and physical worlds.

The understanding of emotions based on counterfactual reasoning was studied (Begeer et al. 2014). Children were presented with eight stories about two characters who experienced the same positive or negative outcome, either due to their own action or by default. Relative to the comparison group, children with high-functioning autism spectrum disorder were poor at explaining emotions based on downward counterfactual reasoning (i.e. *contentment* and *relief*). There were no group differences in upward counterfactual reasoning (i.e. *disappointment* and *regret*). In the comparison group, second-order false-belief reasoning was related to children's understanding of second-order counterfactual emotions (i.e. regret and relief), while children in the high-functioning autism spectrum disorder group relied more on their general intellectual skills.

All scenarios involved two characters who experienced the same outcome (i.e. both either achieve or do not achieve what they desire). For the target character, a counterfactual alternative was available that would have resulted in a better (upward) or worse (downward) outcome. In the simple stories, emotions were yielded by demonstrating that the target character nearly achieved a positive or negative outcome. The near attainment of the outcome was intended to yield disappointment (when a positive outcome was avoided) or contentment (when a negative outcome was avoided). In the second-order emotion stories, a target character always made an active decision that led to the avoidance of a positive or negative result. This was intended to yield regret or relief. At the end of each story, children were reminded of the outcome and of the critical element of the story that differentiated the characters involved. Following this, children were asked whether one character would feel "better," "worse," or "the same" about the results compared to the other character and explain why.

6.3.1 Example Relief Story and Questions

Bill and Pete are going on a school trip. They are allowed to choose between going on a sports day in the playing fields or to a kids' museum. Bill wants to go to the museum. Pete chooses the sports day. When the teacher asks them what they chose, Bill says he wants to go to the museum. Pete changes his mind and also says he wants to go to the museum. On the day of the trip, it is pouring with rain. Children who chose to go to the sports day in the playing fields have to stay at school.

Questions Who is happier about choosing the museum, Bill, who chose the museum right away, or Pete, who changed his mind, or do you think they are both equally happy? Why?

6.3.2 Example Regret Story and Questions

Miriam and Susan go to the same school. Miriam usually takes the bus. Susan usually goes on her bike. Today, Susan decides to take the bus. Both Susan and Miriam are waiting at the bus stop but the bus does not come, and they have to wait a long time for the next bus. They both arrive at school very late.

Questions Who is more annoyed with being late for school, Miriam, who usually takes the bus, or Susan, who usually goes by bike, or do you think they are both equally annoyed? Why?

6.4 Autistic Planning and Adjustment of Action to a New Environment

Current studies of autistic reasoning overlooked such aspect of reasoning as operating beyond strict rule-following. Everyday reasoning requires more than applying literal rules since most all rules are associated with exceptions. Most rules in the real life are *defeasible* and can be modified as new information comes. For example, we put on our own shoes to go out and assume it will fit. However, we will withdraw this assumption if it turns out that someone put a small ball in the shoe. Since one has to adjust a conclusion when the context changes, some flexibility in reasoning is required to handle cases with exceptions.

Although reasoning about the physical world of autistic patients is corrupted in a lesser degree than reasoning about mental world (Galitsky 2002), it still has serious limitations and needs to be substantially improved. Various reasoning domains that are the subjects of explorations in traditional logical Artificial Intelligence, such as space, time, and probabilities are explored in the context of autism. It turns out that each of these domains is affected of autistic development in one way or another. In this section we focus on autistic way to adjust actions to a new environment, employing a formalism of default logic (Brewka et al. 1995; Bochman 2001). The finding here is that while people with autism may be able to process single default rules, they have a characteristic difficulty in cases where multiple default rules conflict. Even though default reasoning is intended to simulate the reasoning of typical human subjects, it turns out that following the operational semantics of default reasoning in a literal way leads to the peculiarities of autistic behavior observed in the literature (Peterson and Galitsky 2004).

6.4.1 Triangulation Structure

We first introduce the concept of triangulation by way of an illustrative scenario:

> *Arthur habitually follows a route to school which involves walking straight down a particular pavement. One day this pavement is blocked by a puddle. Should Arthur walk straight through the puddle, or walk round it?*

What Arthur needs to do in this example is to depart temporarily from his standard route to school, in response to a passing circumstance. He does not need to jettison or revise this standard route: tomorrow, when there is no puddle, he can follow it without interference. But today his actions need to reflect a compromise between the standard route and the additional circumstance. This structure can be represented as follows. The basic unit of knowledge (in this case, the standard route to school) we call the *source* (S). The default, usual, normal action (such as walking straight ahead) that can be performed when the source is as usual, or considered in isolation, is called the *generic action* (G). The additional factor (the presence of a puddle) that indicates a modification, adjustment of this norm, we call the *context*

(C). And when the context causes us to select an adjustment of the generic action G (to walking round the puddle), we call this a *triangulated action* (T). Thus we have the following structure:

> S: *the standard route to school*
> G: *walk straight*
> C: *today there is a puddle in the way*
> T: *walk round it.*

In such situations two separate perspectives, the source and the context, bear on the same issue of action. The agent is thus faced with the cognitive task of coordinating these demands, in a process of practical reasoning which we call *triangulation*:

> S, so do G, but C, so do T

This kind of task can be encountered by any cognitive system, whether natural or artificial, but our present concern is with people with autism. We therefore turn to a series of tendencies found in autism, in each case using the triangulation structure identified above to analyze an illustrative example. This serves two purposes:

1. It reveals a pattern common to some of the tendencies found in autism, thus advancing our conceptualization of the syndrome.
2. It provides a systematic basis for computer support which allows users to navigate and experiment with these structures.

It is worth emphasizing from the outset that we are dealing here with tendencies: people with autism do not follow these patterns all of the time (and people without autism do not always avoid them). Rather the point is that where these tendencies do occur, their structure can be identified.

6.4.2   Triangulation Cases

Case 1: Performance of Routines People with autism show an inflexible relationship with routines. On an occasion when it seems that the best thing is to alter, abbreviate or terminate the performance of a routine, the person with autism may step through a standard procedure in a manner which is 'rigid', 'formal', 'obsessive', or 'ritualistic' (Kanner 1943, DSM C). A typical example follows.

> *Arthur's routine for getting up in the morning takes 30 minutes and involves a shower, washing, drying and brushing his hair, eating a breakfast of muesli, toast and tea, and brushing his teeth for 2 minutes. He begins this at 8.00 am, so as to be ready for the school bus at 8.32 am. One day, when Arthur is in mid-routine, his mother receives a phone call saying that the school bus will arrive 10 minutes early, so she tells this to Arthur through the bathroom door. Should Arthur continue to enact his routine as usual, or should he omit or accelerate parts of it so as to catch the bus on time?*

We have here a routine which is perfectly reasonable, but an occasion on which an adjustment is needed. One solution, for example, would be to omit breakfast, and eat a sandwich on the bus instead. (Another solution would be to do everything more quickly than usual.) This gives the following pattern of reasoning:

S: the usual routine
G: enact it all as usual
C: but today time is short
T: omit part of it

The inflexibility found in autism in this regard consists in a tendency to choose the generic action (G) rather than the triangulated action (T) in such structures. The routine is enacted in a manner that is unresponsive to special circumstances: faithful to one perspective rather than two. Furthermore, the person may become upset and agitated when asked to adjust, indicating that this is not easy to do. This is not to say that routines are bad, or that this one is in need of revision. Routines serve as labor-saving devices, and this one promotes hygiene, nourishment and dental care. Rather, the problem in the example scenario is that the routine and its goals constitute one of two frames of reference, and a compromise is needed. Again, this is not to say that accommodation of a second perspective is necessarily a good thing: Arthur might have decided that he is tired of being messed about by an unreliable bus service and so he will let things go wrong. However, in the cases typically seen in autism the second perspective is not rationally rejected, but is simply unengaged.

Case 2: Informing We now turn to another area of the symptomatology of autism in which, despite superficial differences, the same structural features operate. Among the communication difficulties found in autism are tendencies to *over-inform*. That is, where only part of a story is relevant to a particular audience or topic of conversation, the person with autism may nevertheless recite the story from beginning to end and in all its detail. (Equally, where expansion and extra explanation are needed, there is a tendency in autism to *under-inform*). There can be many reasons for editing the telling of a story: perhaps only part of a story is relevant to the current conversation, perhaps the audience was present during most of events described, perhaps one of the audience becomes visibly upset as we start to tell the story. There follows an illustrative example:

> *Earlier in the year, Arthur took a trip in which he travelled by bicycle from York to London, visiting museums along the way, and on arriving in London he happened to eat a hamburger. One day, Arthur meets some people who ask him about the quality of hamburgers in London. Should he tell the whole story of his trip, or just the part about the hamburger?*

The story of Arthur's trip is a data structure whose default execution is step-by-step recitation starting at the beginning. This might be just what is needed, for example when recording it in a diary. However in the present context what is needed is a compromise in which the part about the hamburger is selected and the rest only briefly mentioned, as follows.

S: the story of my journey
G: tell it exhaustively from beginning to end
C: but we are talking about hamburgers
T: tell that part only

The over-informing found in autism consists in a tendency to choose G rather than T in such structures. One point which this characterization brings out is that this tendency concerns the use of knowledge rather and simply its existence (Peterson and Bowler 2000). In our example, Arthur knows the story of his trip, and he knows that he has been asked about hamburgers: what is missing is a coordinated response to the two. This tendency may cause trouble, since the capacity to adjust the presentation of information is central to communication, rhetoric and tact, all of which show deficit in autism. No general value judgment is forthcoming here: whether we prefer the charm of smooth talking to a grave and comprehensive recitation of facts will vary from case to case. However, as above, in the cases typically seen in autism the grave recitation is due to insulation rather than judgment.

Case 3: Tunnel or Jump In conversation, CwA tend either to 'tunnel' on one subject, or suddenly to 'jump'—change the subject—destroying narrative coherence.

> *S: a new subject occurs to me*
> *G: change the subject to this*
> *C: but the conversation's theme is ...*
> *T: stick to the theme*

Case 4: Interpretation of Ambiguity Homonyms are the words in written form that have two (or more) meanings with different associated pronunciations. Autistics are unreliable in choosing the one that is indicated by sentence context.

> S: 'tear' can mean X or Y
> G: take either
> C: but the sentence context indicates Y
> T: use Y

There is a class of social interactions that involve our predicting and/or explaining the actions of other participants, but in which the relevant predictions and explanations seem to develop without us having to attribute propositional attitudes. These social interactions rest on what social psychologists call "scripts" ("frames" in artificial intelligence), that is, complex information structures that allow predictions to be made on the basis of the specification of the purpose of some social practice (for example, eating a meal at a restaurant), the various individual roles, and the appropriate sequence of moves.

Case 5: Social Scripts Brittleness & amalgamation of exceptions

> *Arthur is told not to speak to strangers in the street. Some policemen address him, and he ignores them and gets into trouble.*
>
> *S: ignore strangers in the street, and these are strangers*
> *G: ignore them*
> *C: but these are policemen*
> *T: talk to them.*

Case 5': Social Scripts 2

> *Arthur was taught a conversation routine involving sitting near a person and nodding. He got on the underground late at night, entered a carriage with just one old lady in it, and began his routine. She panicked.*

S: this is my conversation routine
G: do it
C: but this is an old lady and she looks frightened
T: stop

Case 6. Executive Function People with autism show poor performance on clinical tests of executive function (Sect. 2.5.2). In the experiment on the proper timing of actions, the participant is asked to grab a marble from a box, <u>after</u> pushing a switch.

S: grab the marble
G: do it now
C: the switch needs to be pushed first
T: do it (grab the marble) afterwards

Autistics show 'pre-potency' (in relation to C). In the Wisconsin Card Sort Test they show 'perseveration' (in relation to C): they carry on doing something after it has stopped serving its purpose.

Case 7: Generalization There exist situations in which the main point or purpose is not stated explicitly, and so constitutes an implicit context.

> *Arthur is asked by his father to empty all the waste paper baskets in the house. When he has finished, his father asks why he has not emptied two receptacles. Arthur replies that these are bins, not baskets.*

Once the context has been detected it can be applied as follows.

S: I am emptying baskets, and these two are bins
G: ignore them
C: but the goal is to remove rubbish, and they contain rubbish
T: empty them too.

In several of the cases given so far, the context serves to narrow our range of actions, causing us to omit certain possibilities or at least select a partial case of them. In the above case the opposite is true: apprehension of the context broadens our understanding of the situation and extends our range of actions.

Case 8′: Controlling the Scope of Actions

> *Arthur is found pulling up flowers on the north side garden. His mother says 'please don't do that'. So Arthur then goes to the south side of the garden and carries on pulling up flowers there.*

The main point or objective here was not stated explicitly by Arthur's mother. Unless Arthur detects it or makes a guess at it, it will seem reasonable to do as he does.

S: I am no longer on the north side of the garden, and here are some flowers
G: pull them up
C: but the point of the previous request was to preserve the flower beds in the garden
T: don't pull them up.

Case 8: Alternative Contexts Another case in which we need to project possible contexts is when we try to think of alternative uses for an object. In which new contexts could the object serve a useful function?

Arthur is asked 'think of lots of uses for a brick'. He refers to standard examples, as indicated by the definition of a brick, rather than connecting with alternative contexts so as to give alternative uses.

S: bricks are for building
G: give examples of building
C: but I need an ashtray (imagined), and bricks have appropriate indentations
T: give example of ashtray

Case 9: Suppression of Irrelevant Details   A common occurrence in autism is that a person focuses on insignificant or non-functional details in a situation. These can be parts or aspects of objects or situations that would normally be regarded as inconsequential (American Psychiatric Association 2000). This inconsequentiality is not an inherent feature of the detail in question, but rather a relation with a context; it is determined by seeing that the detail is not relevant to the purpose or function expressed in the context. The detail may be inherently interesting, but from the perspective of the context it is not. The context says *ignore such details, we have a job to do*. Therefore, what we need to do (in the current situation) is to subtract or ignore the detail in question. The question is the usual one: S may be correct or interesting, but given C what do we *do* about it now?

Arthur usually has a blue cup for water. When presented with a green one, he refuses to drink at all.

S: my usual cup is blue, and this one is green
G: refuse it
C: but the point is to drink water, and it's OK for drinking
T: accept it (i.e. the colour is unimportant to C)

Arthur gets upset when a minor change is made to the arrangement of furniture in his room.

S: the arrangement of my room has been slightly changed
G: worry about this
C: but the functions of my room are . . .
T: don't worry (i.e. the change is unimportant to C)

During a car trip to LA, Arthur gets upset because his underwear is not exactly as usual, and wants to return to where his usual ones are bought. [from Rain Man]

S: my underwear is different from usual
G: worry about this
C: but our purpose is to drive to LA
T: forget it for the moment

Case 10: Subtraction   One aspect of learning is that we refine our knowledge by removing non-functional elements from our knowledge-structures. In the situation in which we initially encounter something there may be details which are inessential, and so we need subsequently to remove these.

Arthur first hears the word 'impolite' pronounced as 'im-pol-ite'. Thereafter he always pronounces it this way. What is odd about this?

Here the data structure is a correct record of the initial experience (as usual the problem in autism is not simply one of truth or accuracy). However, subsequent context indicates that an element in the data structure is nevertheless in appropriate.

S: pronunciation as 'im-pol-ite'
G: use this
C: frequent experience of hearing alternative pronunciation as 'impolite'
T: subtract the non-functional element

It is likewise notable that autistic routines may have non-functional 'extras' that are maintained despite being non-functional.

Case 11: Dealing with Open Structures   There are cases in which a cognitive system is provided at one time with a data structure (or database) that is incomplete, and at a later time with the details required to fill its open *slots*. The usual approach is to treat this as an issue of time: we have some of what we need now, and we look out to get the rest later, completing our decision 'on the fly'. This is problematic in autism, where such open structures can evoke anxiety due to their indefinite nature.

S: this is currently an incomplete structure
G: worry
C: the gaps will be filled tomorrow
T: use it when they are filled

6.4.3   Discovering Commonalities Between the Triangulation Cases

We proceed with the discussions of how the cases are inter-related. There are many differences between the cases examined above. Some involve understanding of other people while others do not. Some involve language while others do not. Some make greater call on imagination (cases 7 and 8) than others. Our point however is that they are variations on a theme in the following sense:

1. each case presents a task which is of a type well known to present difficulty in autism;
2. each task can be analyzed as a triangulation task;
3. in these terms, the tendency found in autism is a tendency to produce the 'generic' rather than the 'triangulated' response.

This analysis serves as a tool for understanding: the moment when we identify a triangulation structure and its elements can be the moment when we understand another person's actions, the moment when we say *oh, that's where he is coming from*. The analysis serves as a basis for a computer-based therapeutic facility, since it identifies a common structure which people with autism need practice in navigating. Below, we will provide a more formal analysis of the triangulation structure.

The source in the structure gives us a generic or standard action; the context indicates how, when, where or with whom to perform the action, what to change, repeat or omit, when to stop, or whether to do it at all; and the cognitive system needs to work out in each case what the nature of this adjustment should be. These adjustments fall into two broad categories, narrowing and widening of the actions performed, and in each case above there is an established tendency in autism not to make the relevant adjustment.

We attempt to cover these eleven scenarios by five well-known deficiencies of autistic reasoning described in the literature:

1. Non-toleration of novelty of any sort (cases 1, 9, 11).
2. Incapability to change plan online when necessary (cases 1, 2, 5, 6, 11).
3. Easy deviation from a reasoning context, caused by an insignificant detail (cases 2, 3, 4, 5, 5′, 8).
4. Lack of capability to distinguish more important from less important features for a given situation (cases 2, 7, 9, 10).
5. Inability to properly perceive the level of generality of a feature appropriate for a given situation (cases 2, 4, 7, 8, 10).

Note that each deficiency covers multiple cases, and each case is covered by two or more deficiencies. Also, these deficiencies of reasoning can be distinguished from reasoning about mental attitudes, which are usually corrupted in a higher degree in case of autism (Baron-Cohen 2000).

6.4.4   Building a Bridge Between Triangulation and Default Reasoning

Default reasoning is intended as a model of real-world commonsense reasoning in cases which include typical and non-typical features and situations. A default rule states that a situation should be considered as typical and an action should be chosen accordingly unless the typicality assumption is inconsistent. We observe that autistic intelligence is capable of operating with stand-alone default rules in a correct manner most of times.

When there is a system of conflicting default rules, the formal treatment (operational semantics) has been developed so that multiple valid actions can be chosen in a given situation, depending on the order in which the default rules are applied. All such actions are formally accepted in such a situation, and the default logic approach does not provide means for preference of some of these actions over the other ones. Analyzing the behavior of people with autism, we will observe that unlike the controls, CwA lack the capability to choose the more appropriate action instead of a less appropriate. In this respect we will illustrate that the model of default reasoning suits autistic subjects better than controls.

Default reasoning is a particular machinery intended to simulate how human reasoning handles typical and atypical features and situations. Apart from reasoning about mental attitudes which is essential in presenting autism, we apply default reasoning to conceptualize a wide range of phenomena of autistic reasoning presented in Chap. 2, taking advantage of the experience of computer implementation of default reasoning. Peculiarities of autistic reasoning can then be matched against the known possibilities of malfunctioning of artificial default reasoning systems.

In this Chapter we argue that the inability to use default rules properly leads to certain phenomena of autistic reasoning identified in existing experimental studies. Conducting research of human reasoning in AI, the phenomena of autistic reasoning are of particular interest, since they help us to locate the actual significance of formal models of default reasoning. At the same time, we expect this study to shed light on how autistic reasoning may be improved by default reasoning-based rehabilitation techniques.

Abstract default logic distinguishes between two kinds of knowledge: the usual formulas of predicate logic (axioms, facts) and "rules of thumb" (defaults, Antoniou 1997). Corrupted reasoning may handle improperly either kind of knowledge, and we pose the question which kind may function improperly in autistic reasoning. Moreover, we consider the possibility that an improper interaction between the facts and rules of thumb may be a cause for corrupted reasoning.

Default theory (Brewka et al. 1995) includes a set of facts that represent certain, but usually incomplete, information about the world; and a set of defaults that cause plausible but not necessarily true conclusions (for example, because of the lack of a world knowledge or a particular situation-specific knowledge). In the course of routine thinking of human and automatic agents some of these conclusions have to be revised when additional context information becomes available.

Let us consider the traditional example quoted in the literature on nonmonotonic reasoning:

$$\frac{bird(X): fly(X)}{fly(X)}$$

One reads it as *If X is a bird and it is consistent to assume that X flies, then conclude that X flies.* In the real life, if one sees a bird, she assumes that it flies as long as no exceptions can be observed.

$$fly(X):- not\ penguin(X).\quad fly(X):- not\ sick(X).\quad fly(X):- not\ just\_born(X).\ ...$$

Exceptions are the potentially extensive list of clauses implying that X does *not fly*. It would be inefficient to start reasoning based on exceptions; it should be first assumed that there are no exceptions, then verified that this is true and then proceed to the consequent of a default rule.

A penguin (the bird which does not fly) is a *novelty* (it is atypical). Conventional reasoning first assumes that there are no novelties (there is no exception) and then performs the reasoning step, concluding that X flies. If this assumption is wrong (e.g. X-novelty is taking place) then the rule is inapplicable for penguins and it cannot be deduced that X flies. It is quite hard for autistic reasoning to update this kind of belief because it handles typical and atypical situations in the same manner, unlike the default rule machinery suggests. It is quite computationally expensive to handle typical and atypical situations similarly, because a typical situation is compact and most likely to occur, and an atypical situation comprises an extensive set of cases (clauses) each of which is unlikely to occur.

Having outlined the triangulation reasoning pattern, we proceed to a formal treatment of such structure using default logic. The components of triangulation structure can be represented as a pair *<classical rule, default rule>*. If the state S occurs, action G is to be performed. Hence we have a rule

$$\frac{S}{G}$$

However, if C occurs in addition to S (serves as a context of S)

$$\frac{S: C}{T}$$

We simulate autistic reasoning as a formal system where the top rule above always works, and the bottom rule fails either as a stand-alone one or as a combination of some rules with mutual dependence. In accordance to our methodology, a hypothetical autistic reasoning system would then always be capable of producing G but sometimes fails T due to a computational problem of deriving T. We have initially described this problem as enumeration of 11 cases, and then as five higher-level phenomena of autistic reasoning.

6.4.5 Handling a Single Default Rule by Autistic Reasoning

Let us now consider the above examples from the perspectives of five deficiencies. Unlike normal subjects, and similar to software systems, autistic subjects can hardly tolerate the

Additional_features_of_en_do_not_change_routine
     when they have a *Usual_intention* to *Follow_usual_routine*:

$$\frac{Usual\_intention : Additional\_features\_of\_env\_do\_not\_change\_routine}{Follow\_usual\_routine}$$

Table 6.1 Capabilities in revising beliefs and adjusting to new environments

A child knows that birds fly. The child sees observes that penguins do not fly	
Child updates the list of exceptions for not property flying	Child adds new rule that penguins do not fly
The *flying* default rules stays intact	It is necessary to update the existing rule of *flying* and all the rest of affected rules
The process of accepting new exceptions is not computationally expensive	This process takes substantial computational efforts and, therefore, is quite undesirable and overloading
Observing a novelty and remembering exceptions is a routine activity	Observing a novelty is stressful

This default rule schema is read as follows: when there is a *Usual_intention*, and the assumption that

Additional_features_of_env_do_not_change_routine is consistent, then it is OK to *Follow_usual_routine*. There should be clauses specifying the situations where this assumption fails:

Additional_features_of_env_do_not_change_routine:-   not   (alarm(fire)   ∨   desire(DoSometrhingElse) ∨…).

This clause (assumption) fails because of either external reasons or internal ones, and the list of potential reasons is rather long.

In the following Table 6.1 we compare the features of default reasoning for a CC (on the right) and a CwA, once new observation becomes available and beliefs change.

A good example here is that the autistic child runs into tremendous problems under deviation in an external environment which typical cognition would consider to be insignificant.

We proceed to the deficiency of *Incapability to change a plan online when necessary*. A characteristic example is that of an autistic child who does not walk around a puddle which is blocking her customary route to school, but rather walks through it and gets wet as a result. This happens not because the autistic child does not know that she would get wet stepping through a puddle, but because the underlying reasoning for puddle avoidance is not integrated into the process of reasoning. Let us consider the reasoning steps a default system needs to come through.

Initial plan to follow a certain path is subject to application (verification) by the following default rule:

$$\frac{need(Child, cross(Child, Area)) : \ normal(Area)}{cross(Child, Area)}$$

abnormal(Area) :- wet(Area) ∨ muddy(Area) ∨ dangerous(Area).

Here we consider a general case of an arbitrary area to pass by, *Area = puddle* in our example above. The rule sounds as follows: *If it is necessary to go across an area, and it is consistent to assume that it is normal (there is nothing abnormal there, including water, mud, danger etc.) then go ahead and do it.* A control individual would apply the default rule and associated clause above to choose her action, if the *Area* is normal. Otherwise, the companion default rule below is to be applied and alternative *AreaNearBy* is chosen.

$$\frac{need(Child,\ cross(Child,\ Area)),\ abnormal(Area)\ :\ normal(AreaNearBy)}{cross(Child,\ AreaNearBy)}$$

Note that formally one needs a similar default rule for the case when something is wrong with *AreaNearBy: abnormal(AreaNearBy)*. A control individual ignores it to make a decision with reasonable time and efforts. On the contrary, autistic child keeps applying the default rules, finds herself in a loop, gives up and goes across the puddle.

In other words, autistic reasoning literally propagates through the totality of relevant default rules and runs into the memory/operations overflow whereas a normal human reasoning stops after the first or second rule is applied. Therefore it is hard for CwA to make a choice appropriate for a given context (Fig. 6.1).

Fig. 6.1 A child is selecting a direction of movement towards one of two helpers

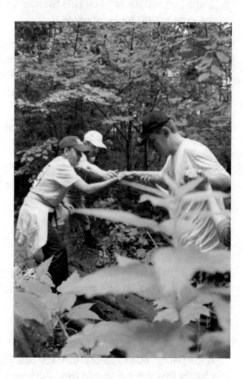

What are the peculiarities of how autistic children apply a newly acquired rule? First of all, they do their best in applying it; however, they follow it literally. Let us consider the following example:

> An autistic girl was advised by her parents not to speak with strangers in the street. On one occasion a policeman approached the girl and started asking questions, but was ignored by her. In spite of his multiple attempts to encourage the girl to communicate, they failed and he became upset.
>
> After the parents were told about the incident they suggested that the girl should not have treated policemen as a stranger. They also confirmed that the girl new who policemen were. The girl required that she needed the new explicit rule overwriting the initial one that a policeman was not a typical stranger and should have been treated differently.

On the basis of the analysis presented here, this anecdote could be given the following interpretation.

1. The subject is doing her best to follow the rule, and readily accepts new rules
2. The girl did know that the approaching man was a policeman, but she did not know him as a person, therefore she categorized him as a stranger in the context of the behavioral rule.
3. In this situation the girl was familiar with who policemen are, as she knew that policemen should not be ignored.
4. However, she was not able to handle a policeman as an exception in the rule for stranger.
5. If she had had the explicit rule for how to respond to strangers who are policemen then she would have followed it.

We conjecture that the girl had sufficient knowledge of the subject and was capable of applying the rules, taken separately. What she was not able of doing was to resolve a conflict between considering the same individual as *a stranger* and as a *policemen* in the context of decision whether to communicate or to ignore.

$$\frac{in\_street(me) :\text{-} stranger(Person)}{not\ talk(me,\ Person)}$$

Usually, strangers do not fall into a special category; however, exceptions are possible:

$$stranger(Person) :\text{-} not\ (policeman(Person) \lor rescue(Person) \lor military(Person \lor \ldots).$$

Indeed, the girl is likely capable of identifying the categories of persons above, but not in the context of a *stranger* rule. The latter is an opposing rule to the one for handling exceptions:

$$talk(me,\ Person):\text{-} not\ (Person).$$

If the parent would incorporate the rule above into the default rule explicitly, then it is likely that the girl would treat the policemen properly.

6.4.6   Handling Conflicting Default Rules

In this section we proceed to the situation where there are multiple (conflicting) default rules, and the results of their execution depend on the order these rules are applied. Here we propose an informal description for such situations, introducing *operational semantics* for default reasoning.

The main goal of applying default rules is to make all the possible conclusions from the given set of facts. This is the bottleneck for autistic reasoning: a child may come to a single conclusion without being aware than other solutions may be as valid. A control subject is usually capable of identifying the totality of conclusions and of applying some kind of preference criteria to select a more appropriate one. Presenting the operational semantics, we bear in mind that in contrast to controls, autistic reasoning follows it literally. Following the operational semantics of default reasoning in case of conflicting rules provides conclusions similar to what autistic subjects produce, because both lack the machinery to apply preference and select a more adequate solutions, taking into account circumstances which are neither expressed by facts nor rules in the default system.

What is the nature of conflict under operational semantics? If one applies only one default, we can simply add its consequent to our knowledge base. The situation becomes more complicated if we have a set of defaults because, for example, the rules can have consequents contradicting each other or, a consequent of one rule can contradict the justification of another one. In order to provide an accurate solution we have to introduce the notion of *extensions* : current knowledge bases, satisfying some specific conditions.

Suppose D is a set of defaults and W is a set of facts (our initial knowledge base). Let Δ be an ordered subset of D without multiple occurrences (it is useless to apply the default twice because it would add no information). We denote a deductive closure (in terms of classical logic) of Δ by $In(\Delta)$: $W \cup \{cons(\delta)|\delta \in \Delta\}$. We also denote by $Out(\Delta)$ the set $\{\neg\psi|\psi \in just(\delta),\ \delta \in \Delta\}$. We call $\Delta = \{\delta_0, \delta_1, \ldots\}$ a process iff for every k δ_k is applicable to $In(\Delta_k)$, where Δ_k is the initial part of Δ of the length k.

Given a process Δ, we can determine whether it is successful and closed. A process Δ is called successful iff $In(\Delta) \cap Out(\Delta) = \varnothing$. A process Δ is called closed if Δ already contains all the defaults from D, applicable to $In(\Delta)$.

Now we can define extensions. A set of formulae $E \supset W$ is an extension of the default theory $<D,\ W>$ iff there is some process Δ so that it is successful, closed, and $E = In(\Delta)$.

Let us consider an example of a *lost toy*; a child needs to decide on which action to choose. Let us suppose that W is empty and D is the set of

$$\delta_1 \quad \frac{true\ :\ not\ toy\_lost(X)}{not\ toy\_lost(X)}$$

$$\delta_2 \quad \frac{true\ :\ toy\_lost(X)}{search(X,\ toy\_lost)}$$

These rules describe a situation when children toys are normally not assumed to be lost if not immediately seen, but, if it's consistent to assume that the toy has been taken by someone, then it is worth searching for.

After we have applied the first rule, we extend our knowledge base by *not toy_lost(X)*:

$$In(\{\delta_1\}) = \{\ not\ toy\_lost(X)\ \},$$
$$Out(\{\delta_1\}) = \{\ toy\_lost(X)\ \}.$$

The second rule is not applicable to $In(\{\delta_1\})$. Therefore the process $\Delta = \{\delta_1\}$ is closed. It is also successful, so $In(\{\delta_1\})$ is an extension. Suppose now we now apply δ_1 first:

$$In(\{\delta_2\}) = \{\ search(X,\ toy\_lost)\ \},$$
$$Out(\{\delta_2\}) = \{\ not\ toy\_lost(X)\ \}.$$

The rule δ_1 is still applicable now, so $\{\delta_2\}$ process is not closed. Let us apply δ_1 to $In(\{\delta_2\})$:

$$In(\{\delta_2,\delta_1\}) = \{\ search(X,\ toy\_lost),\ not\ toy\_lost(X)\ \},$$
$$Out(\{\delta_2,\delta_1\}) = \{\ not\ toy\_lost(X),\ toy\_lost(X)\ \}.$$

Now $In(\{\delta_2,\delta_1\}) \cap Out(\{\delta_2,\delta_1\}) \neq \varnothing$ so $\{\delta_2,\ \delta_1\}$ is not successful and $\{search(X, toy\_lost),\ not\ toy\_lost(X)\}$ is not an extension. This comes in accordance with our intuitive expectations, because if we accept the later statement to be a possible knowledge base, then we conjecture that the toy will be searched always, not only when we suspect that it has been taken by someone.

However, if there are two extensions (possibilities for actions), then more than one action are deemed formally legitimate. In a real-life situation, normal individuals, unlike autistic ones, possess additional machinery to select appropriate actions. On the contrary, autistic children, if capable of using default rule, follow the above methodology literally. They therefore may choose an action inadequate from the perspective of control subjects, but nevertheless correct from the perspective of formal default reasoning.

Due to literal following of the operational semantics, autistic children have significant difficulties understanding natural language sentences and reacting to commands including multiple ambiguous words. Analyzing combinations of meaning, autistic reasoning may produce formally valid but inadequate (from the viewpoint of control subjects) representations.

We conclude this section by the training example we have been using in the autistic rehabilitation Center "Our Sunny World" (Moscow, Russia). The exercise teaches autistic children to operate with multiple possible interpretations of natural language expressions. Indeed, autistic children have problems understanding situations where there are multiple ambiguous words in a query and the totality of overall meaning for a sentence is a combination of meanings of these words. Let us consider the following expression (in Russian):

"Эта *картина* заставила его забыть о своем *состоянии*"

The first ambiguous word, *картина,* has two following meanings:

1. A work of art, a painting;
2. A set of events observable at a certain time.

The meanings of the second word, *состояни*е (normalized), are:

2.1. Monetary assets of an individual;
2.2. Mental and physical state of an individual.

The respective default theory has four extensions with the following meanings:

1.1–2.1. This painting made him forgot about his poverty/wealth;
1.2–2.1. This accident made him forgot about how poor/rich he was;
1.1–2.2. This painting made him ignore his feeling unwell;
1.2–2.2. This accident distracted him from his thoughts.

The children are demonstrated that all above meaning are valid; however, some of them are more appropriate than others in a certain context. This is also the case under disambiguation for question answering (Galitsky 2003).

An easier training example which was attempted by eleven children with autism is depicted at Fig. 6.2. The focus of this exercise is to develop the capability of changing plans online. The user interface represents a decision-making procedure in changing environment via list boxes.

Another form of nonmonotonic reasoning is a closed world assumption. It is based on the statement that is true is also known to be true (Antoniou 1997). At the same time, what is not currently known to be true, is false. Stenning and van Lambalgen (2008, 2012) identified a number of areas to which closed world reasoning is applicable, each time in slightly different form:

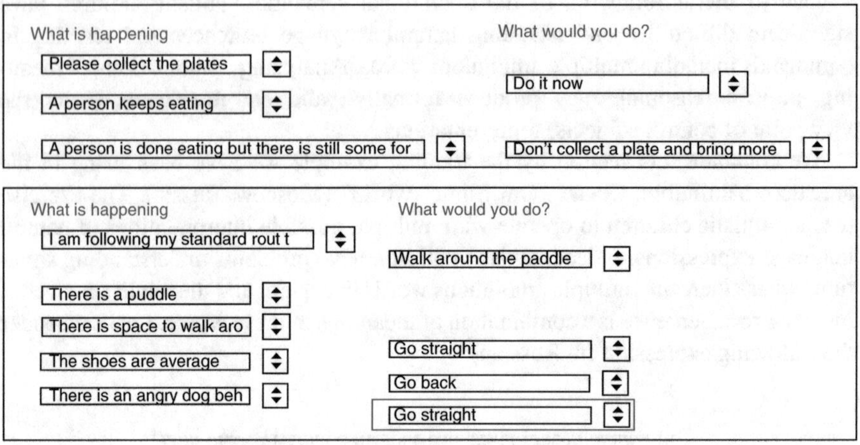

Fig. 6.2 A form to train adjustment of actions

1. lists, sequences, in space and time, train schedules, airline databases, ...;
2. diagnostic reasoning and abduction;
3. analogical reasoning;
4. arbitrary deduction;
5. unknown preconditions and post-conditions;
6. causal and counterfactual reasoning;
7. attribution of beliefs and intentions.

PwA have difficulties with at least items (2), (3), (5)–(7). CwA are pre-occupied with lists, in the sense that they feel lost without lists, such as timetables to organize daily activities; they have great difficulty accommodating unexpected changes to the timetable, and try to avoid situations such as holidays in which rigid schedules are not applicable. One may view this as an extreme version of closed world reasoning, sometimes even applied in inappropriate circumstances. But before one concludes from this that PwA are good at closed world reasoning to the point of over-applying it, one must carefully distinguish several components of closed world reasoning.

On the one hand, there is the inference from given premises which reduces to a computation of the minimal model of the premises and checking whether a given formula holds. Non-monotonic reasoning also involves 'pre-processing' the given situation or discourse, that is, encoding the law-like features of a situation in a particular type of premises.

Laws and regularities always allow exceptions, and a skill to handle exception is required based on identifying and encoding the relevant exceptions, and knowing when "enough is enough". CwA appear to perform significantly worse than CC doing that, although they behave normally with respect to the non-monotonic inferences themselves.

6.5 Discussion and Conclusions

In this Chapter we focused on the reasoning domains of the secondary importance for CwA after the mental world. As we explore the deviation between the conventional (rational, adult) reasoner from the one of the young children, irrational, autistic, we are getting closer to the nature of reasoning about the physical world, choice of action, non-monotonic, probabilistic and counterfactual domains. Whereas in the domain of reasoning about mental world one can localize the exact axioms that are missing, the general observation in other reasoning domains is that CwA cannot *achieve the required level of complexity* to behave and act in the real world. In these domains just learning particular axioms is necessary but not sufficient and more general operations including certain metareasoning patterns, like operations on defaults, are required.

It is well known that it takes significantly less amount of data for a human to learn than for a computer to learn. In machine learning, approaches like deep learning, relying on a high volume datasets and high speed computing, are becoming more available and popular. For CwAs with hyper-sensitivity a capability to maintain high volume of data and perform high efficiency computations may potentially approach deep learning-like architectures for learning from vast data. At the same time, inductive learning from a limited set of examples is a most typical way control humans acquire knowledge.

In this chapter we used default logic to provide a framework for understanding of the elusive phenomena of autistic reasoning. Our thesis is that difficulty arises in autism specifically in those situations where an appropriate default rule should be applied, or conflicts between two default rules are to be resolved. This model of autistic reasoning provides a relatively precise tool for understanding some of the phenomena of autism and autistic behavior. Our model provides an explanation on how the five major problems in autistic reasoning outlined in Chap. 2 and Sect. 6.4.3 arise:

1. Non-toleration of novelty of any sort, because it requires update of the whole commonsense knowledge, since it is not adequately divided into typical and atypical cases, norms and exceptions;
2. Incapability to change plan online when necessary, because it requires substantial computational efforts to exhaustively search the space of all possibilities;
3. Easy deviation from a reasoning context, caused by an insignificant detail, because there is an extremely high number of issues to address at each reasoning step; each such issue is seemed to be plausible and there is no proper feature selection mechanism present;
4. Lack of capability to distinguish more important from less important features for given situation, because feature importance is mainly measured in the context of being a justification of a default rule.
5. Inability to properly perceive the level of generality of features appropriate for a given situation is due to the problem of estimating which generality of a given feature is most typical, and which is less typical to be applied as a justification of a default rule.

We observed that a loss of reasoning efficiency due to improper use of default rules leads to a wide range of decision-making problems reflected in behavioral characteristics of CwA. To teach children how to overcome their decision-making problems, we developed a set or exercises encouraging default reasoning in a number of environments (Chap. 8). We will evaluate how the learners transfer acquired default rules from artificial to real world situations, which is more feasible task for the target category of children with autism than forming new rules to match the real world environment. This step requires the learners to be capable of *transferring* acquired reasoning patterns from simulation to real world environment and their *application* to real-life objects. The evaluation of the developed set of exercises has shown that performance of children with autism in real-world situations can be dramatically increased (Sect. 8.9.3).

Therefore, having an artificial environments for teaching children with autism and other mental illnesses how to adjust their actions in specific domains is beneficial. An alternative to this of postponing such training to the mental age when learners can be expected to form new rules in the real world independently would delay the overall development of learners and therefore seems unacceptable.

Exploration of the peculiarities of autistic reasoning is an emerging area involving logic, linguistic, psychology and philosophy has been conducted by van Lambalgen and Smid (2004). The ideas in this area have just started to contribute to design of rehabilitation software for autistic children, and the current book is one of the first linking these areas. Pijnacker et al. (2008) investigated inference patterns which can be revised as new informaticon is coming. The authors used a behavioral task to investigate conditional reasoning and its suppression. In the suppression task (Sect. 2.5.1, McKenzie et al. 2011) a possible exception was made salient, which could prevent yielding a conclusion. This study confirmed our finding (Galitsky and Peterson 2005) that CwA experience difficulties with yielding conclusions in the environment of exception. This is due to the fact that CwA require a flexibility in thinking to adjust to the context, which is frequently not present. Similar to our earlier studies, Pijnacker et al. (2008) hypothesized that CwA experience difficulties handling exceptions in reasoning sessions, and also discussed the neural underpinnings of reasoning in autism. Conditional reasoning is a high-order cognitive process involving such components as linguistic processing, information access in long-term memory, maintaining and manipulating verbal information in working memory, attention and inhibition of responses. Some of these components belong to executive function (Sect. 2.5.2). Executive functions are possibly regulated by frontal lobes. Studies including (Goel and Dolan 2004) investigated the neural basis of reasoning and found that frontal-temporal and frontal-parietal networks are involved in deductive reasoning.

The model presented here applies techniques of logic to an issue of psychology, and so raises the issue of the relation between the two. Logic is the study of reasoning, and psychology is the study of the mind and behavior, and so one might expect a consonant relationship between the two, since minds (the subject of psychology) use reasoning (the subject of logic) to arrive at decisions, beliefs, and actions. Since the end of the nineteenth century, however, there has been a tendency for work in logic to focus on a particular type of reasoning: one that constitutes a small fraction of the range used in real life. This is 'monotonic' reasoning, in which a conclusion, once inferred from a premise, will not be altered or retracted in light of further evidence.

Our interest to non-monotonic reasoning is motivated by the fact that it is in this area that people with autism show difficulty. Monotonic reasoning patterns, as found for example in arithmetic, seem to be much less problematic in autism (excluding reasoning about mental worlds). This monotonicity is reflected in what has become a standard definition of valid deduction in logic: X follows from Y if it is impossible that Y be true and X false. It would be inadmissible that Y is accepted and X rejected, even given further evidence.

References

American Psychiatric Association (2000) Diagnostic and statistical manual of mental disorders, fourth edition, text revision (DSM-IV-TR). American Psychiatric Association, Washington, DC

Antoniou G (1997) Nonmonotonic reasoning. MIT Press, Cambridge, MA/London

Baron-Cohen S (1995) Mindblindness: an essay on autism and theory of mind. MIT Press/Bradford Books, Boston

Baron-Cohen S (2000) Theory of mind and autism: a fifteen year review. In: Baron-Cohen S, Tagar-Flusberg H, Cohen DJ (eds) Understanding other minds, volume A. Oxford University Press, Oxford, pp 3–20

Baron-Cohen S, Wheelwright S, Skinner R, Martin J, Clubley E (2001) The autism-spectrum quotient (AQ): evidence from Asperger syndrome/high-functioning autism, males and females, scientists and mathematicians. J Autism Dev Disord 31(1):5–1

Begeer S, De Rosnay M, Lunenburg P, Stegge H, Terwogt M (2014) Understanding of emotions based on counterfactual reasoning in children with autism spectrum disorders. Autism 18(3):301–310

Bochman A (2001) A logical theory of nonmonotonic inference and belief change. Springer, Berlin

Brewka G, Dix J, Konolige K (1995) Nonmonotonic reasoning: an overview. CSLI Lecture Notes 73

Ekman P (1992) Facial expression of emotion: an old controversy and new findings. In: Bruce V (ed) The face, Royal Society

Galitsky B (2002) Extending the BDI model to accelerate the mental development of autistic patients. Second international conference on development & learning. Cambridge, MA

Galitsky B (2003) Natural language question answering system: technique of semantic headers. Advanced Knowledge International, Adelaide

Galitsky B, Peterson D (2005) On the peculiarities of default reasoning of children with Autism FLAIRS-05

Galitsky B, González MP, Chesñevar CI (2009) A novel approach for classifying customer complaints through graphs similarities in argumentative dialogues. Decis Support Syst 46(3): 717–729

Gillberg C (1991) Outcome in autism and autistic-like conditions. J Am Acad Child Adolesc Psychiatry 30:375–382

Goel V, Dolan RJ (2004) Differential involvement of left prefrontal cortex in inductive and deductive reasoning. Cognition 93(3):B109–B121

Gopnik AD, Sobel LS, Glymour C (2001) Causal learning mechanisms in very young children: two, three, and four-year-olds infer causal relations from patterns of variation and covariation. Dev Psychol 37(5):620–629

Harris P, Johnson CN, Hutton D, Andrews G, Cooke T (1989) Young children's theory of mind and emotion. Cognit Emot 3:379–400

Harris PL, German TP, Mills PE (1996) Children's use of counterfactual thinking in causal reasoning. Cognition 61:233–259

Johnson S (2000) The recognition of mentalistic agents in infancy. Trends Cogn Sci 4:22–28

Johnson C, Rakison D (2006) Early categorization of animate/inanimate concepts in young children with autism. J Dev Phys Disabil 20:73–89

Kahneman D, Tversky A (1972) Subjective probability: a judgement of representativeness. Cogn Psychol 3:430–454

Kanner L (1943) Autistic disturbances of affective contact. Ner Child 2:217–250

Karmiloff-Smith A (1992) Beyond modularity. MIT Press/Bradford Books, Cambridge

Leslie AM (1987) Pretence and representation: the origins of "theory of mind". Psychol Rev 94:412–426

Leslie AM, Keeble S (1987) Do six-month-olds perceive causality? Cognition 25:265–288

McKenzie R, Evans JSBT, Handley SJ (2011) Autism and performance on the suppression task: reasoning, context and complexity. Think Reason 17(2):182–196

Minsky M (2006) The emotion machine. Simon & Schuster, New York

Mundy P, Crowson M (1997) Joint attention and early social communication. J Autism Dev Disord 27:653–676

Peterson DM, Bowler DM (2000) Counterfactual reasoning and false belief understanding in children with autism. Autism: Int J Res Pract 4(4):391–405

Peterson D, Galitsky B (2004) Handling default rules by autistic reasoning. KES: LNAI 3215, pp 314–320

Piaget J (1953) Logic and psychology. Manchester University Press, Manchester

Pijnacker J et al (2008) Pragmatic inferences in high-functioning adults with autism and Asperger syndrome. J Autism Dev Disord 39(4):607–618

Premack D (1990) The infant's theory of self-propelled objects. Cognition 36:1–16

Randi J, Newman T, Grigorenko EL (2010) Teaching children with autism to read for meaning: challenges and possibilities. J Autism Dev Disord 40(7):890–902

Riggs KJ, Peterson DM (2000) Counterfactual reasoning in pre-school children:mental state and causal inferences. In: Mitchell P, Riggs K (eds) Children's reasoning and the mind, chapter 5, Psychology Press, pp 87–100

Stanovich KE (1999) Who is rational? Studies of individual differences in reasoning. Lawrence Erlbaum, Mahwah

Stenning K, van Lambalgen M (2008) Human reasoning and cognitive science. MIT Press, Cambridge

Stenning K, van Lambalgen M (2012) Human reasoning and cognitive science. MIT Press, Cambridge

Tager-Flusberg H (1989) The development of questions in autistic and down syndrome children. Gatlinburg conference on research and theory in mental retardation. Gatlinburg, TN

Tomasello M (1988) The role of joint-attentional processes in early language acquisition. Lang Sci 10:69–88

van Lambalgen M, Smid H (2004). Reasoning patterns in autism: rules and exceptions. In: Larrazabal JM, Perez Miranda LA (eds) Proceedings 8th international colloquium on cognitive science (Donostia/San Sebastian)

Wason PC (1968) Reasoning about a rule. Q J Exp Psychol 20:273–281

Wilson M, Dupuis B (2010) From bricks to brains: the embodied cognitive science of LEGO robots. Athabasca University Press, Edmonton

Chapter 7
Autistic Learning and Cognition

Boris Galitsky and Igor Shpitsberg

Having explored how reasoning works in mental and physical worlds, and how it can be broken in humans and artificial systems, we now focus on the domains tightly connected with reasoning: automated learning and cognition. In these domains, autistic and engineering learning systems experience substantial difficulties, and we will attempt to understand their nature.

We first describe the peculiarities of autistic cognition and introduce the concept of active learning. We then informally describe the autistic active learning system and explain the appearance of the features of autistic cognition. After that we introduce the active learning system *Jasmine* that is intended to simulate the normal vs autistic cognition and describe the respective cognitive pathways. Finally, we present our experiment with forming and updating hypotheses in *Jasmine* setting by humans and outline the deductive system for reasoning about action based on an extension of *Jasmine*, demonstrating how such hybrid reasoning domain can possible be implemented in the brain and in a robot.

7.1 Autistic Cognition

Autistic peripheral vision is significantly more developed than the central, frontal vision, unlike the vision of CC. Peripheral vision is a part of vision that detects objects outside the direct line of vision. For instance, when one reads a word on a page, she is using her central vision, but it is her side vision that tells her if the word is at the beginning or end of a sentence, or at the top or bottom of a page.

B. Galitsky (✉)
Knowledge-Trail Inc, San Jose, CA, USA

I. Shpitsberg
Center Our Sunny World, Moscow, Russia

© Springer International Publishing Switzerland 2016
B. Galitsky, *Computational Autism*, Human–Computer Interaction Series,
DOI 10.1007/978-3-319-39972-0_7

The peripheral vision also tells one where to look if someone enters the room or if a car is approaching from the side. Most people are not aware of the limitations that would exist without peripheral vision, because they are constantly moving their eyes in order to focus with the central vision.

The difference between central and peripheral vision becomes apparent when one understands the visual function of the eye. The eye works like a camera with two lenses – the cornea at the front of the eye and the natural crystalline lens behind the pupil. The cornea is responsible for about three quarters of the eye's focusing power, while the natural lens adjust the image before it is send on the retina at the back of the eye. Central vision is relatively weak at night or in the dark, when the lack of color cues and lighting makes cone cells far less useful. Rod cells, which are concentrated further away from the retina, operate better than cone cells in low light. This makes peripheral vision useful for seeing movement at night. Since CwA try to perceive the real world with this deficient cognitive system, they mostly hear reflected sounds, and their vision is based on peripheral perception.

Children with autism often have a difficult time answering the question of "Where is it?". Many of the self-stimulatory behaviors that are seen as the problem in CwA are actually the children's own solutions to a problem that they are having. Behaviors such as toe walking, hand-flapping, and rocking back and forth are a child's solution to his problem of answering the question of "Where is it?" in his environment. Children with autism often have a difficult time understanding where something is in space, where they are in space and where things are in relation to themselves (Fig. 7.1).

Another vision problem that leads to repetitive/stereotyped behaviors in children with autism is the poor integration of central visual detail and peripheral visual

Fig. 7.1 Recognizing a person in an unusual outfit requires substantial deviation from learned patterns and multi-modal perception

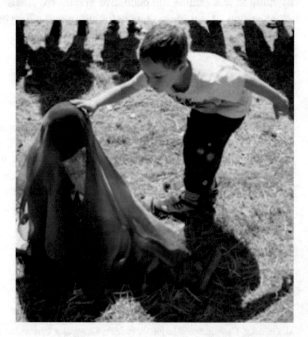

detail. Some people with autism have difficulty understanding the whole because they only seem to notice the part. For example, a child may look at a picture of a garden and focus in on one of the trees, but not understand that there are many other trees in the picture that make up the garden.

Crossing a busy street, a person who can combine central and peripheral visual detail will understand that there are many cars driving by, and that crossing the street before all the cars have passed would be dangerous. At the same time, CwA whose limitations are in using central and peripheral information simultaneously may get stuck on the blue road sign across the street. The child may seem to only notice the blue road sign and will ignore the cars going by. This is the reason why a child may not seem to notice the cars even though it is obvious to the frightened and upset parent.

Face recognition is another day-to-day activity that is affected by poor integration of central and peripheral visual detail. Some people with autism may tend to lock into one part of the face instead of seeing the whole. They will see a nose, an ear or a chin, but not be able to combine this information into forming the entire face. It is like taking pieces of a jigsaw puzzle and spreading them apart rather than placing them all together. Separating the individual pieces makes it more difficult to understand and consistently recognize the picture. Consequently, some children with autism may not be able to consistently recognize even their primary caregiver.

One of the important building blocks in developing social interaction is a skill called joint attention (Sect. 2.5.7, Mundy and Crowson 1997). Joint attention is the ability to look at the same thing at the same time as another person through the use of eye contact and gestures. CwA often have poorly developed joint attention. In particular, children with autism often have a greater deficit in Initiating Joint Attention. The purpose of it is to share interests with others. Naturally, one of the behaviors associated with autism is the lack of spontaneous sharing of likes and dislikes with others.

The ability to perform Initiating Joint Attention is controlled in the brain by four areas, one of which is the Frontal Eye Fields (FEF). In clinical studies that take pictures of the brain during social situations, the part of the brain that is shown to be the most consistently active is the FEF. These pictures of the brain provide neurologic evidence that the FEF and the functions that it is responsible for plays an important role in social interaction.

The FEF is responsible for starting eye gaze movements, fine eye movements and visual attention. Eye gaze movements, or the ability of the brain to accurately move the eyes to an object of interest, is important for joint attention. In turn, joint attention is important in developing social skills. Vision, therefore, plays a vital role in social interaction because eye movements and subsequent visual attention affects the development of joint attention. Children later diagnosed with autism were more likely to repeatedly spin and rotate objects. They were also more likely to explore objects in unusual ways, like glancing sideways at them or starting intently at them for prolonged periods.

The study (Kennedy Krieger Institute 2009) examined patterns of movement as CwA and CC learn to control a novel tool. The findings suggest that CwA learn new actions differently than typically developing children do. As compared to their typically developing peers, children with autism relied much more on their own internal sense of body position (proprioception), rather than visual information coming from the external world to learn new patterns of movement. Furthermore, researchers found that the greater the reliance on proprioception, the greater the child's impairment in social skills, motor skills and imitation.

The study findings also provide support for observations from previous studies suggesting that autism may be associated with abnormalities in the wiring of the brain; specifically, with overdevelopment of short range white matter connections between neighboring brain regions and underdevelopment of longer distance connections between distant brain regions. The findings from this study are consistent with this pattern of abnormal connectivity, as the brain regions involved in proprioception are closely linked to motor areas, while visual-motor processing depends on more distant connections.

7.2   Active Learning in Computer Science

Traditionally, machine learning has focused on the problem of learning a task from labeled examples only. In many applications, however, labeling is expensive while unlabeled data is usually ample. This observation motivated substantial work on properly using unlabeled data to benefit learning, and there are many examples showing that unlabeled data can significantly help. There are two main frameworks for incorporating unlabeled data into the learning process.

The first framework is semi-supervised learning (Zhu 2005), where in addition to a set of labeled examples, the learning algorithm can also use a (usually larger) set of unlabeled examples drawn at random from the same underlying data distribution. In this setting, unlabeled data becomes useful under additional assumptions and beliefs about the learning problem. For example, transductive SVM learning (Yu et al. 2006) assumes that the target function cuts through low-density regions of the space, while co-training assumes that the target should be self-consistent in some way. Unlabeled data is potentially useful in this setting because it allows one to reduce the search space to a set that is a-priori reasonable with respect to the underlying distribution.

The second setting, which is the basis of our model for autistic cognition, is active learning. Here the learning algorithm is allowed to draw unlabeled examples from the underlying distribution and ask for the labels of any of these examples. The hope is that a good classifier can be learned with significantly fewer labels by actively directing the queries to informative examples. One approach is to collect random samples, and another to collect samples which are believed to improve recognition accuracy.

Active learning is typically defined by contrast to the passive model of supervised learning (Fig. 7.2). In passive learning, all the labels for an unlabeled dataset

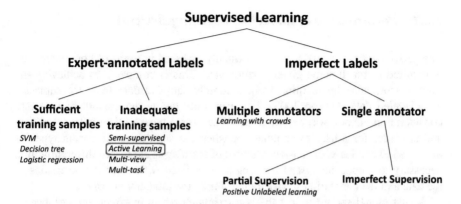

Fig. 7.2 Active learning among the supervised learning family of methods

are obtained at once, while in active learning the learner interactively chooses which data points to label. The great hope of active learning is that interaction can substantially reduce the number of labels required, making learning more practical. This hope is known to be valid in certain special cases, where the number of labels needed to learn actively has been shown to be logarithmic in the usual sample complexity of passive learning; such cases include thresholds on a line, and linear separators with a spherically uniform unlabeled data distribution (Dasgupta 2005). Many earlier active learning algorithms, have problems with data that are not perfectly separable under the given hypothesis class. In such cases, they can exhibit a lack of statistical consistency: even with an infinite labeling budget, they might not converge to an optimal predictor (Dasgupta et al. 2007).

Human learning to recognize the features of external world is active learning by nature. It would be hard to explain the problem of autistic cognition relying on the traditional supervised learning framework, since both CC and CwA have the same external world that contains the fixed training set to operate. We hypothesize that by breaking the framework of active learning, CwA deviate from CC in their cognitive process resulting in faulty recognition system.

Active learning is also used for recommendation systems. The totality of human users then becomes an environment where a learning system picks the elements of its training set. There is an opinion that an active learning from users can be bothersome, intrusive process, but if the items presented to the user are interesting, then it could be both a process of discovery and of exploration. Some recommender systems provide a "surprise me!" button to motivate the user into this explorative process, and indeed there are users who browse suggestions just to see what there is without any intention of buying. Exploration is crucial for users to become more self-aware of their own preferences (changing or not) and at the same time inform the system of what they are. If not properly trained, an active learning-based recommender system may "behave" badly and provide irrelevant results.

7.2.1   Performance of an Active Learning Systems

The performance of active learning is usually assessed in terms of how much data is required to reach some given performance. This is compared to achieving the same performance by learning from randomly sampled data from the same set of unlabeled data (Olsson 2008). However, only taking the amount of data into consideration is not always appropriate. When some types of data is less available and is harder for a user to annotate, or when the acquisition of certain types of unlabeled examples is expensive, the cost of learning is expressed differently. It is necessary to model the cost of learning as associated with other characteristics of the data and the annotation scenario than simply the total amount of data.

A cost model should reflect the constraints currently in effect; for instance, if annotator time is more important than the presumed cognitive load put on the user, then the overall time should take precedence in the evaluation of the plausibility of the method under consideration. If on the other hand a high cognitive load causes the users to produce annotations with too high a variance, resulting in poor data quality, then the user situation may have to take precedence over monetary issues in order to allow for the recruitment and training of more personnel. Using a scale mimicking the actions made by the user when annotating the data is one way of facilitating a finer grained measurement of the learning progress.

7.2.2   Monitoring, Assessing and Terminating the Learning Process

The monitoring, assessing and terminating of the active learning process go hand in hand. The purpose of assessing the learning process is to provide the human annotator with means to form a picture of the learning status. Once the status is known, the annotator has the opportunity to act accordingly, for instance, to manually stop the active learning process. The purpose of defining the stopping criterion is slightly different than that of assessing the learning process. A stopping criterion is used to automatically terminate the learning process, and ideally the realization of the definition, e.g., the setting of any thresholds necessary, should not hinder nor disturb the human annotator.

It should be remembered that there is a readily available way of assessing the process, and thus also to be able to manually decide when the active learning should be stopped; to use a marked-up, held-out test set on which the learner is evaluated in each iteration. This is the way that active learning is usually evaluated in experimental settings. The drawback of this method is that the user has to manually annotate more data before the annotation process takes off. As such, it clearly counteracts the goal of active learning and should only be considered a last resort.

A very common way of monitoring how an active learner behaves is by plotting a learning curve, typically with the classification error or F-score along one axis, commonly the Y-axis, and something else along the other axis. The X-axis is usually

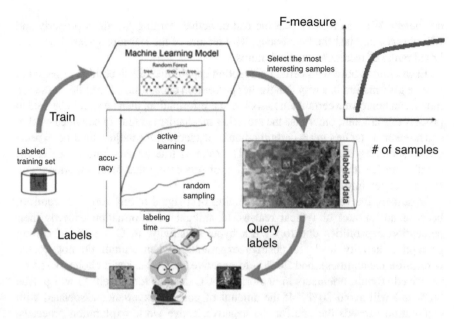

Fig. 7.3 The chart for active learning loop

indicating the amount of data seen – depending on the granularity of choice for that particular learning task it can be for instance tokens, named entities, or sentences – or the number of iterations made while learning. The purpose of a learning curve is to depict the progress in the learning process; few variations of how to measure progress exist, and consequently there are few differences in how the axes of a graph illustrating a learning curve are labeled (Fig. 7.3 on the top-right, Olsson 2008).

7.3   Active Learning and Autistic Development

To demonstrate why a human learning system needs to learn, we employ a paradigm of an active learning system that is rewarded for successful recognition of input stimulus of the real world. Not just the system should be capable of learning, but it needs to decide on which elements of the external world to use to form a training set. In both CC and CwA learning has to be functional, and active, otherwise CwA would not be capable of learning at all.

7.3.1   Hyper-sensitivity

We hypothesize that a root cause of autistic cognition is hyper-sensitivity to input stimuli (Chap. 2). To build as simple model as possible and to observe how many features of autistic behavior can be covered by this model, we select only a single deficiency. We then assume that the rest of active learning functions properly and will observe that just the hyper-sensitivity feature of the learning system leads to a broad range of resultant autistic features.

Each child is born with certain perception capabilities. Each child is expected to receive information in a way that fits her perception capabilities. If a child can see so much, can perceive a certain amount of visual information, then he should be able to process this amount; otherwise the receiving mechanism gradually becomes weaker and weaker. If he can get a certain amount of tactile information, then he expects a corresponding amount of touching. The same is true for any kind of feeling: if a child can feel that much, she is capable of processing that much emotional and feeling-related information.

In autism, the very process of perception of a signal of any sort is discomfort, because an amount of typical real-world amount of information exceeds their perception capabilities due to CwA's hyper-sensitivity. In CC, 80 % of stimuli perception activity leads to positive experience (when stimuli do not exceed perception capabilities), and 20 % – to negative. A CC makes a choice based on perceived stimuli, orienteers in exploration. CC decides for herself: "I will pursue 80 % and will avoid 20 %." If the amount of positive experience associated with exploration exceeds the one for the negative, active world exploration proceeds. Otherwise, if negative experience and failures prevail, then exploration stops and the child chooses a mechanism to avoid exploration (Fig. 7.4). CwA and children with Down syndrome, cerebral palsy, and other mental illnesses experience substantial negative experience from the perception process. Because of the hyper-sensitivity of their perception they fail up to 95 % of perception tasks and succeed in only 5 %. Therefore their interaction with the external world is formed in a way to minimize negative experience.

Hyper-sensitivity leads to a failure to learn to recognize stimuli properly, since the system can only learn to recognize patterns with extremely high similarity (as

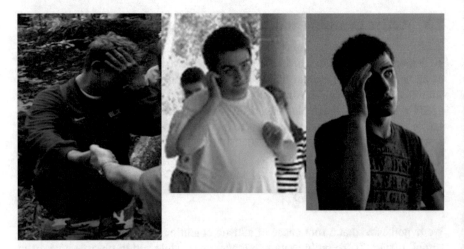

Fig. 7.4 Protecting themselves from the stimuli of the real world

we will show below). This failure leads to a negative experience associated with learning, and as a result CwAs do not investigate the world for the sake of pleasure. Instead they fence themselves from it.

For both CC and CwA, everything that is not recognized is considered dangerous. CwAs tend to consider all new stuff potentially dangerous. For CC clear thought is attractive, but in case of autism a clear thought may cause too strong feeling and can become unattractive. So CwA tries not to fully comprehend anything but instead stays in some proximity to a full understanding of some stimuli or some concept.

7.3.2 Autistic Adaptation

Humans are usually very good at adapting to environments. The human body readily responds to changing environmental stresses in a variety of biological and cultural ways. We can acclimatize to a wide range of temperature and humidity. When traveling to high altitudes, our bodies adjust so that our cells still receive sufficient oxygen. We are also constantly responding in physiological ways to internal and external stresses such as bacterial and viral infections, air and water pollution, dietary imbalance, and overcrowding. This ability to rapidly adapt to varying environmental conditions has made it possible for us to survive in most regions of the world. Humans live successfully in humid tropical forests, harsh deserts, arctic wastelands, and even densely populated cities with considerable amounts of pollution. Most other animal and plant species are restricted to one or relatively few environments by their more limited adaptability.

To adapt, children try to learn. To learn how to learn, there is a genetic mechanism on how to learn most important skills and patterns to recognize. An amount of information coming from the outside world is huge, so we cannot process it all. We select something with a high repetition frequency, primary value for learning. This is phylogenetically set in a way that we learn repetitive events. It does not make sense to learn patterns that do not re-appear because there is no practical value in this kind of knowledge. Only when one learns the patterns that will need to be recognized in the future, one gets reward.

7.3.3 Active Inductive Learning of CwA and CC

If the human learning system exists in a framework of a fixed training sets and not an active learning, a motivational structure of learning would be outside of the system and it is unclear why a human would learn at all and how to *reward* one for successful learning results. In an active learning system we have a notion of reward for a successful recognition session, so a human agent learns, explores the external world so that later he would be rewarded for this, having successfully completed a recognition or prediction task.

In active learning of CC, most of times the exploration experience is positive. A child views, hears, touches, tastes a new object, memorizes its images in various modalities, and next time before perceiving this or other similar object, this child knows what to expect and then confirms his expectations. This happens in most exploration scenarios, unless this child encounters something too hot or cold, sharp or heavy, too bright, smelling bad or tasting bad.

When a child touches a cup of hot coffee and burns his hand, she resets his learning session and tries again after some time. After a certain number of attempts she forms and memories a rule from the data *"brown water and smoke → hot water, may burn me"*

"no smoke above the glass → will not burn me, safe to touch and explore". To form these rules, this child follows the rule of induction, finding the commonalities between the cups where she burns and the ones she does not burn. To form the adequate training set for this induction, it is necessary to diversify these sets, selecting as distinct cups as possible. To form these rules properly, the child should operate in a feature space with limited dimension (size, temperature, shape, and color).

CC's adaption follows the steps:

- Touch a hot cup
- Feel pain – reset (cry)
- Touch it again, until experience is formed and memorized.

Whereas CC takes everything and some day takes a hot cup with smoke, burns himself and eventually is capable of generalizing and avoidance as a result of this generalizing, CwA burns himself from everything, so everything is avoided. Active inductive learning is based on the skill to *generalize* experimental observations.

Being a hyper-sensitive, and possessing higher systemizing skills, a child with autism would be operating in a much higher dimensional feature space (shape of the bottom, shape of handles, shape of cracks, reflection of light, a small bug on a surface, etc). Then it is much harder to form a rule for cold/hot cup because there are too many features involved. Forming invalid, too specific hypotheses, CwA keeps burning his hand, and is overall getting a negative exploration experience. CwA nevertheless keeps exploring, and keeps receiving strong stimuli in the very high dimensional space where it is almost impossible to form correct decision rules. Therefore, CwA keeps receiving negative rewards for his recognition results in the real world.

Why do CwAs, having their negative exploration experience re-occurring, keep exploring? When a normal adult encounters an unpleasantly strong stimulus such as very loud noise or very bright light, she knows it will end soon so no reason for distress. On the contrary, CwA does not know that receiving strong stimuli is something abnormal, and he does not expect different kinds of stimuli, so he keeps receiving them in spite of negative rewards, attempting to minimize these negative rewards.

For both CC and CwA, *switching attention* mechanism allows avoidance of a negative experience. As CC keeps switching to new stimuli instead of focusing

Fig. 7.5 Teaching proper orienteering in space and switching attention

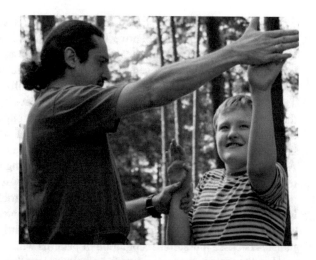

on one and exploring it, he avoids negative exploration experience. For CC a mechanism to explore prevails, but protective mechanism of avoidance is sometimes necessary. And for CwA avoidance becomes a norm (Fig. 7.5).

Let us consider normal and autistic development for children in educational environment. Unlike exploring the real world in early childhood, educational environment is usually explicitly rewarding: a teacher expresses compliments to students upon successful completion of exercises. In normal education, CC starts first grade with optimism because he have been receiving compliments so far. She starts learning with high interest because she believes that she is going to be successful, and she will keep hearing compliments. Sometimes she is not interested in her actual achievements but instead concerned with how her peers and the teacher estimate and value them.

On the contrary, if CC gets an unkind teacher who is always negative in assessing his results, he does some exercises well and some not so well, and he gets negative comment for the latter. His motivation for study goes down, and he stops receiving pleasure from the learning process. His thinking tends to avoid problems; instead he focuses on what he likes, like after-school activities.

With a friendly teacher, CwA can enjoy a school environment. Interacting with the real (hostile for CwA) world or with an unfriendly educational environment, CwA would continue his autistic development.

7.3.4 Learning Repetitive Patterns

In the conditions of hyper-sensitivity and overly strong stimuli, CwA is only capable of recognizing a pattern that is extremely close to an element of the training set. A typical case of high-similarity stimuli is repetitive events.

As an example of such stimuli in visual space, let us consider recognition of (1) child's mother and (2) repetitive TV commercials. Since the perceived image of mother's face varies more significantly (facial expression, face position, condition of illumination) than the perceived image of TV commercials (which are broadcasted over and over again; they essentially the same stimuli), the latter turns out to be a preferred type of stimulus that drives the child development. At the same time, the former stimuli can be filtered out as being too strong (due to its variability and therefore higher recognition efforts). A partial case of stimuli with high similarity is repetitive stimuli, which go through the whole path of autistic development. All children select to use most repetitive stimuli among the other stimuli for their training sets; however, autistic children *only* select most repetitive stimuli and do not proceed beyond them. As a result of this initial problem, CwA stop exploring human behavior and complex behavior of physical objects. Having stopped their explorations, they do not communicate properly with their mothers and other humans because it requires recognition of patterns with a broader range of features.

Usually, most repetitive events for a baby are mothers' behavior. She is always nearby, always saying *"hi"*. Babies get used to their mothers as a typical environment, so they accept the belief *"I need to adopt to my mothers, learn to recognize her."* Children from orphan houses have on average lower intellect (Ghera et al. 2009) because at the very beginning they don't have a source of repetitive objects to learn from, and "learning to learn" occurs much slower. A mother is a calibrating instrument for the building of learning mechanism for a child. Considering re-appearance of the mother as the repetitive event, a baby builds its learning mechanism to properly recognize if an approaching object is the mother or not. The baby develops an adaptation rule that is essential for pattern recognition:"If I do too many false positives, increase the threshold. Otherwise, if I do too many false negatives, decrease the threshold."

Mother's reappearance has its own accuracy in terms of new positions, illumination, sounds and frequency, which becomes the set of patterns for a child to optimize her recognition threshold. The mother would never say "hi" in exactly the same way, so the baby should be able to deal with some level of deviation, recognizing the sound. Intonation is different; the mother holds the baby in different ways, wears different clothes, smells differently, etc. The baby can recognize patterns with substantial deviation.

Usually the baby looks for most repetitive events and finds his mother. In the case with a huge amount of advertisement, repetitive things on radio and TV, machines roar in the same way, noise from appliances and images can trigger the choice of the learning source of the best repetitive pattern. After that, the baby stops recognizing the events which have lower precision in their repetition, and looses the skills to do it. Then the mother is rejected because she is too different in appearance.

Repetitions are natural for CC as well, CC repeats the same movement or perception activity, but then proceeds to the exploration of the world to change it and make it better for him. CC applies already developed recognition mechanisms, tuned and tested in repetitions. At the same time, CwA remains in the phase of receiving primary feelings. The role of repetition is not tuning but a reproduction of the same familiar pleasant feelings. By self-stimulation (stereotypy) CwA form feeling directly. Unlike CC playing with a ball, a CwA avoids catching it and passing it over to another player. Instead, CwA would just hold and squeeze a ball. For a CwA the willingness to change the world to make it better is reduced to maintaining it in a current, familiar form, since there is a lack of positive experience in exploring and recognizing it.

7.3.5   Stereotypy

In case of autism, there is a failure to determine what is a repetitive event and what is not. CwA consider repetitive only the events that repeat with ideal frequency. Tremendous volume of external information does not make it into CwA. CwA stops perceiving whole stimuli of real world and only captures elements of these stimuli. This is because the whole stimuli do not fit into the narrow gap formed by autistic cognition trained on the fully repetitive training sets. CwA start to perceive objects and events by their small parts. In these parts, repetitions are most accurate.

At the age of 18 months CwA with their available perception mechanism encounter a necessity to perceive stimulus as a whole. Then the whole pattern is formed not at the level of causal links between parts, like CC, but instead at the level of unordered sets of these parts. CwA are now getting used to perceive individual parts. When it is necessary to perceive the whole object, CwA attempts to combine these individual parts. CwA continues perceive elements, but not the whole stimulus. CwA want to perceive the world as a whole, but lack a mechanism to do that.

In terms of multi-modal perception, visual, speech and auditory patterns are perceived separately and are not coordinated (Figs. 7.6 and 7.7). In autistic brain sensory integration does not occur (Bogdashina 2005). Multi-modal integration is based on amplification of stimuli, but it is unwanted for CwA, since stronger stimuli cause negative feeling. Neither binocular vision nor binaural hearing is developing. Whereas for CC vision prevails, it is not the case for CwA where hearing is more important, since sound is not as intense as light and its perception is associated with fewer failures.

Making efforts to protect themselves from stimuli which are too strong, CwA develop a mechanism to filter out these strong stimuli (which are also more informative) and perceive weaker ones, less informative, but with a higher similarity with each other. Due to the hyper-sensitivity, a child with autism is over-selective to the stimuli of external world. We attempt to simulate the phenomenology of early development of autistic cognition as a choice of perception mode in the conditions of hyper-sensitive sensory system:

1. A child selects, or capable of, recognizing humans such as parents and relatives, which requires multimodal perception, classification of rather distinct images

Fig. 7.6 Example of
avoidance behavior

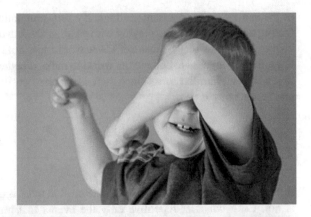

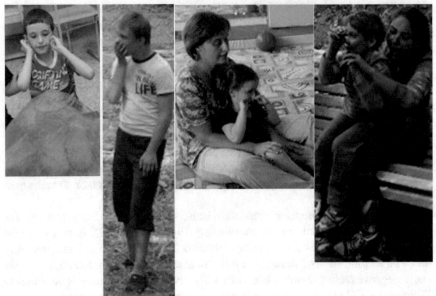

Fig. 7.7 Stereotypy in children with autism

into a single class, and is then capable of further emotional and mental development. Selecting to recognize the subjects of the mental world leads to a normal
adaptation.

2. A child selects to recognize highly repetitive artificial stimuli such as TV
   advertisement, smartphone images and sounds, passing by cars, and other
   subjects of the physical world with extremely high similarity. Being forced to
   recognize the subjects of the *physical world only* leads to *autistic adaptation*.
   Autistic adaptation implies the *avoidance behavior* to ignore stimuli other than
   highly repetitive ones (Fig. 7.8).

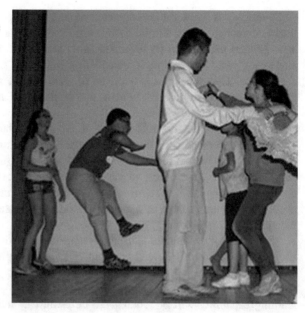

Fig. 7.8 Movement and perception of space in autistic development (Sunny World 2013)

Human and machine intelligence both experience a pleasure from predictability. Control children like to play games, which reflect the world, but reduce its representation to a structured of a limited complexity. Playing games, CC can tolerate a broad range of variability, and wide spectrums of variations are allowed.

On the contrary, CwA will play in a game with zero variability; their doll would say the same expression in the same way. No diversity in behavior can be handled within the comfort zone of CwA. Whereas CC play with many little cars, CwA would arrange cars in rows: they can only handle a simple element of repetition that is familiar, and therefore rewarding. The range of deviation for repetition is different between CwA and CC: under hyper-sensitivity a totally novel signal is almost like pain.

Stereotypy or self-stimulatory behavior refers to repetitive body movements or repetitive movement of objects being held by an individual. This behavior is common in many individuals with developmental disabilities and those who experienced institutional care (Bos et al. 2011); however, it appears to be more common in autism. In fact, if a person with another developmental disability exhibits a form of self-stimulatory behavior, often the person is also labelled as having autistic characteristics.

Stereotypy includes repetitive or ritualistic body movements, posture, or utterance that serves no social function (Rapp et al. 2004). Stereotypies may be simple movements such as body rocking, or complex, such as self-caressing, crossing and uncrossing of legs, and marching in place. Often children with autism engage in these repetitive, restricted, and stereotyped patterns of behavior. Stereotyping is caused by sensory deprivation and lack of afferentation. Stereotypic behaviors can take many unusual forms.

Stereotypy is a natural consequence of autistic adaptation. CwA's cognition is unable to recognize real stimuli of the world and therefore recognizes *auto-created, stereotypical* patterns, to be rewarded as an active learning system. CwA follows an "easier" way of perception, considering only very similar patterns coming as a sequence. Then this child is deprived of mental and emotional development due to his incapability to perceive humans and their mental attitudes (Shpitsberg 2005; Galitsky and Shpitsberg 2015).

Not only CwA demonstrate feature of autistic adaptation, learning the external world. Blind persons sometimes develop self-stimulation, as well as Down syndrome (due to a mental retardation) and cerebral palsy (due to the inability to hold subjects). In all these cases, to get a reward for successful recognition (having a defective recognition system), CwA are forced to pose themselves recognition problems they are capable of handling via stereotypy, creating artificial patterns to recognize.

Notice that if a machine learning system is fed with very similar elements of the training set, it will have a problem of recognizing even very similar objects to the training ones. Moreover, it will be unable to recognize the ones with significant deviation from the elements of the training set, therefore the whole learning capability will be lacking. To be rewarded, such learning system would need to find input stimuli that are alike to be able to recognize them. At the same time, to avoid unsuccessful recognitions, the learning system would need to do without complex stimuli, especially those requiring multiple modality signals to be recognized (visual, auditory, tactile; Fig. 7.9). Selectively blocking of a particular modality allows avoiding a stimulus that is too strong (for a machine learning system, too different to what has been in the training dataset). Hence we conclude that a hyper-sensitivity may lead to a condition where links between perception system for various modalities are not reinforced and therefore become dysfunctional at the next steps of autistic development.

Fig. 7.9 Visual and tactile multi-modal perception (Sunny World 2013)

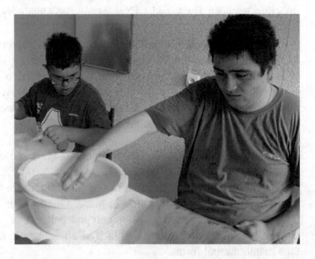

Because autistic sensory and behavior control mechanisms does not fit the real world, children with autism experience failures after failures, forming their behavioral experience, unlike control children which are fairly successful at learning these control mechanism from real world. This is true for autism as well as other disorders, such as tonic regulation under cerebral palsy.

The only way of successful learning from the real world is permanent confirmation that the learned control patterns are adequate to the real world. The control patterns are further advanced and adjusted to changes in the real world if the learner feels a success of newly formed control patterns.

Under normal development, based on success in her own investigative experience, a child builds an adaptive model of behavior. This model is oriented to the consecutive investigation of the real world and successful adaptation. All behavioral forms target receiving various feeling of the real world, and as a result various forms of communication with this world develops, including speech. Also, the experience of social interaction is gained.

Under anomalous development, a child experiences a constant discomfort interacting with the real world. There are many reasons for this: a child with autism cannot grab an object, mentally retarded child cannot understand what an adult wants from him, and a child with autism experiences discomfort from interaction with another person or an object from the real world. Such a child rebuilds his adaptation mechanisms so that feelings come from his internal world, not the real world. This child satisfies his natural desire in feelings by means of stimulus he forms himself. In this case he pleases himself by the successful feelings at the both tactile/sensory and intellectual levels. In the case of infantile type of mental development of children with cerebral palsy we encounter an extensive and saturated world of phantasies. This world of phantasies is intended to replace the negative sentiments associated with the perception of the real world. As a result, the behavior of such child becomes "autistic". The desire to receive feelings from the real world is replaced by the desire to receive feelings that are formed by this child "directly", without physical means. In this case the self-stimulation (stereotypy) of a child with autism, mental retardation and cerebral palsy can be similar.

The purpose of stereotypy is to assure the comfort feelings in the conditions when the feelings from the real world are impossible. Under such development scenario it is impossible to form an adequate adaptation system for the real world. We refer to this scenario as dis-ontogenesis; under this scenario the demand to develop communication skills is minimal down to the total lack of the necessity to communicate.

We suggest the anomaly occurs in the process of early formation if sensory system (before the age of 1.5–2 years), and afterwards, as a result of usage of the improperly formed sensory system, "sensory stereotypy".

Self-stimulation can be of "reinforcing" as well as "substituting" natures, depending on how a child is focused on the feature selection process and his capability on combining stereotypical and arbitrary activities. Hence a child with autism stops at an "autistic" self-regulation mechanism as most adaptive for him.

Stereotypy can involve any individual sensing modality or cover all modalities. For vision, CwA may staring at a light, do repetitive blinking, move his fingers or the palm in front of his eyes, or do hand-flapping. For the auditory modality, CwA can be tapping ears, snapping fingers, or making vocal sounds. In the tactile space, a child may rub the skin with her hands or with another object, or scratch. Vestibular rocking, placing body parts in her mouth and licking as taste stereotypy, and sniffing people as smell stereotypy are all examples in other sensory modalities. The stereotypy behavior can take the form of mouthing objects, hand flapping, body rocking, repetitive finger movements, nonfunctional or non-contextual repeated vocalizations. Other forms include toe walking, spinning objects, requiring order and predictability in routines, immediate or delayed echolalia (repeating things that others have said), running objects across one's visual field, or dropping items and watching them fall.

According to our model, recognition of visual, auditory, tactile, taste and smell patterns occurred with the training set of extremely high, repetitive similarity. As a result the recognition system in all these modalities can only successfully recognize repetitive or same stimuli, and self-stimulation is necessary to feed the recognition system with patterns which can be recognized successfully. Psychological theories confirm that self-stimulation is exhibited to calm a person, to adapt her in her hypersensitive state. Since the environment is too stimulating and the person is in a state of sensory overload, he engages in these behaviors to block-out the over-stimulating environment; and his attention becomes focused inwardly.

Alternatively, there is a popular opinion that due to some dysfunctional system in the brain, the body calls for stimulation. CwA engages in this form of behaviors to excite or arouse the nervous system. One specific theory states that these behaviors release beta-endorphins in the body (endogeneous opiate-like substances) and provides the person with some form of internal pleasure (Sandman and Kemp 2011). It has been also shown that stereotypic behaviors interfere with attention and learning. Interestingly, these behaviors are often effective positive reinforcers if a person is allowed to engage in these behaviors after completing a task.

There are many possibilities to reduce or get rid of stereotypic behaviors, such as physical exercise. Also, providing a CwA with alternative, more socially-appropriate, forms of stimulation helps such as chewing a gum instead of biting her hand. Drugs are also used to reduce these behaviors; however, it is not clear whether the drugs actually reduce the behaviors explicitly by providing internal arousal or indirectly (e.g., slowing down one's overall motor movement).

Self-stimulation is normal process for CC and adults. A man restores his psycho-emotional balance by receiving a sensory input which is expected. These self-stimulation activities must be accurate, totally predictable, ideal: a person first expects certain feeling and then receives it, being awarded by a positive recognition experience. For different people this may involve smoking, eating sweet, biking, solving a math problem etc. When smoking, it has to be the same cigarette, because all feelings need to be predictable. Humans need to receive known feelings, old feelings, familiar feelings, since new feelings require too many computational/recognition resources. Self-stimulation requires high accuracy: the patterns should be exactly the same: for example, smoking and coffee together works well since remembered by association stimuli. And this pleasure can be associated with any sensory modality.

Self-stimulation can be based on rhythms, stem self-stimulation, reverse breathing, swallowing, rocking. Also, higher-level self-stimulation includes attaching palm to mouth to strengthen the sound, repeating text. Since a necessity to receive similar feeling is physiologically necessary for all humans, auto stimulation is common, but CC spend a fifth part of their time on self-stimulation and the rest on exploration, and CwA vice versa.

7.3.6 Ignoring Important Features

When one observes the behavior of a child with autism 2–3 year old, it is the second stage of the development process. At this second stage, a child tries to interact with the real world based on the anomalous sensory system built on the first stage. This first stage is primarily oriented at the protection of unknown stimulus and at finding familiar stimulus that can be understood.

Two factors lead to this: broken mechanism of interaction with the real world, and decrease of the threshold of affective discomfort caused by this interaction. In other words, the latter factor is connected with the increased sensitivity to sensory signals.

Control children learn to recognize objects of the real world correctly because:

1. improving the technique of focusing at an object, relying on the skills of ignorance of secondary, noisy information.
2. the coordination of sensory signals from various systems and the analysis of various properties of objects being recognized.

Under autistic development, since the majority of sensory signals is perceived as redundant, the child is forced to learn the process of ignoring, decreasing the volume of these signals. As a result, a child with autism learns to avoid the stimuli that are intended for him.

Instead of systematic development and improvement of sensory systems in the direction of better understanding of the real world, a child with autism develops a mechanism to ignore signals from the real world. At the same time, a child with autism develops his sensitivity of the signals that carry minimal sensory information. Instead of the frontal direction, which carries important stimuli, a child with autism perceives the peripheral visual and auditory signals. All bright and powerful stimuli are ignored: eye contacts are avoided, and a child is crying when petted. Sensory mechanisms are built in a way to perceive a minimum of sensory information and nevertheless represent somehow the real world. Hence the capability to merge different sensory systems (visual, auditory) is lacking, binocular vision and binaural auditory systems are not being developed.

Peripheral vision as a way to protect from overwhelming signals has always existed, even in medieval times. One of the examples can be a "puzzled look" of Mona Lisa of Leonardo da Vinci. We hypothesize that it is due to the fact that she uses peripheral vision. If one looks at the painting, it is visible that the face is oriented not along the pupils, but deviates from it. This is typical for people with autism.

If one looks at how an autistic child is tracking a hand of an adult ringing a bell, it is noticeable that this child either watches or hears, but does not do it simultaneously. A merge of sensory stimulus of a child with autism occurs only in the process of the formation of self-stimulation. This process, being fairly intense, is intended to distract the child from other stimuli of the real world.

In fact, the possibility to use a merged perception helps us interact with the external world successfully, building behavioral strategies capable of embedding us in this world. The feature of selectivity of perception, formed by a child with autism spontaneously, to decrease the intensity of the sensory input, leads to the lack of capability of perception of the real world and interaction with it.

Recent studies of autism also show a high capability of children with autism to ignore object in the domains they are not interested in. A child with autism concentrates on an object with high intensity and ignores background objects situated very near it. In case of control, such concentration decreases slowly as the objects are further away from the focus of attention.

One can hypothesize that to implement the mechanism of ignoring objects a child with autism develops and improves the fixation mechanisms. This mechanism achieves maximum annihilation of background objects by the property of the object she is being focused on. A child with autism selects less informative sensory features and directions in the real world as preferred, and at the same time develops the stimulus substitution mechanism, substituting unknown (as possibly dangerous) stimulus with the ones well known, his own (stereotypy). The mechanism of fixation plays the key role in this feature selection process.

In his further life, when the (intense) period of feature selections is over, a child continues to learn the real world with less intensity, relying on his specifically built sensory system. Peripheral sensory directions advance, and the real world is perceived by means of discreet signals, which are correlated neither within a single sensory mode nor synthesizing different signal modalities. Stereotypy occupies a key position in the sensory system of a child with autism, being "reinforcing" and "substituting". The substituting sensory signals almost completely replace the external ones, and reinforcing assure a stable self-perception, preventing to perceive real external stimuli.

A part of active learning is perceiving pleasant stimuli and avoiding unpleasant ones. When most people come across a pleasant scent, such as a nice perfume or freshly baked cookies, they typically take a good long sniff. While walking next to a dumpster, however, a person would most likely shorten his incoming breaths, minimizing the intake of the unpleasant odor. At the same time, CwA don't make this natural adjustment like other people do. In fact, children with autism continue right on sniffing in the same way, no matter how pleasant or awful the scent (Pedersen 2015)

7.3.7   From Hyper-sensitivity to Stereotypy of an Engineering System

People with autism suffer from difficulties in learning social rules from examples, however many remediation strategies have not taken this into account. Therefore an appropriate remediation strategy is to teach not simply via examples (via inductive learning) but instead to teach the appropriate rules (via deduction). The cognitive learning skills of children with autism from the standpoint of active inductive learning are analyzed. We start with the hyper-sensitivity that leads to the broken links between perceptions of different modalities, lack of adequate capability to perceive real world stimuli, which then leads to auto stimulation and autistic cognition. We propose an architecture for a software active learning system which behaves in a similar way, going through the same cognitive steps. The commonalities in deficiencies of autistic and software active learning systems are analyzed. We hypothesize that the autistic learning system, starting with just a hyper-sensitivity feature without other deficiencies, can potentially evolve in a faulty inductive learning system, deviating stronger and stronger from a normally developed systems at each iteration of the learning process. This chapter confirms that the autistic cognitive process is plausible in terms of an abstract computational learning system.

We summarize this section in the chart for the sequence of step towards autistic cognitive development (Fig. 7.10).

Not just humans can evolve into autistic cognition. A number of poorly designed engineering intelligent systems can recognize only patterns that are very similar to the ones being trained.

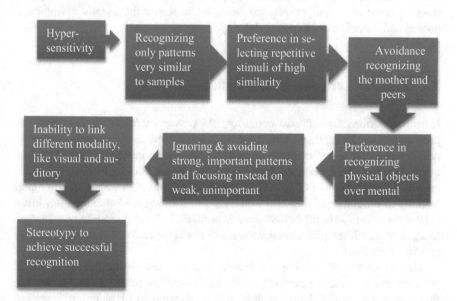

Fig. 7.10 Steps in autistic cognitive development

One such engineering domain is security: because the system architects intend to avoid false positive in as much degree as possible, they configure the system to issue alerts only for the patterns very similar to which has been identified as true attack or intrusion. False positive is any normal or expected behavior that is identified as anomalous or malicious. This can fall into several categories:

- An application not seen in the training stage of an anomaly detection system will likely trigger an alert when the application attempts to run.
- A signature can be written too broadly and thus include both legitimate and illegitimate traffic.
- Anomalous behavior in one area of an organization may be acceptable while highly suspect in another. As an example NetBIOS over TCP/IP traffic is normal in a Windows LAN environment but not generally expected on the Internet.

Since it is hard to find real-life positive sets, the creators of security systems demonstrate their functionality on a very limited set of examples. Only these examples are then demonstrated, so from our view what is happening is self-stimulation. Usually active learning is impossible in the security domain.

Another domain where a poorly designed system can only function if self-stimulation mode is search and recommendation. A number of conversational customer support agents can only repeat very closely the dialogues introduced by the creator. Once there is a deviation from such dialog, the system behavior starts being totally meaningless, and it can learn nothing from user inputs.

We share two examples of customer support agents of financial institutions who function in the mode close to stereotypy (Fig. 7.11).

Table 7.1 shows the delivery log: initially the steps are consecutive but then they evolve into stereotypy with obvious repetitive patterns. It looks like the system cannot get rid of stereotype patterns here, but in reality the agent's reasoning is normal and it is reluctant to do the delivery.

7.4 Hybrid Active Learning System *Jasmine*

Having described the autistic cognition, its development and its features, we proceed to formalizing them. We demonstrate how a hypersensitive technical system developing in an active learning framework can evolve into an autistic cognition mode. We describe a software learning system *Jasmine* configured to imitate the cognitive development of CC and CwA. Originally *Jasmine* was designed to support learning in a number of domains which require learning *explainability*: not just a correct classification or prediction needs to be made, but also it needs to be explained in terms of which samples and which rules were employed in the decision (Galitsky and Spitsberg 2006).

The foundation of learning and cognition is an inductive reasoning pattern. If we want to recognize the mother or distinguish her from other people, we want to find a common feature shared by at least two appearances (or sound, or touch) of

Eric P.: Hi, my name is Eric P.. How may I help you?
Boris : This money transfer was not approved. If you were charged for this money transfer, you will be automatically refunded.
Boris : Can you please check my account and help me to select another option?
Eric P.: I would be happy to help you with that.
Boris : I have valid bank accounts and debit cards
Eric P.: Unfortunately, it's not always possible to authenticate everyone electronically to allow a credit card payment.
Eric P.: We can offer an alternative with our WU® Pay service:
Eric P.: We will e-mail you a bill for the amount of your money transfer, and you pay using your bank's online bill pay service.
Eric P.: Once we receive your payment, your money transfer will be completed.
Boris : ok, I can do that
Eric P.: We apologize for any inconvenience.
Eric P.: Is there anything else I can help you with today?
Boris : can you do this email?
Eric P.: Please clarify and restate your question.
Boris : can you please send me email for bill pay information?
Eric P.: Once you have selected WU Pay as the "Pay With" option and clicked the SUBMIT button, the RECEIPT screen will provide instructions on how to fund the Money Transfer.
Boris : ok, I will try that
Boris : are you an automated agent?
Eric P.: After choosing WU® Pay, you'll receive a bill by email.
Eric P.: Is there anything else I can help you with today?
Boris : can you please answer my previous question?
Eric P.: What question Boris?
Boris : are you an automated agent?
Eric P.: No sir
Boris : It is my right as a customer to know if I am served by an automated or human agent, right?
Eric P.: Yes it is
Boris : which financial institutions can I use to do auto bill pay option?
Eric P.: You pay on your bank's website using online bill pay (just like paying other bills).
Boris : ok, thanks, no more questions
Eric P.: Is there anything else I can help you with today?
Boris : no, thanks

Boris : Can you please reactivate my card which I am trying to use in Nepal?
CS Rep: We value you as a customer... We will cancel your card... New card will be mailed to your California address.

Boris : Can you please give your candy to my daughter who is hungry now and is about to cry?
CwA: No, my mom told me not to feed babies. Its wrapper is nice and blue. I need to wash my hands before I eat it.

Fig. 7.11 Two dialogues with agents where it is hard to judge whether it is a human or software agent (on the top) and a CwA

the mother. This feature should not be present for other patterns (father, siblings, friends, nurses). The principle of induction states that a commonality of features between the patterns (such as mother appearance, with the same *haircut* and *smell of perfume*) causes the target feature (the object being the *mother*). This principle is referred to as the *direct method of agreement*.

Table 7.1 A log of activity for mail delivery showing the system evolving in an "infinite" loop

Sunnyvale, CA, United States	03/22/2016	9:09 P.M.	The receiver has moved. We're attempting to obtain a new delivery address for this receiver./We've contacted the receiver to request additional information
	03/22/2016	5:16 P.M.	The receiver has moved. We're attempting to obtain a new delivery address for this receiver
	03/22/2016	6:43 A.M.	Destination Scan
Sunnyvale, CA, United States	03/21/2016	3:44 P.M.	The delivery change was completed./The address was corrected
	03/21/2016	3:40 P.M.	The delivery change was completed./The package is being held for a future delivery date
	03/21/2016	3:39 P.M.	The street number is incorrect. This may delay delivery. We're attempting to update the address
	03/21/2016	11:24 A.M.	A delivery change for this package is in progress./We've rescheduled this delivery
Sunnyvale, CA, United States	03/15/2016	5:15 P.M.	The street number is incorrect. This may delay delivery. We're attempting to update the address/We've contacted the receiver to request additional information
Sunnyvale, CA, United States	03/14/2016	7:55 P.M.	The street number is incorrect. This may delay delivery. We're attempting to update the address/We're unable to contact the receiver
	03/14/2016	2:34 P.M.	The street number is incorrect. This may delay delivery. We're attempting to update the address
	03/14/2016	3:34 A.M.	Destination Scan
Sunnyvale, CA, United States	03/11/2016	2:50 P.M.	The delivery change was completed./The package is being held for a future delivery date
	03/11/2016	2:50 P.M.	The delivery change was completed./Your delivery has been rescheduled for the next business day
	03/11/2016	2:49 P.M.	Incomplete address information may delay delivery. We are attempting to update this information
	03/11/2016	1:33 P.M.	A delivery change for this package is in progress./We've rescheduled this delivery
Sunnyvale, CA, United States	03/10/2016	11:49 A.M.	Incomplete address information may delay delivery. We are attempting to update this information./We've contacted the receiver to request additional information
	03/10/2016	4:20 A.M.	Destination Scan
	03/10/2016	2:55 A.M.	Arrival Scan
Oakland, CA, United States	03/10/2016	2:08 A.M.	Departure Scan
Oakland, CA, United States	03/09/2016	5:24 P.M.	Arrival Scan
Louisville, KY, United States	03/09/2016	3:42 P.M.	Departure Scan
	03/09/2016	12:58 P.M.	Origin Scan
United States	03/08/2016	10:23 P.M.	Order Processed: Ready for UPS

If two or more instances of the phenomenon under investigation have only one circumstance in common, the circumstance in which alone all the instances agree, is the cause (or effect) of the given phenomenon (Mills 1843).

We will explore how a hyper-sensitivity to cognition of an arbitrary phenomenon leads to faulty recognition capabilities although the direct method of agreement holds.

7.4.1   A Reasoning Schema

Jasmine is based on a learning model called JSM-method (Anshakov et al. 1989, in honor of John Stuart Mill, the English philosopher who proposed schemes of inductive reasoning in the nineteenth century). JSM-method to be presented in this section implements Mill's direct method of agreement stating that similar effects (associated features, target features) are likely to follow common causes (attributes), as well as abduction in the form of explainability. We use the Explanation-based Learning framework to introduce our reasoning schema. Within this framework JSM attempts to solve the problem of *inductive bias*, a means to select one generalization over another. Like for CwA, it is hard for an automated learning system to find a proper generalization level, making decisions in the real world.

The task of *Jasmine* is to predict or recognize a *target feature* (mother or not mother, eatable or not eatable) given observable features (such as color and texture of hairs, smell of perfume or vinegar, sound of steps or cutting material under question). These features are observed in the *objects* of a training set so that a target feature of new, unknown object can be recognized or predicted (Galitsky 2007).

Given the *features* of *objects of a training set*, we intend to obtain *an expression* for the target feature that includes all positive examples and excludes all negative examples, given some initial formalized background knowledge. For the human learning, it can be a genetically set or previously acquired (learned) knowledge, in the form of generalization from training set objects.

In the Explanation-based Learning setting such expression for the target feature is a logical consequence of background knowledge and training dataset; however, this condition is not always viable in a domain of human learning from with experimental observations. Explanation-based Learning is designed to generalize form a single example; however, in human learning domains one would prefer more reliable conclusions from multiple observations. These multiple observations (examples) may introduce inconsistencies; and the desired machine learning technique should be capable of finding consistent explanations linking possibly mutually inconsistent observations with the target feature.

Within *Jasmine* first-order language, objects are atoms, and known features and the target feature are the terms which include these atoms. For a given target feature, a term for a feature of an object can be as follows:

- *Positive*
- *Negative*
- *Inconsistent*
- *Unknown*

An inference to obtain this target feature (satisfied or not) can be represented as one in a respective four-valued logic (Anshakov et al. 1989). The predictive machinery is based on building hypotheses in the form of clauses where *target_feature(O)*

$$target\_feature(O):\text{-} feature_1(O, \ldots), \ldots, feature_n(O, \ldots),\text{ that separate examples,}$$

is to be predicted, and *features* $_1$, . . . ,*feature* $_n \in features$ are the features the target feature is associated with; *O* ranges over objects.

Desired separation is based on the *similarity* of objects in terms of features they satisfy (according to the direct method of agreement above). Usually, such similarity is domain-dependent. However, building the general framework of inductive-based prediction, we use the anti-unification of formulas that express the totality of features of the given and other objects (our features (causes) do not have to be unary predicates; they are expressed by arbitrary first-order terms). We assume the human learning to be as general and flexible as this operation of anti-unification, to be introduced.

Figure 7.12 is an example of a learning setting, where features, objects, the target feature and the knowledge base is given. We keep using the conventional PROLOG notations for variables and constants.

```
features([e1, e2, e3, e4, e5, e6, oa1, oa2, ap1, ap2, ap3, ap4, f1, f2,
    cc4, cc5, cc6, cc7, cb5, cb7]). %% Features and target features
objects([o1, o2, o3, o4, o5, o6, o7, o8, o9, o10, o11, o12, o13, o14,
    o15, o16, o17, o18]).
target_feature [cb5]).
    %% Beginning of knowledge base
e1(o1). oa1(o1). ap1(o1). ap3(o1). f1(o1). cc5(o1). cb5(o1).
e1(o2). oa1(o2). ap1(o2). ap3(o2). f1(o2). cc5(o2). cb5(o2).
e2(o8). oa2(o8). ap2(o8). ap1(o8). f1(o8). cc5(o8). cb5(o8).
e3(o10). oa1(o10). a3(o10). ap2(o10). f1(o10). cc4(o10).
e3(o11). oa1(o11). a3(o11). ap2(o11). f1(o11). cc4(o11). cb5(o11). cb7(o11).
e4(o16). oa1(o16). a1(o16). ap1(o16). f1(o16). cc5(o16). cb5(o16).
e5(o17). oa1(o17). a4(o17). ap2(o17). f1(o17). cc6(o17). cb7(o17).
e6(o18). oa1(o18). a1(o18). ap2(o18). f1(o18). cc4(o18). cb7(o18).
    %% End of knowledge base
unknown(cb5(o10)).
```

Fig. 7.12 A sample knowledge base for high-level mining of protein sequence data

In a numerical, statistical learning similarity between objects is expressed by a number. In deterministic, structured learning with explainability of results similarity is a *structure*. Similarity between a pair of objects is a hypothetical object which obeys the common features of this pair of objects. In handling similarity *Jasmine* is close to Formal Concept Analysis (Ganter and Wille 1999, Section 4.3.5), where similarity is the *meet* operation of a *lattice* (called concept lattice) where features are represented by unary predicates only. For the arbitrary first-order formulas for objects in *Jasmine* we choose the anti-unification of formulas which expresses features of the pair of objects to derive a formula for similarity sub-object. Below we will be using the predicate

similar(Object1, Object2, CommonSubObject) which yields the third argument given the first and the second arguments.

The reasoning procedure of *Jasmine* is shown in Fig. 7.13. Note that the prediction schema is oriented to discover which features cause the target feature and how (the causal link) rather than just searching for common features for the target feature (which would be much simpler, six units on the top). The respective clauses (1–4) and sample results for each numbered unit (1–4) are presented in Fig. 7.13.

Let us build a framework for predicting the target feature V of objects set by the formulas X expressing their features: *unknown(X, V)*. We are going to predict whether $V(x_1, \ldots, x_n)$ holds or not, where $x_1, \ldots, x_n$ are variables of the formula set X (in our example, $X = cb5(o10)$, $x_1 = o10$).

We start with the raw data, positive and negative examples, raw*Pos(X, V)* and *rawNeg(X, V)*, for the target feature V, where X range over formulas expressing features of objects. We form the totality of intersections for these examples (positive ones, U, that satisfy *iPos(U,V)*, and negative ones, W, that satisfy *iNeg(W,V)*, not shown):

$$iPos(U, V):- rawPos(X1, V), rawPos(X2, V), X1\backslash=X2, similar(X1, X2, U), U\backslash=[\,].$$
$$iPos(U, V):- iPos(U1, V), rawPos(X1, V), similar(X1, U1, U), U\backslash=[\,]. \qquad (7.1)$$

Above are the recursive definitions of the intersections. As the logic program clauses which actually construct the lattice for the totality of intersections for positive and negative examples, we introduce the third argument to accumulate the currently obtained intersections (the negative case is analogous):

```
iPos(U, V):- iPos(U, V, _).
iPos(U, V, Accums):- rawPos(X1, V), rawPos(X2, V), X1\=X2, similar(X1, X2, U),
         Accums=[X1, X2], U\=[ ].
iPos(U, V, AccumsX1):- iPos(U1, V, Accums), !, rawPos(X1, V),
         not member(X1, Accums), similar(X1, U1, U), U\=[ ],
         append(Accums, [X1], AccumsX1).
```

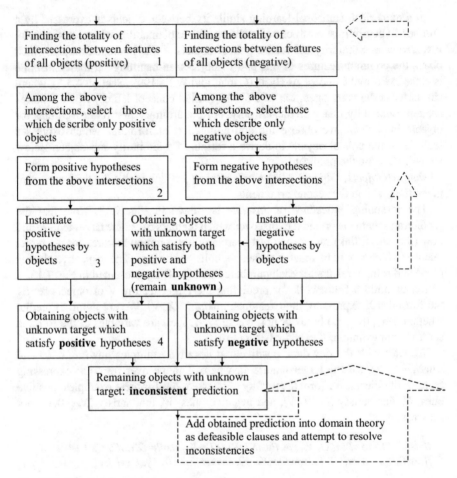

Fig. 7.13 The chart for reasoning procedure of *Jasmine*

As one can see, there is a "symmetric" treatment of positive and negative examples and hypotheses: *Jasmine* uses negative examples to falsify hypotheses that have counter-examples. On the contrary, a simplified Explanation-based Learning uses only positive examples and can be viewed as just the "left half" of Figure ....

To obtain the actual positive *posHyp* and negative *negHyp* hypotheses from the intersections derived above, we filter out the inconsistent hypotheses which belong to both positive and negative intersections *inconsHyp(U, V)*:

$$inconsHyp(U, V):- iPos(U, V), iNeg(U, V).$$
$$posHyp(U, V):-iPos(U, V), not\ inconsHyp(U, V).$$
$$negHyp(U, V):-iNeg(U, V), not\ inconsHyp(U, V). \qquad (7.2)$$

Here U is the formula expressing the features of objects. It serves as a body of clauses for hypotheses V :- U.

The following clauses deliver the totality of objects so that the features expressed by the hypotheses are *included* in the features of these objects. We derive positive and negative hypotheses *reprObjectsPos(X, V)* and *reprObjectsNeg(X, V)* where X is instantiated with objects (V is positive and negative respectively). The last clause (with the head *reprObjectsIncons(X, V)*) implements the search for the objects to be predicted so that the features expressed by both the positive and negative hypotheses are included in the features of these objects.

$$reprObjectsPos(X, V):- rawPos(X, V), posHyp(U, V), similar(X, U, U).$$

$$reprObjectsNeg \ (X, V):- rawNeg(X, V), negHyp(U, V), similar(X, U, U).$$
$$reprObjectsIncons(X, V):-unknown(X,V), \ posHyp(U1, V), \ negHyp(U2, V),$$
$$similar(X, U1, U1), \ similar(X, U2, U2). \tag{7.3}$$

Two clauses above (top and middle) do not participate in prediction directly; their role is to indicate which objects deliver what kind of prediction.

Finally, we approach the clauses for prediction. For the objects with unknown target features, the system predicts that they either satisfy these target features, do not satisfy these target features, or that the fact of satisfaction is inconsistent with the raw facts. To deliver V, a positive hypothesis has to be found so that the set of features X of an object has to include the features expressed by this hypothesis, and X should not be from *reprObjectsIncons(X, V)*. To deliver $\neg V$, a negative hypothesis has to be found so that a set of features X of an object has to include the features expressed by this hypothesis and X is not from *reprObjectsIncons(X, V)*. No prediction can be made for the objects with features expressed by X from the third clause,

$$predictIncons(X,V).$$
$$\mathbf{predictPos(X,V):- \ unknown(X, V), posHyp(U, V), similar(X, U,U),}$$

$$\mathbf{not \ reprObjectsIncons(X, V).}$$
$$predictNeg(X,V):- unknown(X, V), negHyp(U, V), similar(X, U,U),$$
$$not \ reprObjectsIncons(X, V).$$
$$predictIncons(X,V):- unknown(X, V), not \ predictPos(X, V),$$
$$not \ predictNeg(X, V), not \ reprObjectsIncons(X, V). \tag{7.4}$$

The first clause above (shown in bold) will serve as an entry point to predict (choose) a given target feature among a generated list of possible target features that can be obtained for the current state. The clause below is an entry point to *Jasmine* if it is integrated with other applications and/or reasoning components

predict_target_feature_by_learning(GoalConceptToBePredicted,S):-
findAllPossibleGoalConcepts (S, As), loadRequiredSamples(As),
member(EffectToBePredicted, As),
predictPos(X, GoalConceptToBePredicted), X\=[ ].

Predicate *loadRequiredSamples(As)* above forms the training dataset. If for a given dataset a prediction is inconsistent, it is worth eliminating the objects from the dataset which deliver this inconsistency. Conversely, if there are an insufficient number of positive or negative objects, additional ones are included in the dataset. A number of iterations may be required to obtain a prediction, however the iteration procedure is monotonic and deterministic: the source of inconsistency/insufficient data cases are explicitly indicated at the step where predicates *reprObjectsPos* and *reprObjectsNeg* introduced above are satisfied. This is the solution to the so called *blame assignment* problem, where by starting at the erroneous or inconsistent conclusion and tracking backward through the explanation structure, it is possible to identify pieces of domain knowledge that might have caused an error or inconsistency (Galitsky 2007).

When the set of obtained rules *posHyp* and *negHyp* for positive and negative examples (together with the original domain theory) is applied to a more extensive (evaluation or exploration) dataset, some of these rules may not always hold. If at the first run (1–4) *Jasmine* refuses to make predictions for some objects with unknown target features, then a repetitive iteration may be required, attempting to use newly generated predictions to obtain objects' target features which are currently unavailable. The arrows on the right of Fig. 7.13 illustrate this kind of iterative process.

For example, for the knowledge base Fig. 7.12 above, we have the following protocol and results (Fig. 7.14).

Hence *cb5(o10)* holds, which means that the sequence o10 has the length of loop of 5 amino acids.

7.4.2   *Computing Similarity Between Objects*

The quality of *Jasmine*-based prediction is dramatically dependent on how the similarity of objects is defined. Usually, high prediction accuracy can be achieved if the measure of similarity is sensitive to object features which determine the target feature (explicitly or implicitly). Since most of times it is unclear in advance which features affect the target feature, the similarity measure should take into account all available features. If the totality of selected features describing each object is expressed by formulas, a reasonable expression of similarity between a pair of objects is the following. It is a formula which is the least common generalization of the formulas for both objects, which is anti-unification, mentioned in the previous section. Anti-unification is the inverse operation to the unification of formulas in

---

1. Intersections
Positive: [[e1(_),oa1(_),ap1(_),ap3(_),f1(_),cc5(_)],
[ap1(_),f1(_),cc5(_)],[ap1(_),f1(_)],[oa1(_),f1(_)], [oa1(_),ap1(_),f1(_),cc5(_)],
[e2(_),e3(_),oa2(_),ap1(_),ap2(_),f1(_)],[e3(_),ap2(_),f1(_)],[e4(_),oa1(_),ap1(_),
f1(_),cc5(_)]]
Negative: [[oa1(_),ap2(_),f1(_),cb7(_)]]
Unassigned examples:

2. Hypotheses
Positive:[e1(_),oa1(_),ap1(_),ap3(_),f1(_),cc5(_)],[ap1(_),f1(_),cc5(_)],
[ap1(_),f1(_)],[oa1(_),f1(_)],[oa1(_),ap1(_),f1(_),cc5(_3B60)],
[e2(_),e3(_),oa2(_),ap1(_),ap2(_),f1(_)], [e3(_),ap2(_),f1(_)],
[e4(_),oa1(_),ap1(_),f1(_),cc5(_)]]
Negative: [[oa1(_),ap2(_),f1(_),cb7(_)]]
Contradicting hypotheses: []
    The clauses for hypotheses here are:
cb5(X)>-e1(X),oa1(X),ap1(X),ap3(X),f1(X),cc5(X);ap1(X),f1(X),cc5(X);ap1(X),f1(X).
cb5(X)>- not (oa1(X),ap2(X),f1(X),cb7(X)).   Note that all intersections are turned into
hypotheses because there is no overlap between positive and negative ones

3. Background (positive and negative objects with respect to the target feature cb5)
Positive:
[[e1(o1),oa1(o1),ap1(o1),ap3(o1),f1(o1),cc5(o1)],[e1(o2),oa1(o2),ap1(o2),ap3(o2),f1(o2
),cc5(o2)],
[e2(o7),e3(o7),oa2(o7), ap1(o7),ap2(o7),f1(o7),cc5(o7)],
[e2(o8),e3(o8),oa2(o8),ap1(o8),ap2(o8),f1(o8)],
[e3(o11),oa1(o11),ap2(o11),f1(o11),cc4(o11),cb7(o11)],[e4(o15),
oa1(o15),ap1(o15),f1(o15),cc5(o15)],
[e4(o16),oa1(o16),ap1(o16),f1(o16),cc5(o16)]]
Negative:
[[e5(o17),oa1(o17),ap2(o17),f1(o17),cc6(o17),cb7(o17)],[e6(o18),oa1(o18),ap2(o18),f1(
o18),cc4(o18),cb7(o18)]]]
Inconsistent: []
4. Prediction for cb5 (objects o10)
Positive: [[e3(o10),oa1(o10),ap2(o10),f1(o10),cc4(o10)]]
Negative:[]
Inconsistent: []
Uninstantiated derived rules (confirmed hypotheses)
cb5(O):- e3(O), oa1(O),ap2(O), f1(O), cc4(O).

Fig. 7.14 The *Jasmine* prediction protocol. Steps are numbered in accordance to the units at
Fig. 7.15

logic programming. Unification is the basic operation which finds the least general
(instantiated) formula (if it exists), given a pair of formulas. Anti-unification was
used as a method of generalization; later this work was extended to form a theory of
inductive generalization and hypothesis formation.

For example, for two formulas $p(a, X, f(X))$ and $p(Y, f(b), f(f(b)))$ their anti-
unification (least general generalization) is $p(Z1, Z2, f(Z2))$. Conversely, unification
of this formulas, $p(a, X, f(X)) = p(Y, f(b), f(f(b)))$ will be $p(a, f(b), f(f(b)))$. Our logic

```
similar(F1, F2, F):- antiUnifyFormulas(F1, F2, F).
  antiUnifyFormulas(F1, F2, F):- clause_list(F1, F1s), clause_list(F2, F2s),
    findall( Fm, (member(T1, F1s), member(T2, F2s),
       antiUnifyTerms(T1, T2, Fm)), Fms), %finding pairs
       %Now it is necessary to sort out formulas which are not
       % most general within the list
    findall( Fmost, (member(Fmost, Fms),
      not ( member(Fcover, Fms), Fcover \= Fmost,
         antiUnifyTerms(Fmost, Fcover, Fcover)) ), Fss),
    clause_list(F, Fss). % converting back to clause


antiUnifyTerms(Term1, Term2,Term):-
    Term1=..[Pred0|Args1],len(Args1, LA),% make sure predicates
    Term2=..[Pred0|Args2],len(Args2, LA),% have the same arity
    findall( Var, ( member(N, [0,1,2,3,4,5,6,7,8,9,10 ]), % not more than 10 arguments
    [! sublist(N, 1, Args1, [VarN1]), %loop through arguments
       sublist(N, 1, Args2, [VarN2]),
     string_term(Nstr,N), VarN1=..[Name|_],        string_term(Tstr,Name),
     concat(['z',Nstr,Tstr],ZNstr),   atom_string(ZN, ZNstr) !],
       % building a canonical argument to create a variable
       % as a result of anti-unification
    ifthenelse( not (VarN1=VarN2),
    ifthenelse(( VarN1=..[Pred,_|_],VarN2=..[Pred,_|_]),
       ifthenelse( antiUnifyConst(VarN1, VarN2, VarN12),
         %going deeper into a subterm when an argument is a term
           (Var=VarN12),   Var=ZNstr) ),
    %OR domain-specific code here for special treatment of certain arguments
    % various cases: variable vs variable, or vs constant, or constant vs constant
         Var=ZNstr),Var=VarN1)        ), Args),        Term=..[Pred0|Args].
```

Fig. 7.15 The clauses for logic program for anti-unification (least general generalization) of two formulas (conjunctions of terms). Predicate *antiUnify(T1, T2, Tv)* inputs two formulas (scenarios in our case) and outputs a resultant anti-unification

programming implementation of anti-unification for a pair of conjunctions, which can be customized to a particular knowledge domain, is presented in Fig. 7.15.

Although the issue of implementation of the anti-unification has been addressed in the literature, we present the full code to have this book self-contained. In a given domain, additional constraints on terms can be enforced to express a domain-specific similarity. Particularly, certain arguments can be treated differently (should not be allowed to change if they are very important, or should form a special kind of constant). A domain – specific code should occur in the line shown in bold.

There are other *Jasmine*-compatible approaches to computing similarities except the anti-unification. In particular, it is worth mentioning the graph-based approach of finding similarities between scenarios (Sect. 4.3.6). The operation of finding the maximum common subgraphs serves the purpose of anti-unification in such the domain. This operation was subject to further refinement expressing similarities between scenarios of multiagent interaction, where it is quite important to take into account different roles of edges of distinct sorts.

Novice users of *Jasmine* are advised to start building the similarity operation as an intersection between objects' features (unordered set of features) and obtain an initial prediction. Then, when the explanations for predictions are observed, the users may feel that less important features occur in these explanations too frequently, and anti-unification expression should be introduced so that less important features are nested deeper into the expressions for objects' features. Another option is to build a domain-specific Prolog predicate that computes unification, introducing explicit conditions for selected variables (bold line in the Fig. 7.15).

7.4.3   *Normal and Autistic Development Pathways for* Jasmine

For a benchmarking face recognition problem, we select a feature of a face and form a sample recognition knowledge base.

An image can be represented as a set of vectors where each vector contains gray levels of a sub-image (this is usually referred to as local representation) (Fig. 7.16). Also a feature set can be obtained by varying the size and position of each type of Haar-like features. Object detection using Haar feature-based cascade classifiers is an effective object detection method proposed by (Viola and Jones 2001). A Haar-like feature considers adjacent rectangular regions at a specific location in a detection window, sums up the pixel intensities in each region and calculates the difference between these sums. This difference is then used to categorize subsections of an image. For example, let us say we have an image database with human faces. It is a common observation that among all faces the region of the eyes is darker than the region of the cheeks. Therefore a common Haar feature for face detection is a set of two adjacent rectangles that lie above the eye and the cheek

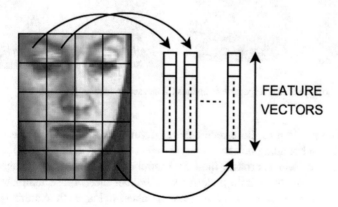

Fig. 7.16 vector based local representation for image features

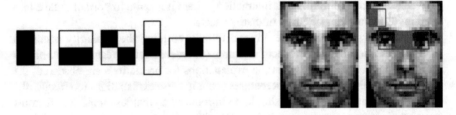

Fig. 7.17 Haar approach to extracting features from images

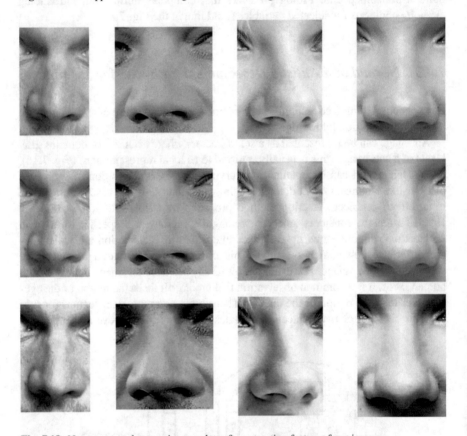

Fig. 7.18 Nose types and respective templates for extracting features from images

region. The position of these rectangles is defined relative to a detection window that acts like a bounding box to the target object (the face in this case) (Fig. 7.17).

Besides the Haar approach, there is a number of templates for image features used to recognize the whole pattern like a human face. These templates can be averaged image areas for a nose, ears, or cheeks. For each feature (part of a face) there are multiple templates corresponding to each type, such as nose type (Fig. 7.18). Hence these features have multiple values.

To summarize, feature extraction from an image occurs as follows:

1. All templates are formed in advance.
2. For a given image (object), each template is applied in the way of computing similarity between the pixels of an image and this template. The template is positions in all locations in an image to identify the first feature and then in a number of restricted locations once the first feature is identified. For example, once a nose area is identified we position each mouth template below to compute pixel similarity with the image.
3. A maximal consistent number of templates is applied and a maximum number of types of features is identified.
4. For an image *o* we obtain the list of expressions for the feature type, such as

> *nose(o, aquiline), ear(o, size(large), shape(tilted)), mouth(o, lips(thin), teeth(even))* ...

This way we form an element of a training set or an unknown image object to be recognized. Then Jasmine machine is applied in the way described above.

Imagine now that multiple observation of the mother images gave the following training set:

> *nose(o, aquiline), ear(o, size(medium), shape(tilted)), mouth(o, lips(thick), teeth(even))* ...
> *nose(o, aquiline), ear(o, size(large), shape(long)), mouth(o, lips(thin), teeth(even))* ...
> *nose(o, aquiline), ear(o, size(large), shape(tilted)), mouth(o, lips(thick), teeth(even))* ...

And multiple observations of the father

> *nose(o, straight-edged), ear(o, size(large), shape(short)), mouth(o, lips(fallen), teeth(uneven))* ...
> *nose(o, straight-edged), ear(o, size(medium), shape(short)), mouth(o, lips(oomph), teeth(uneven))* ...
> *nose(o, snub), ear(o, size(large), shape(short)), mouth(o, lips(fallen), teeth(uneven))* ...
> *nose(o, straight-edged), ear(o, size(large), shape(short)), mouth(o, lips(oomph), teeth(uneven))* ...

As we build intersections between these observations (pair-wise anti-unifications) we observe that these intersections are distinct for the mother and the father. There is a totally different situation if the number of features are extremely high and the number of samples is the same: this is the case of hyper-sensitivity:

Mother:

> *nose(o, aquiline(high), color(pink, grade5), ear(o, size(medium), hole_shape(type1, overall_shape(tilted), thickness(low), color(pale)), mouth(o, lips(thick, color(red(grade3)), teeth(even, color(white(grade2), yellow(grade4))...*
>
> *nose(o, aquiline(low), color(red, grade1), ear(o, size(large), hole_shape(type3, overall_shape(non-tilted), thickness(high), color(red)), mouth(o, lips(thin, color(red(grade1)), teeth(even, color(white(grade5), yellow(grade3))...*
>
> *nose(o, aquiline(medium), color(pink, grade4), ear(o, size(medium-large), hole_shape(type2, overall_shape(hawk), thickness(high), color(light-pale)), mouth(o, lips(medium-thick, color(pink(grade2)), teeth(uneven, color(white(grade4), yellow(grade2))...*

Father:

> *nose(o, straight-edged (low), color(pink-yellow, grade1), ear(o, size(large), hole_shape(type3, overall_shape(oval), thickness(medium-low), color(pale)), mouth(o, lips(fallen, color(red-pink(grade1)), teeth(uneven, color(white(grade1), yellow(grade2))...*
>
> *nose(o, straight-edged (low), color(pink-yellow, grade1), ear(o, size(large), hole_shape(type3, overall_shape(oval), thickness(medium-low), color(pale)), mouth(o, lips(fallen, color(red-pink(grade1)), teeth(uneven, color(white(grade1), yellow(grade2))...*

The reader can see that given a limited number of samples with specific, detailed information yields an empty expression in intersection for both the mother and the father. Since the learning system is unable to find commonalities for each class, it is unclear whether these classes are distinct in terms of these samples. Statistical approach to learning would not work either since the training dataset is so limited. And CwAs do not have many years to collect a richer dataset that would match the learning dimension since they are growing and expectations from the recognition system are increasing as well.

In case of hyper-sensitivity, when the representation is rich but the number of stimuli in real life is limited, a learning engine is unable to build a rule to recognize the mother since all here appearance are distinct. The only way to build a rule now is to intersect each of these formulas with itself. The resultant rule is going to be very specific and only appearance of the mother in certain location, posture and illumination conditions.

Under normal sensitivity, a face can be recognized for multiple angles (Figs. 7.19 and 7.20).

But with hyper-sensitivity, only the same position is recognizable, and only the recognition areas can be varied.

Finally, we present the overall architecture of the active learning system which is evolved into autistic adaptation under hyper-sensitivity (Fig. 7.21).

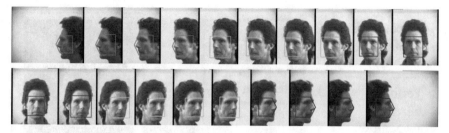

Fig. 7.19 Face recognition at various angles

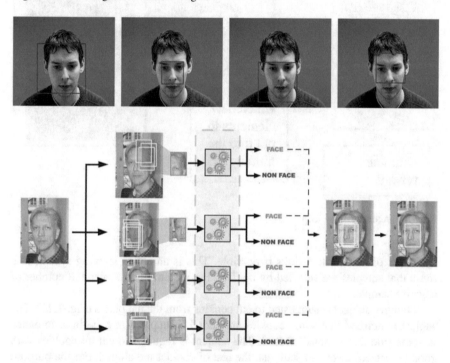

Fig. 7.20 Showing selecting an area at an image, extracting features from it, and then deciding whether it is a face or not. When the system is hypersensitive, it forms very high number of patterns

7.5 Exploring Forming and Updating Hypotheses in Human Learning

Our accumulated experience of teaching autistic children how to behave properly has contributed to the design of a rule-based machine learning system which automatically generates hypotheses to explain observations, verifies these hypotheses by finding the subset of data satisfying them, falsifies some of the hypotheses by revealing inconsistencies and finally derives the explanations for the observations

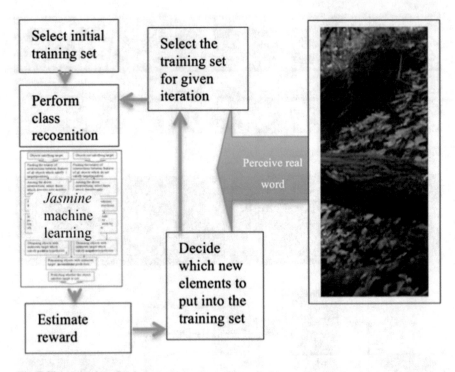

Fig. 7.21 Active learning loop

by means of cause-effect links if possible. This is an active learning system in a sense that samples are selected by the learning system to minimize the number of negative samples.

A hungry subject is suggested to eat cookies from the ten plates (Fig. 7.22). The subject is notified that some cookies are added an unpleasant taste in accordance to some rule that is not disclosed. The subject is required to eat all cookies with good (expected) taste and state that the rest of cookies are altered. For the purpose of verification, a subject is encouraged to formulate the formed rule when done with cookies.

When a trainee tries all cookies one-by-one, she discovers that cookies from plates 1,3,5,6,7,10 are normal and those from plates 2,4,8,9 are added an unpleasant taste (Fig. 7.23). The objective of this experimental environment is to come up with an algorithm of forming, confirming and defeating hypotheses such that the least number of cookies with unpleasant taste is eaten. This environment approximates the real world where human attempt to optimize their behavior. Since it is hard to make CwA act in an artificial environment, this experiment is designed to involve children who are hungry at the beginning of the experimental session. Since children are eager to satisfy their appetite they don't need to be motivated to participate in cookie-eating session and they genuinely attempt to avoid altered cookies.

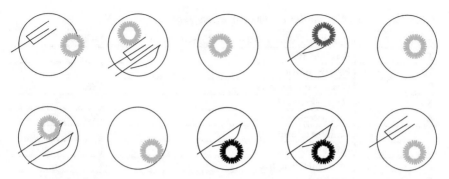

Fig. 7.22 The environment for active learning and hypotheses formation as seen by a subject

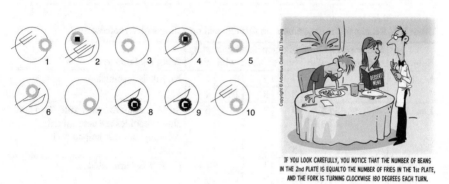

IF YOU LOOK CAREFULLY, YOU NOTICE THAT THE NUMBER OF BEANS IN THE 2nd PLATE IS EQUAL TO THE NUMBER OF FRIES IN THE 1st PLATE, AND THE FORK IS TURNING CLOCKWISE 180 DEGREES EACH TURN.

Fig. 7.23 Labeled samples

A good way to do it, invented by some children, is to find the common property of all good cookies and that of the bad cookies. These common properties should not overlap between positive and negative sets. Applying inductive procedure to positive and negative examples turns out to be a good advancement of both inductive logic programming and explanation-based learning (these methods generalize positive examples only).

A subject is expected to start with simple hypothesis such as "where there is a fork, the cookie is normal or altered" or "where there is a knife, the cookie is normal or altered". Once a new cookie is encountered, the current hypothesis can be updated or removed in favor of the new one. One of the proper session is shown in Table 7.2 where we start with the hypothesis that a fork is associated with a normal cookie, then update this hypothesis adding "no knife" clause. Then the subject discovers that '*fork*' is a redundant condition and continues acquiring new samples till she has to transition to *"no single knife"* instead of *"no any knife"* condition. *Jasmine* is capable of producing a similar learning session.

The experimental results of hypotheses formation for six subjects are shown in Table 7.3. Only one out of six subjects produced an optimal scenario (on the bottom).

Table 7.2 The log of hypotheses forming and revising session

Sample	Hypothesis formed as a result of given sample	Altered
1	Fork → normal	
10	Fork → normal	
2	Fork –knife → normal	Yes
3	–knife → normal	
4	–knife → normal	Yes
7	–knife → normal	
5	–knife → normal	
6	–one knife → normal	
8	Predicted	Yes
9	Predicted	Yes

Table 7.3 Results of the experiment on forming and operating with hypotheses

Subject	Successful completion	Order of object testing (starting with 1 and finishing with 10)					Additional remarks
Masha Z	–	5	7	2	6	1	No rule is formulated
		9	3	8	10	4	
Lena B	–	4	9	7	8	6	Some attempt to state a rule. Two last altered cookies are determined correctly, but was helped with advices
		3	5	2	10	1	
Valya V	–	7	6	1	9	10	No rule is formulated
		5	4	3	8	2	
Alina Z	–	6	5	9	10	4	Failure to formulate a rule; ate all cookies including altered
		3	8	2	7	1	
Serge T	–	1	3	5	8	6	A wrong rule is suggested: no cutlery – no alterations; also, forks – no alterations. Multiple hypotheses were evaluated but neither is correct
		9	4	7	10	2	
Sofia S	+	1	10	2	3	4	Independently achieved the correct rule
		7	5	6	8	9	

The experiments have indicated that selected high-functioning autistic subjects are the best and most precise means to judge on human intelligence from the perspective of algorithmic decision making. CC strategy selection behavior would be rather multi-dimensional: they would involve information about cookies, intent of an experimenter, the role of cutlery and their inter-relations with cookies, etc.

7.6 Deductive Reasoning About Actions

In this section we introduce a reasoning engine about generic actions based on deductions. Analyzing its limitations, we will keep in mind that CwA with developed deduction but limited induction experience similar difficulties (Chap. 6).

A series of formalisms, developed in the logic programming environment, have been suggested for reasoning about actions in robotics applications. Particularly, the system for reasoning about dynamic domains, GOLOG, suggested in (Levesque et al. 1997), has been extended by multiple authors for a variety of fields. Involvement of sensory information in building the plan of multiagent interaction has significantly increased the applicability of GOLOG (Lakemeyer 1999).

However, a deduction-based logical framework is still not well suited to handle the multiagent scenarios with lack of information concerning the actions of opponent agents, when it is impossible to sense them (acquire additional features online). A strong progress in the efficient implementation of reasoning about action in many ubiquitous applications has been achieved; however such implementations deal with explicit set of pre-conditions and effect axioms. Clearly, the formalism of reasoning about actions does not target situations with uncertainty such as multiagent conflict scenarios, where full knowledge reflects only the perspective of a particular side. In particular, uncertainty is often unavoidable in medical practice, where additional techniques are applied to GOLOG, including Bayesian networks (Levesque and Pagnucco 2000). A series of GOLOG extensions have been built for processing information from noisy sensors for applications in robotics (Bacchus et al. 1999), as well as a theoretical framework concerning situation calculus operating in probabilistic conditions.

Incomplete knowledge about the world is reflected as an expression for non-deterministic choice of the order in which to perform actions, non-deterministic choice of argument values, and non-deterministic repetition. These settings are adequate for the selected robotics applications, where the designer uses a particular approximation of the external world. In a general setting, an agent that performs reasoning about actions is expected to learn from the situations, where the actual sequence of actions has been forced by the environment to deviate from the initially obtained plan, using the current world model.

A generic environment for reasoning about actions is not well suited for handling incomplete data, where neither totality of procedures, nor action preconditions, nor successor state constraints are available. Evidently, situation calculus by itself does not have a sufficient predictive power and needs to be augmented by a learning system capable of operating in the dynamic language. Abstraction of reasoning about action in the way of GOLOG assumes that action preconditions, successor state expressions and ones for complex actions are known, or at least that the respective probabilities can be estimated.

However, scenarios of multiagent interactions cannot be efficiently handled by the traditional deterministic machine learning (an attribute value learning system), because of the high dimension, sparseness of the feature space and a lack of an important body of commonsense knowledge. A knowledge discovery system that is based on inductive logic programming or similar approaches is insufficient, taken alone, because it is incapable of performing necessary commonsense reasoning about actions and knowledge in accordance to heuristics available from domain experts. Neglecting this knowledge would dramatically decrease the extent of possible predictions. Also, a generic knowledge discovery system is not oriented

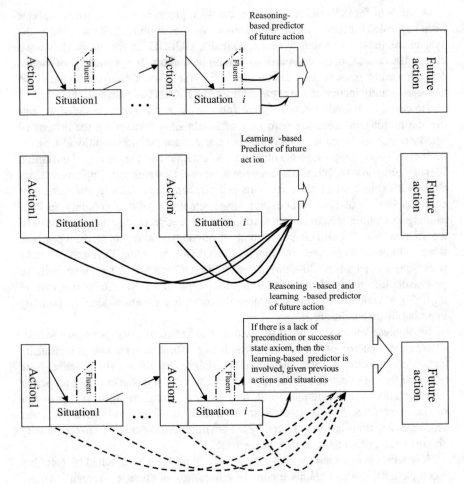

Fig. 7.24 Illustration for the merging reasoning about action-based and learning-based machinery for performing the prediction of future (or unknown) actions in dynamic domain. *On the top*: reasoning about action, *in the middle*: machine learning, *on the bottom*: our hybrid approach that is the results of merge between the two above

to handle dynamic kinds of data, which include such a complex structure of interdependencies as multiagent scenarios. Therefore, we intend to merge reasoning about action-based deductive and learning-based inductive systems to form the environment to handle dynamic domains with incomplete information (Fig. 7.24). Teaching CwA, one should clearly communicate that these two forms of reasoning should be merged, having explained stand-alone reasoning about action and stand-alone deterministic machine learning (Sect. 7.4).

We outline two basic methodologies for predicting the future action or a set of possible actions:

1. By means of reasoning about actions. Following this methodology, one specifies a set of available basic and combined actions with conditions, given a current situation, described via a set of fluents. These fluents in turn have additional constraints and obey certain conditions, given a set of previous actions. Action possibilities, pre-conditions and successor state axioms are formulated *manually*, analyzing the past experience. This methodology can fully solve the problem if the complete formal prerequisites for reasoning about actions are available.
2. By means of supervised learning of the future action from the set of examples. Given a set of examples with a sequence of actions and fluents in each, a prediction engine generates the hypotheses of how these fluents are linked to future actions. Resultant hypotheses are then applied to predict these future actions. Such kinds of learning require the actions and fluents to be explicitly specified, as in the methodology of reasoning about actions. However, the learning itself is performed automatically. This supervised learning methodology is worth applying in a stand-alone manner if neither explicit rules for agents when to perform an action nor action pre-conditions are available.

Our experience in the implementation of reasoning in the selected application domain demonstrates that the above methodologies are complementary. The following facts contribute this observation:

- Almost any prediction task, particularly in a deterministic approach, is some combination of manually obtained heuristics and automatically extracted features, which characterize an object of interest;
- If an attempt is made to predict all actions using learning, the problem complexity dramatically increases and, therefore, the accuracy of any solution under possible approximation drops.
- On the other hand, if an attempt is made to explicitly construct the required totality of pre- and post-conditions of actions for the deductive settings, we run against a frame problem that may need a unique solution for a specific situation (Shanahan 1997). Moreover, some other difficulties are associated with the search of inference (building of a plan), not assisted by the considerations involving the past experience.
- Considering a sequence of actions in a dynamic domain, the longer this sequence is, the more inductive reasoning comes into play relatively to the deductive one.

Note that above considerations are valid when the choice of action does not occur in a pure mental world, i.e. the world where the situations are described in terms of belief, knowledge and intention (Sect. 4.2). Choosing an action that is to be performed in a given mental state occurs in accordance to quite different laws, unlike ones for physical states we are talking about in this report.

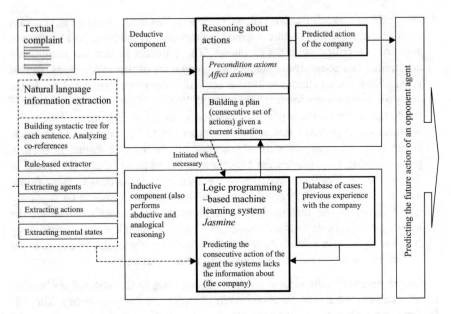

Fig. 7.25 Overall architecture of the system for prediction of a consecutive action in a multiagent conflict

7.6.1 The Architecture of a Hybrid System

Hence we choose the GOLOG and *Jasmine* environments for deterministic reasoning about action and inductive machine learning respectively because of their flexibility and power (Fig. 7.25). Using the above approaches to illustrate our methodology, we keep in mind that our architecture of merging deductive and inductive components is independent of the choice of particular formalism and better models real-world domains than these approaches taken separately.

Overall architecture of the system for prediction of a consecutive action in a multiagent conflict is presented in Fig. 7.25. The natural language information extraction unit (on the left) provides the deductive component (on the top right) with the extracted actions. If the *reasoning about action* component determines a lack of information concerning the opponent agent, the *inductive component* (on the bottom right) is initiated. The *inductive* component loads the set of accumulated complaints for the given company (its name is extracted by NL component) and predicts the following action given the state, obtained by the *reasoning about action* component. If the multiagent scenario is rather complex, the simulation by means of NL_MAMS is required to predict the following mental state. The units with bold frame are the focus of this chapter.

7.6.2   *Merging Deductive and Inductive Reasoning About Action*

Based on the motivations, which were presented in the Introduction, we have the following methodology to predict an action of an agent in an environment where we do not have complete information on this agent. If we are unable to derive the actions of this agent given the preconditions of his actions and successor state axioms to sufficiently characterize his current state, learning-based prediction needs to come into play. Instead of just taking the current state into account, as reasoning about action would do, learning-based prediction takes into account the totality of previous actions and states. It is required because there is a lack of knowledge about which previous actions and situations affect the current choice of action.

Situation calculus is formulated in a first-order language with certain second-order features (Reiter 1993). We briefly repeat our definitions from Sect. 4.2. A possible world history that is a result of a sequence of *actions* is called *situation*. The expression *Do(a,s)*, denotes the successor situation to *s* after action *a* is applied. Also, situations involve the *fluents,* whose values vary from situation to situation and denote them by predicates with the latter arguments ranging over the situations,

Effect axioms express the causal links between the domain entities. We refer the reader to (Levesque et al. 1997) for the further details on the implementation of situation calculus.

As one can see, the methodology of situation calculus is building a sequence of actions given their pre- and post-conditions. To choose an action, we verify that the preconditions are dependent on the current fluents. After an action is performed, it affects these fluents, which in turn determine the consecutive action, and so forth. In the traditional situation calculus pre- and post-conditions are manually coded. In this work we use machine learning to acquire pre-conditions of actions from each complaint. However, since our current complaint representation stores actions but not intermediate states, here we do not learn action post-conditions.

The *frame problem* (Shanahan 1997) comes into play to reduce the number of effect axioms that do not change (the common sense law of inertia). The successor state axiom resolves the frame problem:

$$poss(a,s) \supset [\, f(\hat{y}, Do(a,s)) \equiv \gamma_f^+(\,\hat{y},\, a,s) \ \vee \ (f(\hat{y},s) \ \& \ \neg\gamma_f^-(\,\hat{y},\, a,s)\,)\,],$$

where $\gamma_f^+(\hat{y},\, a,s)$ $(\gamma_f^{--}(\hat{y},\, a,s))$ is a formula describing under what conditions doing action a in situation s makes fluent f become true (false, respectively) in the successor situation $Do(a,s)$.

GOLOG extends the situation calculus with complex actions, involving, in particular, *if-then* and *while* constructions. Macros $do(\delta, s, s')$ denotes the fact that situation s' is a terminating situation of an execution of complex action δ starting in situation s. Here we present the case of complex actions performed by an agent with intentions and beliefs. If $a_1, \ldots, a_n$ are agents' actions, then

- $[a_1: \ldots : a_n]$ is a deterministic sequence of actions. We know that an agent may only perform actions in a given order either because of external constraints or because of her intentions.
- $[a_1\# \ldots \# a_n]$ is a non-deterministic sequence of actions for an agent, any sequence of actions is plausible, given our knowledge about intentions of this agent.
- *ifCond(p)* is checking a condition expressed by p by an agent. This is the case of an explicit condition for agent's choice of action; the condition is available for the reasoning system.
- *star(a)*, nondeterministic repetition.
- *if(p, a_1, a_2)*, if-then-else conditional, applied by an agent in accordance to our knowledge of his rules.
- *while(p, a_1, a_2)*, iteration.

We proceed to the GOLOG interpreter. The last line below is added to the conventional GOLOG interpreter to suggest an alternative choice of action by means of learning from the previous experience, if the other options to determine the following action are exhausted:

> $do(A1 : A2,S,S1) :- do(A1,S,S2), do(A2,S2,S1)$.
> $do(ifCond(P),S,S) :- holds(P,S)$.
> $do(A1 \# A2,S,S1) :- do(A1,S,S1) ; do(A2,S,S1)$.
> $do(if(P,A1,A2),S,S1) :- do((call(P) : A1) \# (call(not P) : A2),S,S1)$.
> $do(star(A),S,S1) :- S1 = S ; do(A : star(A),S,S1)$.
> $do(while(P,A),S,S1):- do(star(call(P) : A) : call(not P),S,S1)$.
> $do(pi(V,A),S,S1) :- sub(V,\_,A,A1), do(A1,S,S1)$.
> $do(A,S,S1) :- proc(A,A1), do(A1,S,S1)$.   % a complex action
> $do(A,S,do(A,S)) :- primitive\_action(A), poss(A,S)$.
> **$do(A, S, do(A, S)):- predict\_action\_by\_learning(A, S)$.**

The last clause with the body **$predict\_action\_by\_learning(A, S)$**, yielding action **A** at the state **S**, can be thought of as an online acquisition of facts of action possibilities, $(poss(A,S))$.

Figure 7.26 depicts the problem of finding a plan as a theorem-proving in situation calculus.

Axioms $|= (\exists \delta,s) Do(\delta, S_0, s) \& Goal(s)$, where plan $Goal(s)$ is synthesized as a side effect while satisfying *Goal*. In our case planning is reduction the number of possible actions of an opponent.

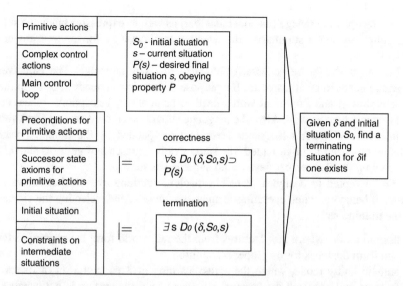

Fig. 7.26 Methodology for deriving a plan in the settings of situation calculus. To predict an action of an opponent agent, we simulate the planning process for this agent to plan his future actions

Below we present the samples of post-condition (effect, successor state) axioms for fluents *unsatisfied, disinformed* and *company_untrusted:*

> holds(unsatisfied, Do(E,S)):- E = wrongDoC;
> E = customerServiceIgnoreWhy; E = explainWrong;
> E = findUnreasonableCauseForCustComplain;
> (holds(unsatisfied,S), not member(E, [agreeToFixCS,
> agreeToCompensateCS, convinceToBeActingAsRequiredCS])).
> holds(disinformed, Do(E, S)):- E = explainWronglyCS.
> holds(company_untrusted, Do(E, S)):- holds(disinformed,S),
> E = followWrongAdviceNoResult.

7.7 Discussion and Conclusions

How can performance of such systems as inductive logic programming and explanation-based learning be improved by taking into account observations concerning operations with hypotheses by children with autism? We will outline the experimental settings and observations.

Adjustment of action technique teaches CwA that his actions carry meaning and elicit a response from her peers. Also learning adjustment of actions increases

CwA's receptive language (its understanding) as well as expressive language skills. The following items summarize the teaching methodology for the adjustment of actions:

Meanings should be necessarily attached to CwA language. The caregiver's language needs to be adjusted for the purpose of learning: it needs to be simplified, spoken slowly, and important words need to be stressed. Receptions, visual cues and gestures help as well. Also, the language should be tailored around CwA focus of interest, and CwA's language needs to be expanded by the trainer. Focused stimulations need to be provided: the same words, phrases and gestures should be repeated up to 20 times per days for all suitable situations.

We attempted to design a plausible machine learning system that shows two forms of behavior, when operating in an active mode of auto selecting the elements of the training set:

1. normal mode, where new features from the real world form the training dataset and form the basis for its proper recognition
2. autistic faulty mode, where the active learning evolves to the set of irrelevant features and although the learning sessions occur, the system is not capable of recognizing the real world.

Hence given the operational learning system, once it becomes hypersensitive in an active learning mode, it displays the number of features inherent to autistic cognition:

- Broken multi-modal links
- Stereotypy
- Blocking the strong stimuli of the real world
- Distinguishing important from unimportant features.

We proposed a concrete design of a machine learning system reproducing the phenomenology of the studies of children with early autism. In our future studies we will attempt to form the methodology of rehabilitation of autistic cognition, based on the model built in this Chapter.

References

Anshakov OM, Finn VK, Skvortsov DP (1989) On axiomatization of many-valued logics associated with formalization of plausible reasoning. Stud Logica 42(4):423–447
Bacchus F, Halpern JY, Levesque H (1999) Reasoning about noisy sensors and effectors in the situation calculus. Artif Intell 111(1–2)
Bogdashina O (2005) Communication Issues in Autism and Asperger Syndrome: do we speak the same language? Jessica Kingsley Publishers, London
Bos K, Zeanah CH, Fox NA, Drury SS, McLaughlin KA, Nelson CA (2011) Psychiatric outcomes in young children with a history of institutionalization. Harv Rev Psychiatry 19(1):15–23
Dasgupta S (2005) Coarse sample complexity bounds for active learning. In NIPS

Dasgupta S, Hsu D, Monteleoni C (2007) A general agnostic active learning algorithm. Technical Report CS2007-0898 Department of Computer Science and Engineering University of California, San Diego

Galitsky B (2007) Handling representation changes by autistic reasoning. AAAI fall symposium – technical report FS-07-03, pp 9–16

Galitsky B, Shpitsberg I (2015) Evaluating assistance to Individuals with autism in reasoning about mental world. Artificial intelligence applied to assistive technologies and smart environments: papers from the 2015 AAAI workshop

Galitsky B, Spitsberg I (2006) How one can learn programming while teaching reasoning to children with autism AAAI Spring Symposia Stanford CA

Ghera M, Marshall P, Fox N, Zeanah C, Nelson CA, Smyke AT (2009) The effects of foster care intervention on socially deprived institutionalized children's attention and positive affect: results from the BEIP study. J Child Psychol Psychiatry 50:246–253

Kennedy Krieger Institute (2009) Difference in the way children with autism learn new behaviors described. ScienceDaily, July 10. Retrieved February 25, 2016 from www.sciencedaily.com/releases/2009/07/090706113647.htm

Lakemeyer G (1999) On sensing in GOLOG. In: Levesque HJ, Pirri F (eds) Logical foundations for cognitive agents. Springer, Berlin

Levesque HL, Pagnucco M (2000) Legolog: inexpensive experiments in cognitive robotics. In: 938 proceedings of the second international cognitive robotics workshop, Berlin, Germany, August 939 pp 21–22

Levesque HJ, Reiter R, Lesperance Y, Lin F, Scherl RB (1997) GOLOG: a logic programming language for dynamic domains. J Log Program 31:59–84

Mill JS (1843) A system of logic 1843. Also available from University Press of the Pacific, Honolulu, 2002

Mundy P, Crowson M (1997) Joint attention and early social communication. J Autism Dev Disord 27:653–676

Olsson, F (2008) Bootstrapping named entity annotation by means of active machine learning – a method for creating corpora. Ph.D. dissertation., Department of Swedish, University of Gothenburg

Pedersen T (2015) Children with autism Don't adjust sniffing time for bad smells. Psych Central. Retrieved on December 8, 2015, from http://psychcentral.com/news/2015/07/03/children-with-autism-dont-adjust-sniffing-time-for-bad-smells/86412.html

Rapp JT, Vollmer TR, St Peter C, Dozier CL, Cotnoir NM (2004) Analysis of response allocation in individuals with multiple forms of stereotyped behavior. J Appl Behav Anal 37(4):481–501

Reiter R (1993) Proving properties of states in the situational calculus. J Artif Intell 64:337–351

Sandman CA, Kemp AS (2011) Opioid antagonists may reverse endogenous opiate. Dependence in the treatment of self-injurious behavior. Pharmaceuticals (Basel) 4(2):366–381

Shanahan M (1997) Solving the frame problem. MIT Press, Cambridge, MA

Shpitsberg I (2005) Sensory system correction for Choldrten with autism (Коррекция особенностей развития сенсорных систем у детей с синдромом раннего детского аутизма». Альманах ИКП РАО – M.) in Russian

Viola P, Jones M (2001) Rapid object detection using a boosted cascade of simple features, conference on computer vision and pattern recognition

Yu K, Bi J, Tresp V (2006) Active learning via transductive experimental design. In Proceedings of the International Conference on Machine Learning (ICML). ACM Press, pp 1081–1087

Zhu X (2005) Semi-supervised learning literature survey. Computer Sciences Technical Report 1530, University of Wisconsin-Madison

Chapter 8
Rehabilitating Autistic Reasoning

Having outlined what are the deficiencies of autistic reasoning on one hand, and what kinds of reasoning and learning is required to control the behavior on the other hand, we proceed to how the issues of autistic reasoning can be cured. We will dive into a broad range of technique improving autistic reasoning, both computer training-based and human training-based. These techniques are the conjecture of the reasoning deficiencies we defined formally or computationally in the previous chapters. The goal of reasoning rehabilitation is twofold: teach CwA to *think soundly* and judge righteously about various aspects of life, and properly chose and control *behavior* based on reasoning and rationality (Fig. 8.1).

8.1 Training Environment

A few versions of the web-based user interface for NL_MAMS have been developed for a number of environments, including describing of mental states of scene characters. A variety of interface components were designed for specifying mental states, including natural language and drop-down box-based.

The one-to-one rehabilitation strategy (NL_MAMS – independent), conducted by a member of rehabilitation stuff, includes the following components:

- direct introduction of the basic mental entities *want-know-believe* using real-world examples;
- explanation of derived mental entities using the basis *want-know-believe*;
- introduction of the derived mental entities by means of real-world examples;
- conversations that heavily rely on a discourse with mental focus;
- conversations that are based on a pictorial representation of interaction scenarios (Figs. 8.3 and 8.6);
- involving the trainees into actual interactions with other children and asking them to verbally represent these interactions;

© Springer International Publishing Switzerland 2016
B. Galitsky, *Computational Autism*, Human–Computer Interaction Series,
DOI 10.1007/978-3-319-39972-0_8

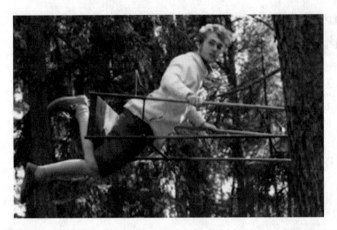

Fig. 8.1 Therapy should leverage available skills such as tolerance to height and fast motion

- encouraging the parents and rehabilitation personnel to demonstrate a special awareness of mental entities in the real world (Galitsky 2000; Galitsky 2001)
- "picture-in-the-head" and "thought-bubbles" techniques, using "physical" representation of mental attitudes (Swettenham et al. 1996, Fig. 8.3).

NL_MAMS-based training is intended to assist in all of the above components. Initially a trainer shows how to represent mental states from the above components via NL_MAMS, and discusses yielded scenarios with a trainee. The plausibility and appropriateness of actions yielded by NL_MAMS require special attention from trainees. Then the trainer specifies other initial mental states and asks a trainee to come up with plausible scenarios originating from these mental states.

After a certain number of demonstrations, the trainees are encouraged to use NL_MAMS independently, applying it to real-world mental states the trainees have experienced, as well as abstract mental states. Trainees are presented with both natural language and structured input and output of NL_MAMS, and they are free to choose their favourite way of user interface.

Trainees are children with high-functioning autism 6–10 years old, selected so that they are capable of reading simple phrases and communicating mental states in one or another way.

An exercise introducing the mental action of *offending* and *forgiving* is depicted at Fig. 8.2. This is a partial case of NL_MAMS training of yielding a scenario given an initial mental state: it is adjusted to the definition of *offending*. Expected resultant scenario is just the actions of *offending* or *forgiving* with appropriate parameters for agents and subjects of these actions. These parameters are specified via drop-down boxes; their instances are expected to show the trainees how to generalize the instances of *offending* or *forgiving* towards different agents. Also, multiple ways to express these generalizations are shown: *friend, parent, brother/sister, they/them,*

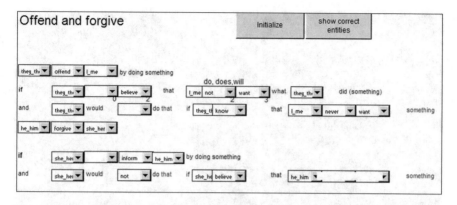

Fig. 8.2 The form to introduce a mental entity (here, to offend and to forgive). After an entity is explained via examples and verbal definition is told, a trainee is suggested to choose the proper basic entities with negations when necessary to build a definition

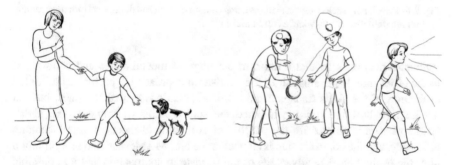

Fig. 8.3 A visualization of interaction scenario: a situation with conflicting goals (on the left). The children are asked the questions about who is hiding where, who wants to find them, and about their other mental states. On the right: "picture-in-the-head" and "thought-bubbles" techniques are used, based on "physical" representation of mental attitudes

he/she, him/her etc. After the trainees learn how to derive a single-step scenario for a fixed mental action, they are given tasks to compose a scenario with two or more mental actions they have already learned (Fig. 8.3).

8.1.1 Short-Term and Long-Term Training Settings

We performed the NL_MAMS-assisted training and its evaluation at two levels: short-term and long-term. The *short-term approach* includes the theory of mind training with and without NL_MAMS for two groups of 12 autistic children of similar mental age and IQ. The evaluation is based on passing the set of tests including the seeing-leads-to-knowing (first-order) and Sally-Anne false belief

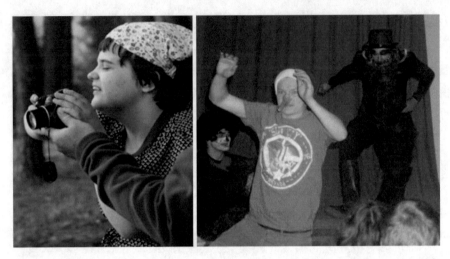

Fig. 8.4 Developing such complex skills as using a photo-camera and doing a performance require integral rehabilitation strategy and a substantial support

(second-order) ones so that a uniform coverage of mental states and actions (up to the order three) is evaluated. In the short-term approach we performed a limited evaluation of the skills transfer from artificial situations to real life ones, but did not analyze how the training affected the socials skills of trainees. The short-term approach is utilized for the purpose of evaluation of theory of mind teaching efficiency, and the control group is subject to the NL_MAMS-assisted rehabilitation after the evaluation. The advantage of the short-term approach is that it is possible to ignore other factors affecting the theory of mind performance of both groups.

The *long-term approach* is applied over 3 years, where manual and NL_MAMS-assisted teaching of the theory of mind is combined with rehabilitation strategies of various natures. The goal of our long-term approach is to teach theory of mind reasoning not just for the reasoning skills per se, but also for improvement of social behavior (Figs. 8.4 and 8.5). Therefore, the evaluation criteria are based on tests of decision-making in the real world as well as tests of reasoning and choosing actions in artificial situations (below we include the quantitative results for the latter).

When our training occurs over a relatively long period, it is important to verify whether performance improvement is simply due to natural development and other rehabilitation procedures over that time. For this reason a control group with neither one-to-one nor NL_MAMS-based training, matched for mental age, IQ and severity of autism, was subject to examinations at the beginning and the end of the set long-term training period. The control group was selected from another autistic rehabilitation center, where there is a lack of human resources to provide a focused theory of mind training by rehabilitation personnel.

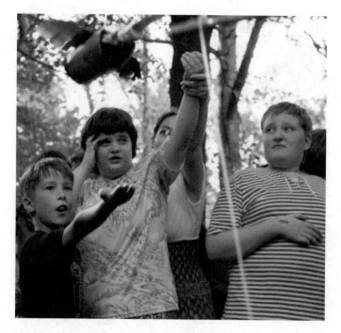

Fig. 8.5 Assisted discovery of unknown objects

8.2   Exercising Scenarios

There are two children, A and B, who are subject to detection and/or training of the corrupted reasoning about mental states and actions. Correct answers follow the question, wrong answers are enumerated in the parenthesis, where presented (Fig. 8.6).

8.2.1   Mental State of Another Person

There is a table in a room with two boxes on it. The experimenter (E) is keeping a token in his hands. Child A is in the room, and child B is outside the room. E is asking A:

1) *You see the token in my hands. Do you know which box I am going to put the token to?*
   A: I don't know that box/nobody knows. (A is confused: I don't know the answer).
2) *E: As you see, I put the token into the left box. Do you know, where B will look for the token: in the right box, in the left one or in both boxes?*
   A: In both boxes. (In the left box, where the token actually is).
3) *E: And do you know where the token is?*
   A: I know where is the token.

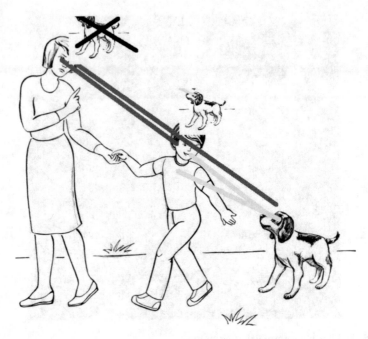

Fig. 8.6 A bubble-thought approach to introduction of mental states

4) *E: Does B know where the token is? If we ask him, what would he respond:*
       A: I don't know where the token is. (I know where it is. I know it is in the left box).
5) *E: If we ask B about his opinion, do you (A) know whether B knows where the token is?*
       A: B knows that I know that he does not know where the token is. (B knows where the token is, B does not know where the token is, B knows that I know where the token is, B knows that I know that B knows where the token is.)
6) *E: Can we achieve a situation, when B will know where the token is?*
       A: Yes, we can tell him or show him (A is confused: I don't know).
       B enters the room. Now all the questions are repeated; B's responses, predicted by A, are actually evaluated.
7) *E, After A showed (or told) B the location of the token: How do you (B) think, did A know whether you knew the location of the token while out of this room?*
       B: A knew that I did not know where the token is.
8) *E, interrupting B: what do you (A) think, what will B say?*
       A: B will say that B knew that I knew that he B did not know where the token was.
9) *E: Now you (B) know where the token is, because A have shown you. Do you think he (A) wanted you to know where the token was?*
       B: Yes, A wanted myself (B) to know where the token is.
10) *E: Do you (A) know whether B knows that you (A) wanted him (B) to know where the token was?*
       B : Yes, I know that I wanted B to know where the token was.

8.2.2 A Wrong Mental State

1) *E: Now I want to tell you the following. I believe, that B still does not know where the token is. Who is wrong: myself (E) or B?*

    A: You are wrong telling us that B still does not know where the token is. (B is wrong, now he does know where the token is).

8.2.3 Mental State Transmission

This is a mirror test to the *mental state of the other person* one.

E keeps the blank piece of paper. A is next to E, and B is in the other room.

1) *E: I am going to plot a geometric sketch on a piece of paper. I'm about to start the drawing. Do you know what I am going to draw; do I know, if myself knows what will be drawn?*

    A: I don't know, and you do.

    E finishes the picture.

2) *E: Now you know, what I've drawn. Does B know that?*

    A: B does not know what is drawn.

3) *E: How can you let him know what is drawn?*

    A: Either show him or tell him (describe the picture).

4) *E: You mentioned two ways of letting B know about this picture. Do both these ways require your knowledge of what is actually drawn?*

    A: No, to show him, I do not necessarily have to know (have seen) the picture. To describe the picture, I have to know its content. (Yes, I have to know the picture content for both telling and showing).

5) *E: If we call B into the room and ask him if he knows what is on the paper, what would he (B) respond? What would he respond if we ask him after we show him the picture?*

    A: Before we show him (B) the picture, he will tell that he does not know what it is about. After we show or tell him (B) about the picture, he will tell he knows it.

6) *E: if we ask B concerning his opinion, do you (A) know that he (B) does not know what this picture is about right now, before we informed him about the picture?*

    A: B knows that I know that he does not know the drawing. (A is confused: I don't know. B does not know that I know that he does not know. B does not know that I don't know that he knows).

7) *E: I guess, I want your friend to know what is on the picture. Is it true? If so, does B know that you wanted to let him know about the picture? Does B know that you want him to know the picture?*

    A: I'm not sure. After I informed him about the picture, he would know that I wanted him to know what is on the picture. I don't know if he (B) knows that I want him to know the picture.

Thereafter E calls B in and asks A to actually inform B about the picture. All the questions above are posed for B as B's prediction of mental state of A.

8.2.4 Temporal Relationships Over the Mental States. To Forget and to Recall

There are the toys on the table: a bear, a fox and a rabbit. Experimenter is asking the child about his/her mental states.

1) E: As you see, the bear is watching the rabbit. Does the bear know that the rabbit is on the table?
   A: Yes, The bear knows that the rabbit is on the table.
2) E: Now the rabbit leaves the table. The bear knows that the rabbit is not on the table any more. Does the bear know that the rabbit was on the table before?
   A: Yes, he knows that he was on the table before.
3) E: Then, after a while, when the fox asks the bear if the rabbit had been on the table, the bear is saying that the rabbit has not been there. Trusting the bear, what do you think, does the bear know that the rabbit was on the table?
   A: The bear does not know that the rabbit was on the table.
4) E: OK, the bear forgot that the rabbit was on the table. Does the rabbit know that he earlier knew that the rabbit had been on the table?
   A: No, the rabbit does not know that he earlier knew that the rabbit had been on the table.
5) E: Now the fox wants the bear to recall that the rabbit has been on the table. What will she do?
   A: She (the fox) will tell the bear that the rabbit was on the table, and that the bear has seen him there.
6) E: Then, assuming, that the bear trusts the fox, what is the knowledge of the bear?
   A: Now the bear knows that the rabbit was on the table.
7) E: OK, so the bear recalls that the rabbit was on the table. Does the bear know that before the recollection he did not know that the rabbit had been on the table? Analogously, does the bear know that he(bear) knew that the rabbit had been on the table, while (bear) was watching the rabbit?
   A: Yes, the bear knows that he did not know that the rabbit has been on the table, as well as the bear knows that he knew that the rabbit has been on the table while watching the rabbit.

8.2.5 Pretending

There is a table, and a book on it. The experimenter teaches the child A to pretend that it is soap.

1) E: As you see, there is a book on the table. Do both of us know that it is a book?
   A: Yes, both of us know that it is a book.
2) E: Now let us pretend that it is soap. Both of us will still know, that it is the book. However, if I ask you, what that is, what will I respond?
   A: You respond that it is soup.
3) E: If you ask me, what is on the table, what will I respond?
   A: That there is soap on the table.

4) E: *When one asks you if you know what is on the table, what will you respond?*
   A: *I do know what is on the table.*
5) E: *Now let us stop pretending. Both of us still know that this is actually a book. If one asks me what is on the table, what will I respond?*
   A: *You will respond that it is the book.*

8.2.6 Exercising Results

Twenty autistic children of the age 4–18 participated in the testing and training and 20 control children of the age 8 participated in the testing.

Note that the questions above cover the majority of mental formulas complexity 1–4, involving *want* and *know* (*believe* is identified with know for simplicity). The manifold of tested mental state achieves the real world complexity. Therefore, the trained children are expected to behave properly in the real conditions, if they are able to transfer artificial mental states to the real ones.

Each question with the mental formula complexity below three was successfully answered by every control child.

– Each question of complexity 4 was failed by at least one autistic kid.
– For each question the autistic child failed, it was possible to perform training such that the question is successfully answered after fifth attempt.
– If to replace the mental states by physical states, the questions will be easier answered by the autistic children, than the questions above. It will not make a significant difference with the control children.

8.3 Construction of Mental Formulas

Teaching the exhaustive set of mental formulas in a labor-intensive yet efficient way towards a proper reasoning about mental world. Starting from the simplest formulas for intention, a caregiver proceeds to complex mental states involving contradicting beliefs (Table 8.1). The codes for mental formulas are in seven columns on the left.

Once the totality of mental formulas is acquired by a trainee, he can proceed to formalizing a scenario. Given a story (essay, anecdote), he is expected to formalize it via mental formulas and feed into NL_MAMS (Fig. 8.7).

Once the totality of mental formulas is explored and CwA is capable of formalizing some simple scenarios, the trainer can proceed to more complex mental entities (Figs. 8.7 and 8.8). The definitions of more complex mental concepts: *to offend*, *to forgive* and *to reconcile* are as follows.

Table 8.1 Encoding for the approach of building the mental formular for the exaustive set of mental formulas

Not	Want	Not	Know	Not	Believe	Embed	Definitions of the constructed expressions	Semantic comments
	1					1	want (Agent, do(Agent, Action))	Agent wants to commit an action
	1					2	want (Agent, do(DAgent, Action))	Agent wants another agent to commit an action
	1		2			2	want(Agemt, know (Agent, What)):-(believe(Agent, know (KAgent, What)), ask(Agent, KAgent, What))	Agent wants (himself) to know
	2		3		1	3	believe (Agent, want(WAgent, know (Wagent, What))):-prefer(Agent, tell(Agent, Wagent, What), Other Action)	Believe that other agent wants to know
	2		3		1	3	believe (Agent, inform(WAgent, KAgent, What)). believe(Agent, want(WAgent, know (KAgent, What))):- not know (KAgent, want(WAgent, know (KAgent, What))), inform(Agent, KAgent, ask(KAgent, WAgent, What))	Believe that someone wants to know -> inform believe that someone else wants the third person to know
	2,4		3		1	4	believe(Agent, want(WAgent, know (KAgent, want(Agent, What))):-believe(Agent, inform(WAgent,KAgent, want(Agent, What)))	Believe that someone else wants the third person to know what I want

8.4   The Literature Search System

Once a trainee is familiar with mental formulas and is capable of forming simple scenarios from it, he should proceed to formulating questions in the mental world. A rich and extensive domain in the mental world is the one of the fictional characters in a narrative work of art (such as a novel, play, television series or film). In this section we propose a reasoning exercise based on formulating queries and searching

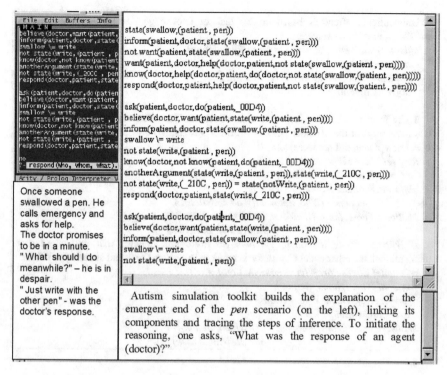

Fig. 8.7 NL_MAMS processing a joke, formalized by a trainee

for works of literature (WOL). This is the most computational intelligence-intensive application in HCI domain among other assistive technologies, along with NL_MAMS.

The methodology and abstraction of such search are very different from those for database querying, keyword-based search of relevant portions of text, and search for the data of various modalities (speech, image, video etc.). Clearly, the search that is based on mental attributes is expected to be semantically accented: using just the author or title name is trivial. Also, using temporal (historical) and geographical circumstances of the characters reduces WOL search to the relatively simple querying against the relational database of WOL parameters.

Focusing on the mental component of WOL plots is rewarding from the prospective of building the compact and closed (in terms of reasoning) vertical natural language question-answering (Q/A) domain. It is important that a user is aware of the lexical units and knowledge that is encoded in a domain to ensure the robust and accurate Q/A system. Division of the commonsense knowledge into mental and non-mental (physical) components introduces a strict and explicit boundary between the "allowed" and "not allowed" questions, that is a key to success of NL Q/A application in the field of education (Galitsky 2000).

Unintentional offend is based on the lack of knowledge that the offending action *do(Who, Action)* is unwanted:

offend(Who, Whom, Action) :- want(Who, Action),
   not want(Whom, Action),
   not know(Who, not want(Whom, Action)),
   do(Who, Action).

To be forgiven, the offender has to demonstrate that the offense is indeed unintentional. It is necessary for the offender *Who* to inform *Whom* that *Who* would not *do* that *Action* if *Who* knew *Whom* did not like (*want*) it.

forgive(Whom, Who, Action) :-
  offend(Who, Whom, Action),
  inform(WhoElse, Whom,
              not know(Who, not want(Whom, Action))),
  believe(Whom, (know(Who, not want(Whom, Action))→
                   not do(Who, Action))).

If *Who* is unable to convince *Whom* (to make him believe) that the *offend* was unintentional, the other agent *Counselor* is required to *explain* the actual situation to *Whom*:

reconcile(Counselor, Who, Whom, Action) :-
  offend(Who, Whom, Action),
  not forgive(Whom, Who, Action),
  explain(Counselor, Whom,
  believe(Whom, (know(Who, not want(Whom, Action))→
                   not do(Who, Action))).

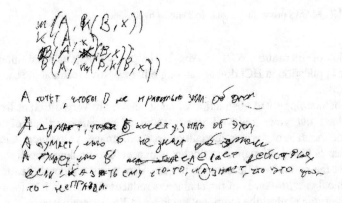

Fig. 8.8 A trainee writes a formal definition for *cheating* followed by its definition in plain words (Russian)

What is the role of mental states of fictional characters in the classification and schematization of the works of literature? We have built the dataset of WOLs, which includes the manually extracted mental states of their characters. We collected as many WOLs as it was necessary to represent the totality of mental states, encoded by logical formulas of the certain complexity (Galitsky 2002). Below are the features of this dataset:

1. As a rule, the main plot of a WOL deals with the development of human emotions, expressible via the basic (*want-know-believe*) and derived (*pretend, deceive*, etc.) mental predicates. A single mental state expresses the very essence of a particular WOL for the small forms (a verse, a story, a sketch, etc.). When one considers a novel, a poem, a drama, etc., which has a more complex nature, then a set of individual plots can be revealed. Each of these plots is depicting its own structure of mental states that is not necessarily unique. Taken all together, they have the highly complex forms, appropriate to identify the WOL.
2. Extraction of the mental states from a WOL allows us to clarify psychological, social and philosophical problems, encoded by this work. The mental components, in contrast to the "physical" ones are frequently expressed implicitly and contain some forms of ambiguity.
3. The same mental formula may be a part of different WOLs, written by the distinguishing authors. Therefore, it is impossible to identify a certain WOL or author when we take into consideration just a single mental formula. However, the frequency of repetition of certain mental formulas shows us the importance of the problem raised by a WOL.
4. The sets of mental formulas are sufficient to identify a WOL. The possibility to recognize a certain author according to a collection of mental states of his or her WOLs is beyond our current considerations.

8.4.1   Architecture and Implementation

We enumerate the tasks that have to be implemented for the literature search system based on the scenario reasoning settings

1. Understanding a natural language query or statement (Galitsky 2003). This unit converts a NL expression in a formalized one (mental formula), using mental metapredicates and generic predicates for physical states and actions.
2. Domain representation in the form of semantic headers (Galitsky 2000), where mental formulas are assigned to the textual representation (abstract) of WOLs.
3. NL_MAMS-supported reasoning that builds the hypothetical mental states, which follow the mental state, mentioned in the query. These generated hypothetical mental states will be searched against WOL knowledge base together with the query representation (in unit 5).
4. Synthesis of all well-written mental formulas in the given vocabulary of basic and derived mental entities.
5. Matching the mental formula, obtained for a query against mental formulas, associated with WOLs. We use the approximate match in case of failure of the direct match.
6. Synthesis of canonical NL sentence based on mental formula to verify if the query was properly understood.

Figure 8.9 presents the chart for interaction between the respective components (1)-(6) of the WOL search system. Suggested system architecture allows two functioning options: WOL search and extension of WOL dataset. When a user wishes to add a new WOL to the current dataset, mental formulas associated with text are automatically build by unit 1 and are multiplied for semantically different phrasings by Unit 3.

Rather complex semantic analysis (unit 1) is required for exact representation of input query: all the logical connectives have to be properly handled. Unit 3 provides the better coverage of the WOL domain, deductively linking mental formula for a query with mental formulas for WOLs. Unit 4 is based on NL_MAMS to handle the totality of all mental formulas, representing the real-life situations.

We rely on NL_MAMS to extract the plausible mental formula from the totality of all well-written mental formulas, represented via metapredicates. In addition, introduction of the classes of equality of mental formulas are required for the approximate match of mental formulas (Unit 5) that is also inconsistent with the traditional formalizations of reasoning about knowledge and belief. NL synthesis of mental expression (Unit 6) is helpful for the verification of the system's deduction. A trainee needs this component to verify that she is understood by the system correctly before starting to evaluate the answer. NL synthesis in such

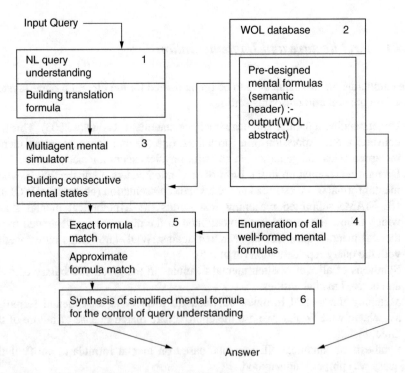

Fig. 8.9 The chart of the WOL search and mental reasoning system

strictly limited domain as mental expression is straightforward and does not require special considerations. Note that semantic rules for the analysis of mental formulas require specific (more advanced) machinery for complex embedded expressions and metapredicate substitutions.

The special question-answering technique for the weakly structured domains has been developed to link the formal representation of a question with the formal expression of the essential idea of an answer. These expressions, enumerating the key mental states and actions of the WOL characters, are called *semantic headers of answers* (Galitsky 2000). The mode of knowledge base extension (automatic annotation), where a customer introduces an abstract of a plot and the system prepares it as an answer for the other customers, takes advantage of the flexibility properties of the semantic header technique.

The mode of knowledge base extension (automatic annotation), where a trainee or a caregiver introduces an abstract of a plot and the system prepares it as an answer for the other trainees, takes advantage of the flexibility properties of the semantic header technique.

To summarize, The WOL architecture is as follows. NL query that includes mental states and action of WOL characters is converted into mental formula (1). Multiagent mental simulator (3) yields the set of mental formulas, associated with the query to extend the knowledge base search. Obtained formulas are matched (5) against the totality of prepared semantic headers (mental formulas) from the WOL database (2). If there is no semantic header (mental formula attached to text) in the dataset component that satisfies the mental formula for a query, the approximate match is initiated. Using the enumeration of all well-formed mental formulas (4), the system finds the best approximation of the mental formula for a query that matches at least single semantic header (mental formula for an answer) (Fig. 8.10).

How would a person pretend to another person that she does not want that person to know something?

When would a person want another person not to pretend that he does not know something?
When would a character pretend about his intention to know something?
Why would a person want another person to pretend about what this other person want?
How can a person pretend that he does not understand that other person does not want?
Is it easy for a person to believe that another person does not pretend what she wants?
How can a person believe that another person might pretend that he wants something?
She wanted to believe that he pretended that he was not a prince.
Can she believe that he does not pretend that he committed the murderer of her spouse because of his love to her?
A person believes that the husband does not want him to love his wife.
A wife wishes not to confess to her husband that she was not faithful.

Fig. 8.10 Sample questions for the literature search

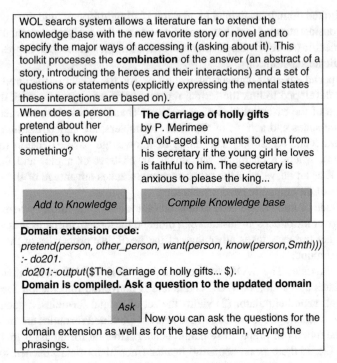

WOL search system allows a literature fan to extend the knowledge base with the new favorite story or novel and to specify the major ways of accessing it (asking about it). This toolkit processes the **combination** of the answer (an abstract of a story, introducing the heroes and their interactions) and a set of questions or statements (explicitly expressing the mental states these interactions are based on).

When does a person pretend about her intention to know something?

The Carriage of holly gifts
by P. Merimee
An old-aged king wants to learn from his secretary if the young girl he loves is faithful to him. The secretary is anxious to please the king...

Add to Knowledge

Compile Knowledge base

Domain extension code:
pretend(person, other_person, want(person, know(person,Smth)))
:- do201.
do201:-output($The Carriage of holly gifts... $).
Domain is compiled. Ask a question to the updated domain

Ask

Now you can ask the questions for the domain extension as well as for the base domain, varying the phrasings.

Fig. 8.11 Autistic child learns the mental interaction with the characters (participants of the scene), using suggested system

8.4.2   HCI Aspects and Query Examples

Interaction with the literature characters is demonstrated to be a novel educational and entertainment area, appealing to adults as well as to children, interacting with the characters of the scenes in NL (Fig. 8.11). Since the players are suggested to both ask questions and share the literature knowledge, the system encourages the cooperation among the members of the players' community. In the demo we have built, the system only recognizes the questions and statements, involving the terms for mental states and actions. This way we encourage the players to stay within a "pure" mental world and to increase the complexity of queries and statements we expect the system to handle properly. Observing the game players, we discovered that they frequently try to obtain the exhaustive list of WOLs, memorize the querying results and enjoy sharing WOL plots with the others.

The demo encourages the users (players, students) to demonstrate their knowledge of classical literature, from medieval to modern, asking questions about the mental states of the characters and compare the system results with their own imagination. The system stimulates the trainees to extract the mental entities, which can be formalized, from the totality of features of literature characters. After an

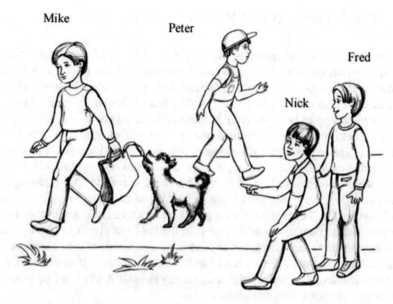

Fig. 8.12 A scene that is a subjects of questions about mental states

answer is obtained, it takes some efforts to verify its relevancy to the question. It takes a little variation in the mental expression to switch from one WOL to another. More advanced users are offered the option of adding new WOL. For mental intervention (particularly, autistic children) certain visualization aids are useful in addition to the WOL search system (Fig. 8.12, Galitsky 2000).

Examples of questions the children may ask the system about, while watching the scene, are shown in Fig. 8.10. Involving more and more complex mental states helps the playing children to develop creativity and imagination of thinking, as well as the communication skills of understanding other's mental states.

1.	Does Mike see that the dog is eating the sausages?
2.	Does Peter see what is happening with Mike and the dog?
3.	Does Nick know what is happening with Mike and the dog?
4.	Which way does Nick express his emotions?
5.	Does Fred know whether Peter knows what is happening with sausages?
6.	Does Nick want to keep the dog from eating the sausages?
7.	What would Fred do if he wants to let Peter know what is happening?

8.5   The Action Adjustor Training System

Having acquired various reasoning patterns, regrettably, CwA experience difficulties transferring these patterns from one domain to another, from home to street environment, from behavior while on holiday or in the class etc. Therefore, although the default reasoning patterns per se are formulated as domain-independent, the same patterns have to be repetitively introduced in each domain.

Adjustment of action can be initiated in a pre-verbal age. It is important to give meanings to CwA actions. Some CwA do not yet use their behavior for communication with others, but a parent or trainee can respond to CwA behavior as if it were a communication. It teaches her that her actions have meanings. For example, if CwA makes sounds without an intent to communicate anything, a parent should respond as if the sounds have a goal, such as a request for some objects. The caregiver should then pronounce "here it is, the toy" and give it to CwA. Also, if CwA reaches up in the air without any intent or associated meaning, react as if he wants to be picked up. Attach a meaning to CwA's play even if she handles a toy in an unusual or odd way. If a child arranged toy animals in a row, a trainer can say "You arranged your animals in a Zoo".

Teaching children with autism proper reasoning patterns concerning selection of actions in a context should be conducted in *all* domains one would expect to make children's behavior more adequate. Hence a separate component for each behavioral domain is required, including home, school, outdoor, sports and other activity. We build a sample interactive form for the "going to school" domain, keeping in mind that similar forms are required for different domains. In the future we expect such forms will be developed (possibly, built by automated tools) by a number of educational content providers.

The generic interactive form that includes two exercises is shown at Fig. 8.13. The form specifies the initial conditions and default actions (drop-down boxes on the left) and also current circumstances with adjusted actions (drop-down boxes on the right); actions are chosen by trainees. Selecting the items on the left, trainees imitate respective sequence of (changing) circumstances/contexts, and the appropriate action adjustment (correct action) should be selected on the right. The link between the selections on the left and those on the right is implemented via default rules.

In Fig. 8.14 we present two interactive forms for organizing a party (on the top) and a route to school (on the bottom). The initial state is randomly set. Then

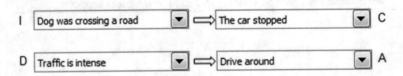

Fig. 8.13 Interactive form to train the adjustment of action to representation change

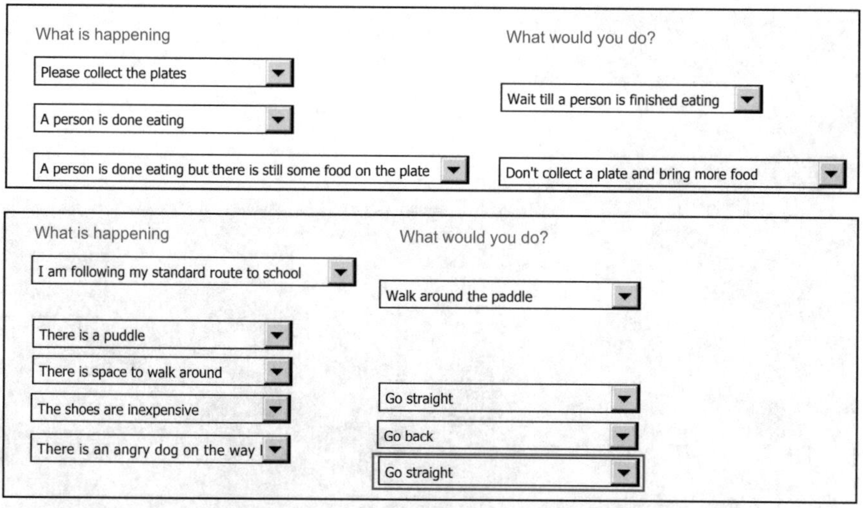

Fig. 8.14 Two interactive forms for training selection of actions

the trainee needs to select an appropriate action in response to the auto-selected circumstances. Alternatively, the trainee can select these circumstances herself to browse through all possibilities. Once the choice is done, the system corrects the selection if the choice was erroneous.

8.6 Emotional Remediation

It is hard for CwA to recognize facial expressions of different emotions. Children who have trouble interpreting the emotional expressions of others are taught about emotional expressions by looking at pictures of people with different facial expressions or through identifying emotional expressions of others in structured exercises. CwA are missing an intuitive, almost automatic sense of another person's affect (Fig. 8.15). This is the feature people rely on to appreciate an emotional state of a peer. In other words, understanding of emotions of other people is supposed to happen very rapidly through a personal, non-logical, emotional reaction. One can often respond to the person's affect before it even consciously accepted. Thus, we flirt back, look embarrasses, puzzled or display anger as part of our intuitive, affective response. Once we have experienced, at the intuitive level, the other person's emotional signal, we can also reflect on it in a conscious and deliberate manner. People may determine that other people are unhappy angry, or puzzled and to do that they are relying on their own affective response, not just on facial expression of an opponent (Fig. 8.16).

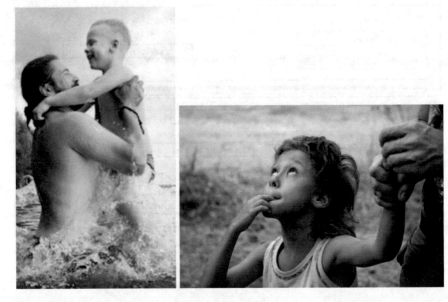

Fig. 8.15 Attempting to cause positive emotions without scaring

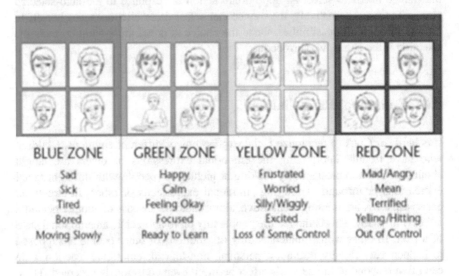

Fig. 8.16 Classes of emotions (Hergott 2016)

During a regular course of events, such as attending a cocktail party or trying to establish relationships with other children at a birthday party, there is a high volume of affect signals being exchanged. If a child or adult consciously tries to figure out each separate one, they will be doomed to failure and confusion.

Therefore, the way to help CwA to recognizing and learn affect signals is to provide him or her extra practice in experiencing and reading those signals. A trainee should start in rather simpler social situations involving lots of reciprocal, affective interactions, initially with one-on-one caregiver and other children. After that CwA should gradually proceed towards more complex situations with other people.

It is not enough to teach child recognize emotions on a computer game. A trainee must proceed talking about emotions in real-world interactions (Fig. 8.15). Since CwA cannot learn this affect on their own; they must be guided. The "practice" needs to involve the personal inner experiences of someone else's affect, as well as one's own, in a series of reciprocal interactions. Similarly, children who have theory of mind problems are often provided with cognitive exercises involving figuring out other people's perspectives, rather than working at the primary level of affective signaling, which is often compromised and at the core of these children's problems.

Our experience in rehabilitation tells that children with autism or Asperger's Syndrome are not able to learn to feel their own and someone else's affect and, therefore, can only learn to read facial expressions through pictures or perform theory of mind tasks in a conscious, deliberate manner (Fig. 8.15).

Although a number of research suggests the opposite, with a program focusing on relating and affect cueing, the majority of children made progress in understanding and showing emotions (Greenspan and Wieder 1998). In general, the missing piece in many intervention programs is a lack of understanding of the developmental steps involved in acquiring certain cognitive, social, and emotional skills (Fig. 8.17). By understanding these steps, which often involve transformations of affect, intervention strategies can help the child master the critical foundations for cognitive and social skills.

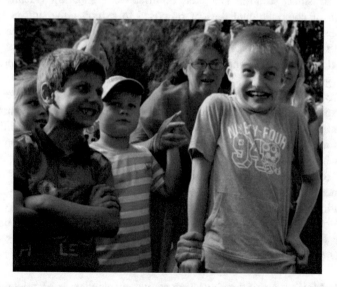

Fig. 8.17 Children express distinct emotions observing something that causes a surprise

Greenspan (1997) worked with children on their skills to interact by means of affective gestures. The first step was simple interaction scenarios including back and forth negotiations (Rosenschein and Zlotkin 1994) such as put a book on the table or get a hat. The author found that CwA can mostly achieve a continuous flow of affective interaction. As children are involved in interactions, their repetitive, idiosyncratic, un-reciprocal and stereotypical forms of behavior were altered. They begin using their gestures, available language and thinking skills in a more purposeful, creative and abstract manner.

For children who start this training at age eight, they need a number of years to develop the basic capability for reciprocal affective gesturing since this skill was omitted at the appropriate age. When this training starts at earlier age, CwA develop these skills more quickly and fully (Greenspan and Wieder 1998). Many children benefit from a balanced intervention program which involves both spontaneous reciprocal affective interchanges and problem solving training with certain structure. When goals are posed in a semi-structured way, the training needs to be offered in a way that initiates enthusiastic affect and a continuous flow of back and forth interaction while solving a problem. An example of such semi-structured problem would be teaching a child to "open" in the context of his trying to open the door to get his favorite toy that has been deliberately placed behind the door.

8.6.1 Emotions in Conversational Agents

Computers need to be programmed emotions from scratch to display affect in response to some stimuli. The area of affective computing (Picard 1997) is the design of computational devices proposed to exhibit either innate emotional capabilities or that are capable of convincingly simulating emotions. With CwA, we target both these directions, giving them rules to reason about emotions as a part of the mental world on one hand, and teach them direct rule when it is appropriate to express a given emotion.

A more practical approach for the case of computers, based on current technological capabilities, is the simulation of emotions in conversational agents in order to enrich and facilitate interactivity between human and machine. While human emotions are often associated with surges in hormones and other neuropeptides, emotions in machines and CwA should be associated with states associated with progress (or lack of progress) in autonomous learning systems, or cognitive development. In this view, affective emotional states correspond to time-derivatives (perturbations) in the achieved recognition accuracies of an arbitrary learning system. Both computer scientists and CwA teachers pose the question on how far can their subjects go in terms of doing a good job handling people's emotions and knowing when it is appropriate to show emotions without actually having the feelings.

Marvin Minsky, one of the pioneering computer scientists in AI, relates emotions to the broader issues of machine intelligence, stating in his book "The Emotion

Machine" that emotion is "not especially different from the processes that we call 'thinking' (Minsky 2007). He explains that the distinction between emotions and other kinds of thinking is rather vague. His main argument is that emotions are "ways to think" for different "problem types" that exist in the world. The brain has rule-based mechanisms, implemented as switches or selectors, that initiate emotions to tackle various tasks. Minsky's approach backs up our intervention strategy based on the rule-based assistance with understanding and reproducing emotions.

In his book "Descartes' Error" (Damasio 2004) argued that, thanks to the interplay of the brain's frontal lobe and limbic systems, our ability to reason depends in part on our ability to feel emotion. Too little like too much of this system would cause bad decisions. The simplest example: It is an emotion – fear – that controls one's decision not to go into a forest in the dark at night to avoid wolves. Most AI experts aren't interested in the role of emotion, preferring to build systems that rely solely on rules. Another AI pioneer John McCarthy believes that we should avoid affect in computational models, arguing that it isn't essential to intelligence and, in fact, can get in the way. Others, like Aaron Sloman, think it's unnecessary to build in emotions for their own sake. According to Sloman, feeling will arise as a "side effect" of interactions between components required for other purposes. In terms of our model of the mental world, once mental states are properly trained, emotions will follow since they obey similar definition framework.

Picard (1997) believes that computers should be designed to take into account, express and influence users' feelings. From scheduling an appointment to picking a spouse, humans follow their intuition and listen to their gut feelings. According to Picard, computers that are not capable of understanding and generating emotion are like an autistic ski resort service guy who says, "I remember you! You're the dude who gave me a bad tip."

The pragmatics of autistic intervention of emotional development helps to resolve the disagreement between Picard and her opponents. On one hand, *interactional approach* to affective computing adopts a notion of emotion as constituted in social interaction. This is not to neglect the fact that emotions have neural aspects, but it is to confirm that emotion is "culturally grounded, dynamically experienced, and to some degree constructed in action and interaction". When a CwA is taught to choose an action, once it affects other people or a feeling of himself, a rule needs to be introduced for an associated emotion. When you either step into a puddle or go around, in addition to physical results of either action CwA needs to be explained the feeling of the mother once she observes the pair of wet shoes.

Also, the interactional approach does not seek to enhance the affect-processing capacities of computer systems. Rather, it seeks to help people to understand and experience their own emotions, which is important for CwA. Furthermore, the interactional approach accordingly adopts different design and evaluation strategies than those described by the Picardian research program. Interactional affective design supports open-ended, inter-individual processes of affect interpretation. It recognizes the context-sensitive, subjective, changing and possibly ambiguous character of affect interpretation. Interactional approach considers these efforts to make sense of emotions and that it may be difficult to formalize affect.

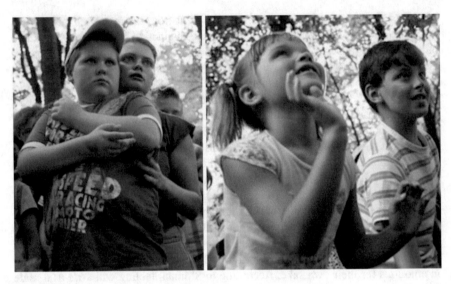

Fig. 8.18 A training to properly express emotions

Picard and her followers pursue a *cognitivist measuring approach* to users' affect, while the interactional followers prefer a pragmatic approach that views (emotional) experience as inherently referring to social interaction (Boehner et al. 2007). While the Picardian approach focuses on human-machine relations, the goal of the interactional affective computing approach is to facilitate computer-mediated inter-personal communication. And while the Picardian approach is concerned with the measurement and modeling of the neural component of the emotional processing system, interactional affective computing considers emotions as complex subjective interpretations of affect, arguing that emotions instead of not affect are at stake, from the point of view of technology users.

Picard uses the state transition diagram to simulate transitions between emotions. The state (here: *interest (I), distress (D)*, or *joy(J)*) of a person cannot be observed directly, but observations which depend on a state can be made (Fig. 8.19). The Hidden Markov Model shown here characterizes the probabilities of transitions among three "hidden" states, (I,D,J), as well as probabilities of observations (measurable eccentric forms, such as features of voice inflection, V) given a state. Given a series of observations over time, an algorithm such as (Viterbi's 1967) can be used to computer the sequence of states which provide the best explanation for observations. These diagrams should be used as an educational aid for trainers to explain how one emotion can grow into another (Fig. 8.18).

For example, if one is *interested* in something, but is denied access or information, she transitions into *distress*. Once the access is granted or information is obtained, she can further transition to *joy*. These transitions can also be illustrated by modifying an schematic image of an agent, an animal or a human (Sect. 8.6.5).

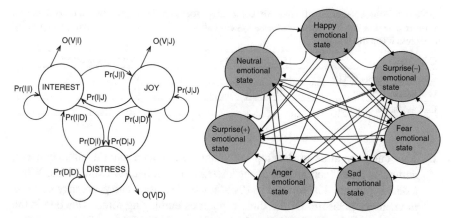

Fig. 8.19 State transition diagram to simulate transitions between emotions (from Jain and Asawa 2015)

This probabilistic algorithm is good to teach a machine to recognize emotions, but for a teaching a CwA a deterministic rule-based approach is necessary, like *always* show a joy once you satisfied your interest, not randomly. In general, random, probabilistic behavior, as observed by others, as associated with autism and therefore needs to be cured. Even if deterministic system does not behave as close to a natural emotional system as a probabilistic one, it is still a step forward in terms of teaching CwA.

Although most computer models for imitating mental activity do not explicitly consider the limbic response, a surprisingly large number implicitly consider it. (Werbos 1994) explains that his original idea of the backpropagation learning algorithm, extensively used in training artificial neural networks, was inspired by trying to mathematically translate an idea of Freud. Freud's model began with the idea that human behavior is governed by emotions, and people attach emotional energy to things Freud called "objects."

According to Freud's theory, people first of all learn cause-and-effect associations; for example, they may learn that "object" A is associated with "object" B at a later time. And his theory was that there is a backwards flow of emotional energy. If A causes B, and B has emotional energy, then some of this energy flows back to A. If A causes B to an extent W, then the backwards flow of emotional energy from B back to A will be proportional to the forwards rate. That really is backpropagation.... If A causes B, then you have to find a way to credit A for B, directly. ... If you want to build a powerful system, you need a backwards flow."

What are the cases that arise in affective computing, and how might we proceed, given the scenarios above? Table 8.2 presents four cases:

I. Most computers and some CwA fall in this category, having rather limited affect recognition and expression. Such computers and humans are neither personal nor friendly.

Table 8.2 Four categories of affective computing, focusing on expression and recognition. Another question can be posed whether a system can act based on emotion, having a capability to express it (on the bottom)

Computer	Cannot express affect	Can express affect
Cannot perceive affect	I.	II.
Can perceive affect	III.	IV.
Can act based on emot. | . . .		

II. This category aims to develop computer voices with natural intonation and computer faces (perhaps on agent interfaces) with natural expressions. When a disk is put into a laptop and its disk-face smiles, users and peers may share its momentary pleasure. Of the three categories employing affect, this one is the most advanced technologically, although it is still in its infancy. This case is also represented by CwA which need to be trained to perceive affect and emotions.

III. This category enables a computer or a CwA to perceive your affective state, enabling it to adjust its response in ways that might, for example, make it a better teacher and more useful assistant. It allays the fears of those who are uneasy with the thought of emotional computers, in particular, if they do not see the difference between a computer expressing affect, and being driven by emotion.

IV. This category maximizes the meaningful communication between human and computer, potentially providing truly "personal" and "user-friendly" computing. It does not imply that the computer would be driven by its emotions. This is the goal of emotional rehabilitation of CwA.

Also it is worth adding the rows "Computer can/can't induce the user's emotions" as it is clear that computers already influence our emotions, the open questions are how deliberately, directly, and for what purpose.

It has to be clearly explained to a CwA what is the difference between feeling, emotion and affect. Feelings are *personal* and *biographical*, emotions are *social*, and affects are *pre-personal* (Shouse 2005).

We can define a feeling as a *sensation that can be recognized* given the previously accumulated training set (of feelings). It is personal and biographical because every person has a distinct training set of previous sensations. An infant does not experience feelings because he lacks such training set. At the same time, parents are confident that their children have feelings (which are indeed affects) and express them regularly.

An emotion is a *display* of a feeling, a means to show feeling to the public. Unlike feelings, the display of emotion can be either genuine or fake (Oatley and Johnson-Laird 1987). We broadcast emotions to the world:

1. an expression of our internal state;
2. in order to fulfill social expectations.

Infants do display emotions although they do not have a training set to experience feelings. The emotions of the infant are direct expressions of affect.

CwA need to be explained that for a given feeling, there are multiple way to express respective emotion. When $feeling = 'upset'$ the emotion $\in$ {'yell', 'throw object', 'tantrum', 'being quiet', 'drop into tears', 'complain'}. A caregiver should give an example first and then make a trainee display one emotion after another, given a particular feeling. Also, CwA needs to be capable of recognizing genuine (sincere, real) emotions versus fake (*cheating, pretending*, trying to *impress* someone with her specific feeling to achieve a goal).

Affect can be defined as the *body's way of preparing itself for action* in a given circumstance by adding a quantitative dimension of intensity to the quality of an experience.

An affect is a non-conscious experience of intensity; it is a moment of unformed and unstructured potential. Affect cannot be fully realized in language, and it is outside of consciousness). The body has a grammar of its own. CwA need to be trained to imitate affect by their bodies, and differentiate it from emotions. According to (Massumi 2002), affects include coordinated responses involving the facial muscles, the viscera, the respiratory system, the skeleton, autonomic blood flow changes, and vocalizations that together produce an analogue of the particular gradient or intensity of stimulation influencing the person's body.

8.6.2   Tuning Emotional Response

Children should be capable of defining emotions and telling a caregiver about a time they feel, experience this emotion. A definition of a particular emotion needs to be provided if a child is unable to produce an appropriate explanation. A trainer must ensure that the children are aware of the meaning of each term referencing emotion as they are asked to discuss their personal experience.

An important class of exercises targeting reasoning that supports understanding and expressing emotions is recalling a prior personal experience. High-functioning individuals with autism also seem able to discuss experiences with simple emotions but usually have trouble with more complex or self-conscious emotions such as *pride* and *embarrassment*. The form-based approach where a child picks a combination of himself or his proponent or opponent in the mental state, is fruitful (Fig. 8.20, Galitsky and Shpitsberg 2015). In the rightmost column the trainees are to give example of cases from their personal experience.

Whereas simple emotions are associated with distinct facial expressions, exhibit little cultural variation in antecedents or expression, and are typically recognized and understood relatively early in development, self-conscious emotions necessarily involve complex attribution processes relying on later developmental achievements, such as the capacity for reflecting upon experiences and evaluating them in relation to sociocultural norms and expectations, as well as the appraisals of others (Lewis et al. 2010, Fig. 8.21). According to Cooley 1902)

proud	I		person
	you		person's action
	he		person A's action towards person B
	they	with	myself
embarrassed	I		my action
	you		my action towards person B
	he		
	they		

Fig. 8.20 A form for being proud and being embarrassed

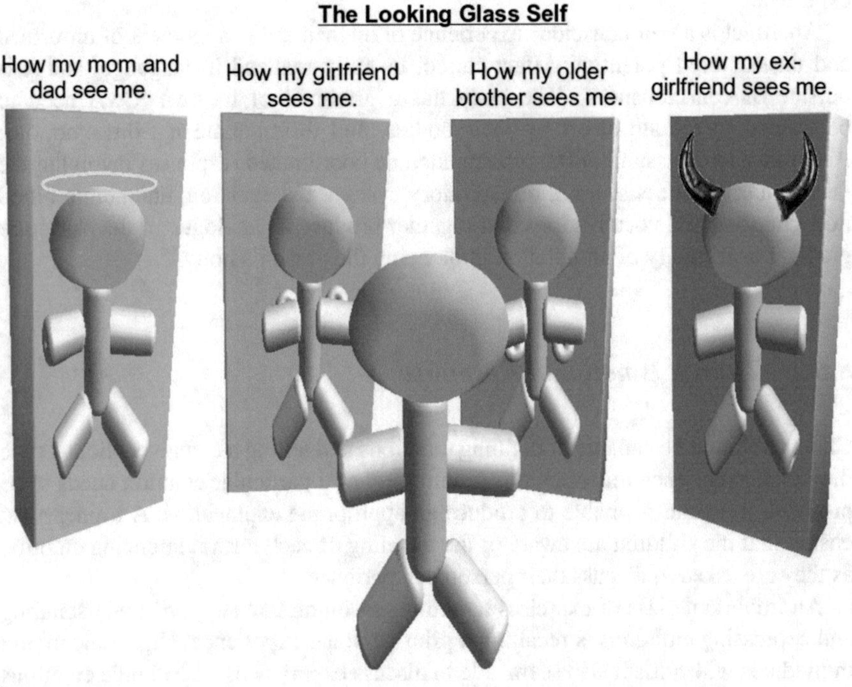

The Looking Glass Self

How my mom and dad see me.   How my girlfriend sees me.   How my older brother sees me.   How my ex-girlfriend sees me.

Fig. 8.21 This drawing depicts the looking-glass self. The person at the front of the image is looking into four mirrors, each of which reflects someone else's image of this person

the thing that moves us to pride and shame is not merely mechanical reflection of ourselves, but an imputed sentiment, the imagined effect of this reflection upon another's mind.

When the children are unable to recall a personal experience, a trainer describes a scripted personal experience of her own involving the term in question, followed by the prompt "Have you ever felt that way?" Once children began their accounts, however, such advising should be limited to requests for elaboration and clarification in response to children's excessive pauses, trailing off, and incoherent remarks.

There are two kinds of issues in understanding and expressing emotions while children recount their emotional experience:

1. Involving inappropriate contexts, actions and events that, without further explanation, would not typically elicit the emotion/or non-emotion in question (e.g., "I was embarrassed once time when I was asked to assist with carrying a bag").
2. Involving episodes that would tend to elicit feelings of appropriate sentiment polarity but did not contain sufficient details or explanation for distinguishing the specific emotion/non-emotion from the feeling expressed in language by a verb of the same class (feelings with the similar patterns). (e.g., "I was proud when I received an acceptance letter in the mail").

These issues are cured by learning correct, concise definitions of emotional entities.

Only describing unambiguously evocative contexts (e.g., "I was not happy when my parents took my brother instead of me to watch a movie") and/or that include explanations clarifying the reasons the particular actions or events were associated with the feeling in question (e.g., "I felt proud when I earned an award for running fast") can be considered as successful understanding of emotion.

8.6.3   Autism and CwA Expression of Feelings

Despite many difficulties, CwA can acquire social skills over a period of time, given appropriate intervention. Attempting to teach people with autism about emotions using conventional strategies, such as trying to make them understand a viewpoint of another person, is rarely successful. A more concrete approach is required.

In this chapter we present a method to teach CwA to understand and acknowledge the thoughts and feeling of others via *social stories*. These short stories describe scenarios that enable individuals to improve their understanding of themselves and others. These stories prompt both children and adults to ask questions about other people and attempt to recognize that different people may think differently.

If one distinguish a child's capacity for deep, joyful relating from the capacity for affective, reciprocal interchanges, one can observe that CwA are capable of the full range of warmth, love, and closeness. This intimacy is relatively easy to observe in families who focus on promoting relaxed interactions for hours and hours and attending to all the subtle ways the children have of showing their intimacy. In the review of 200 cases, over half the children evidenced a deep rich capacity for intimacy and over 90 % showed a continuing growth in this pattern (Greenspan and Wieder 1998) (Fig. 8.22).

When teaching individuals with autism about emotions, it is important to describe each feeling pictorially, using pictures with clear outlines, and with minimal detail. Relate the emotion to what can be seen, such as facial expression or body language.

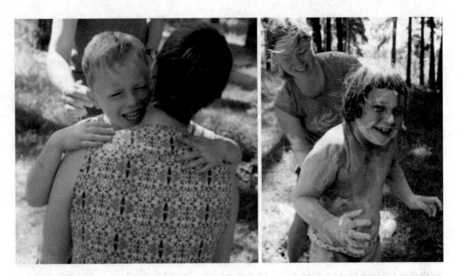

Fig. 8.22 Stimulation via novel unfamiliar patterns to enhance tolerance to unexplored feelings

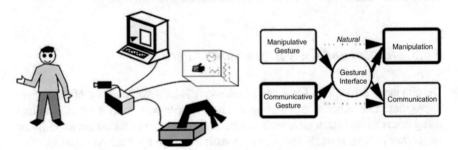

Fig. 8.23 Applications of gestural interface for HCI. Unlike the gestures in a natural environment, both manipulative and communicative gestures in HCI can be employed to direct manipulations of objects or to convey messages

8.6.4 Teaching Gestures

CwA need to be taught gestures as an efficient way of communication.

The taxonomy that seems most appropriate within the context of HCI was recently developed by (Quek 1995). A slightly modified version of the taxonomy is given in Fig. 8.24 and Fig. 8.23. All hand/arm movements are first classified into two major classes: gestures and unintentional movements.

Gestures themselves can have two modalities: communicative and manipulative. Manipulative gestures are the ones used to act on objects in an environment (object movement, rotation, etc.) Communicative gestures, on the other hand, have an inherent communicational purpose. In a natural environment they are usually accompanied by speech. Communicative gestures can be either acts or symbols.

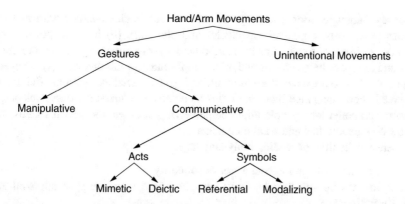

Fig. 8.24 A taxonomy of hand gestures for HCI. Meaningful gestures are differentiated from unintentional movements. Gestures used for manipulation (examination) of objects are separated from the gestures which possess inherent communicational character

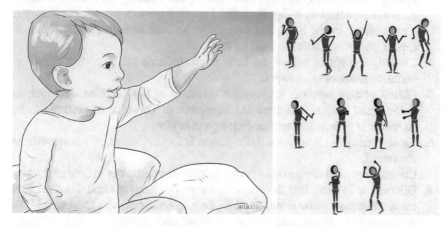

Fig. 8.25 Using gestures for communication

Symbols are those gestures that have a linguistic role. They symbolize some referential action (for instance, circular motion of index finger may be a referent for a wheel) or are used as modalizers, often of speech ("Look at that wing!" and a modalizing gesture specifying that the wing is vibrating, for example). In HCI context these gesture are one of the most commonly used gestures since they can often be represented by different static hand postures (Fig. 8.25).

CwA have trouble reading body language, which makes it increasing difficult for them to interact with others. The good news is that it is possible to learn how to read body language through practice and role-playing.

Noticing the signals that people send out with their body language is a crucial social skill. A few of CwA can read it naturally, but most of us are notoriously oblivious. Fortunately, with a little extra attentiveness, you can learn to read body language, and with enough practice it can become second nature.

Body language often encompasses (a) how our bodies connect with material things (e.g., pens, cigarettes, spectacles and clothing), (b) how we position our bodies, (c) how we touch ourselves and others, (d) our breathing, (e) our closeness to – and the space between – us and other people and how this changes, (f) our eyes – especially how our eyes move and focus, and (g) our facial expressions. Being able to "read" body language therefore helps us greatly to understand ourselves better, understand better how people might be perceiving our own non-verbal signals, and know how people feel and what they mean.

Here are the tips for reading body language:

1. A clenched fist can indicate anger or solidarity.
2. A thumbs up and thumbs down are often used as gestures of approval and disapproval.
3. Blinking is natural, but you should also pay attention to whether a person is blinking too much or too little. People often blink more rapidly when they are feeling distressed or uncomfortable. Infrequent blinking may indicate that a person is intentionally trying to control his or her eye movements. For example, a card player might blink less frequently, because he is purposely trying to appear unexcited about the hand he was dealt.
4. Clasping the hands behind the back might indicate that a person is feeling bored, anxious, or even angry.
5. Closed posture involves keeping the obscured or hidden often by hunching forward and keeping the arms and legs crossed. This type of posture can be an indicator of hostility, unfriendliness, and anxiety.
6. Crossed arms might indicate that a person is feel defensive, self-protective, or closed-off.
7. Crossed legs can indicate that a person is feeling closed off or in need of privacy.
8. Dilated pupils mean that the person is interested. Keep in mind, however, that many substances cause pupils to dilate, including alcohol. So a CwA should not do a mistake of having a few drinks for attraction.
9. If people purposely touch their feet to yours, they are flirting!
10. If someone mimics your body language, this is a very genuine sign that they are trying to establish a communication channel with you. Try changing your body position here and there. If you find that they change theirs similarly, they are mirroring.

Substantial interest in gestural interface for HCI is stimulated by a vast number of potential applications. Hand gestures in connection with human-computer interface can simply enhance the interaction in "classical" desktop computer applications by replacing the computer mouse or similar hand-held devices. Hand gestures can also replace joysticks and buttons in the control of computerized machinery or be used to help the individuals with special needs and physically impaired to communicate more easily with others. Nevertheless, the major impulse to the development of gestural interfaces has come from the growth of virtual environments (Uras and Verri 1995). Hand gestures in natural environments are used for both manipulative actions and communication. However, the communicative role of gestures is limited, since hand gestures tend to be a supportive element of speech (with the exception of deictic gestures, which play a major role in human communication). Manipulative aspect of gestures is fairly important for HCI. Some applications have emerged recently that take advantage of the communicative role of gestures.

8.6.5 Modifying Emotions in an Image

A set of exercises where CwA is asked to modify a schematic image or a photo to substitute an emotion turned out to be fairly fruitful. Modifying certain areas in an image, CwA learn that emotions are expressed by a number of facial features. This helps them to eventually learn to recognize these facial features and then emotions in the real world.

Using a touch-pad or a mouse for drawing emotion-related features helps to develop a tactile reinforcement with visual perception of emotion. A trainee should select features in an image and modify them to convert a sad face into a happy one and other way around. The eyes and the mouth can be altered, using rotations or mirror mappings, or having their elements re-positioned (Fig. 8.26).

These exercises demonstrate that emotions are instant states, not permanent, and external factors can change them. They also help to understand pre- and post conditions of actions which change emotions, and resultant emotional states.

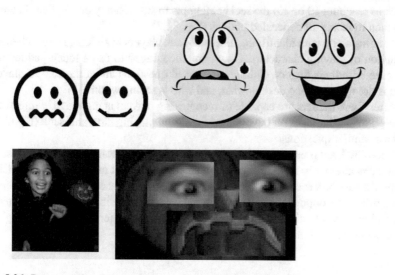

Fig. 8.26 Demonstrating that emotions can change and can be affected from outside

8.7   Teaching Hide-and-Seek Game

One of the important steps in learning the mental world is the hide-and-seek game. This game requires a substantial reasoning about mental states and actions, in both rule-based mental and emotional domain. A child needs to understand the pre- and post-conditions for searching as a desire to identify where the peers are located. A concept of *hiding* needs to be explained as an *opposite* desire of not being found. Children need to be aware that searching may lead to finding, and hiding – to not being found. If one does not search then nobody can be found, and if one does not hide she will be found immediately. It is a game of deception, which requires acknowledgment that other people may have different beliefs. Therefore, many CwA avoid it and/or are not capable of participating in it. Playing hide-and seek requires understanding and handling third-order mental states such as *"I know that he wants me not no know where he is"*.

In the emotional space, a hide-and-seek player is expected to express appropriate emotions when he finds another child, or when he is found by someone else. A rule should be taught that an emotion is appropriate when there was a desire and at the given moment it succeeds. Some emotional expressions are suitable when a child is hiding, he is being looked at but not found.

Another import skill is to conceal yourself in an environment. A child needs to be taught to position himself in the location of a seeker and track his potential gaze to avoid being found. A seeker needs to be able to close his eyes and count to a predetermined number while the other players hide. After reaching the number (such as reaching 10 or 20) the seeker attempts to say, "Ready or not, here I come!" and then to locate all concealed players (Fig. 8.27).

Training starts with identifying hide-and-seek players in an image with schematic depiction of playing characters. CwAs are encouraged to use a touch-pad to track the gaze with their fingers. Children are asked questions about the role of players, who is doing what, who desires what, and who is seeing whom.

After CwA trainers are capable of recognizing players at an image, a trainer can proceed to similar tasks on the photos of children playing hide-and-seek (Fig. 8.28) and ask similar questions:

Once CwA are prepared to play hide and seek, having completed the exercises, a trainer can attempt to involve them in an actual game, first indoor and then outside. To play a role of a seeker or to hide, a CwA needs to be accompanied by a trainer, and a role of an opponent can be performed by a parent, sibling or another trainer. The trainer needs to hide together with CwA and explain her the goal of hiding and the object they are hiding behind.

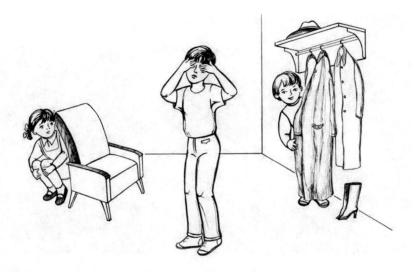

Fig. 8.27 The hide-and-seek training starts with schematic depiction of a seeker and two concealed players

What game do the children play?
Which objects from the environment are used to be hiding behind?
Do those who hiding want the seeker to find them?
Does the seeker want to find those hiding?
Do the hiding children see the seeker? Do they know where he is?
Does the seeker see the hiding children? Does he know where they are?
Why does the seeker have to close his eyes?

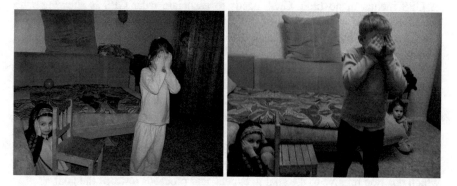

Fig. 8.28 After CwA is confident with schematic depiction of hide-and-seek game, a trainer can proceed to photos. The seekers close their eyes and are counting

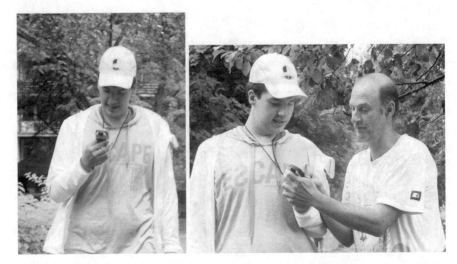

Fig. 8.29 An older trainee finding a direction using GPS (on the left). Some young adults become fairly skillful once the introduction to orienteering with GPS is completed (on the right)

8.7.1   Orienteering Exercise

For most children, orienteering is the next logical step after the hide-and-seek game. However, some children are good at orienteering even if their emotional skills for hide-and-seek are rudimentary and they cannot play independently.

The reason orienteering is not too hard for CwA is that no reasoning about other human is required. CwA usually memorizes the commands and navigation of GPS menus in no time. CwA needs to associate what GPS is showing with what is observed in the real world (Fig. 8.29). Doing that, formulating, adjusting and rejecting of hypotheses of such association is required, based on hypotheses management exercise Sect. 7.5.

The main focus of how orienteering activity supports reasoning is hypotheses management. Looking at a GPS, the child obtains the direction to and distance to the goal. Then observing the landscape, the child selects an object such as a tree and forms an estimate for how far it is from this tree to the goal (Fig. 8.30).

Once the tree is reached, CwA observes her position relative to the goal and possibly updates the hypothesis on where she was relative to the goal. CwA now needs to form a new hypothesis on which direction in the landscape to chose and which position relative to the goal to expect, and proceeds towards the goal.

What this exercise teaches is the skill to maintain hypotheses, revise it when appropriate, and expect it to be wrong again and again. This is opposite to a conventional autistic reasoning which sticks to a given hypothesis once it is formed. After that, CwA will be reluctant to revise this hypothesis, and an observation that it does not fit the real world would be very stressful and unproductive: CwA would give up on the exercise.

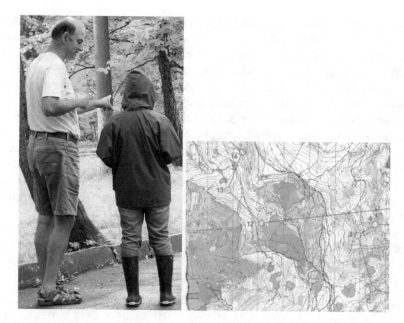

Fig. 8.30 A trainee is being helped to link the GPS indication with the real world spatial references. An orienteering map (on the right) may assist in this activity

8.8 Language Improvement

For language development, a trainer is recommended to use a language that is insignificantly more complex than the current language of a child. Once a given round of training is completed, the trainer should observe how the child communicates on his own. Once the previous trainer level of language is achieved, it can be taken to the next step.

In a CwA does not use words yet, a caregiver should try to model stand-alone words. If single words are used by a child, then the trainer can use two-word phrases. Once the level of two word phrases is achieved, the trainer can proceed to a simple phrase-based speech, followed with the one with descriptors, and then move towards the speech with complex phrases and compound sentences.

Some CwA can imitate long phrases but do not use them on their own without hearing them first. In this case, the trainer is expected to increment the complexity by one element such as an extra word, new word, actions, descriptions, attributes etc. This should be added to a spontaneous communication of CwA. It is advised to simplify the language grammar ("give candy" instead of "please give this candy to your sister").

Speech rate should be slowed down. Then it is easier for the child to learn the important words. These important words should also be stressed. To increase the teaching efficiency, the trainer should use the same language over and over. Specific important words should be repeated, such as physical and mental actions. Visual cues like gestures support the language learning as well. A caregiver should point to an object, animate or inanimate, introducing its name and referring to it. This is critical for nonverbal CwA. Also, it is worth talking about the objects CwA is paying attention to; this will increase the chance the child would borrow the trainers' language for his experience. It can be achieved by a parallel talk and self-talk. The caregiver should comment on, or describe during the process of CwA is seeing, hearing or doing. The trainer's language should be linked to CwA language to be meaningful. A selective set of actions should be chosen for commenting, since an information overload needs to be avoided. For example, when CwA is feeding a stuffed dog, he should say "dog" pointing towards it, or "dog eat". For self-talk, a trainer should talk about what she is doing while CwA watches; short, repetitive sentences should be used.

A caregiver can expand on child's own language by focusing new words or more appropriate grammar or syntax. By adding new terms, the caregiver revises and completes CwA speech and adds information at the same time. When CwA is saying "toy" the trainer can say "give toy", "push toy", "feed toy".

8.8.1 Reading Comprehension

There is a growing body of literature guiding the teaching of reading comprehension including (McNamara 2009) who describes the intervention methodologies linked to theories of readers' cognitive processes. Given the wide variety of strengths and weaknesses exhibited by children on the spectrum, it seems reasonable that reading comprehension interventions targeted for typically developing children who struggle with the complexities of reading comprehension may also benefit children with ASDs. Poor comprehenders are typically adept at phonological processing and word recognition, but are less skilled at handling semantic representations. CwA may focus on word recognition and neglect semantic processing.

Cartwright (2006) described cognitive flexibility exercises, which classroom teachers, parents, and intervention professionals could use to assist children in developing reading-specific cognitive flexibility. The exercises consist of word sorts, in which readers are asked to sort a set of word cards, first based on phonological rules, such as initial consonant sounds, and then again, based on semantic categories, such as foods and non-foods.

"Meaning-focused" remediation such as collaborative learning activities in which peers quizzed each other on vocabulary and factual recall or played games based on reading materials turned out to be efficient. Instructional approaches that consist of reviews and rote activities focus on *practicing* skills, including anaphoric cuing and reciprocal questioning, rather than *learning* skills to build the framework for the cognitive processes involved in reading for meaning.

Trainees are encouraged to read passages under four conditions: answering pre-reading questions, completing sentences, identifying anaphoric references, and reading only. In the anaphoric cuing procedure, students were given a passage with the anaphora or "shortcuts" underlined and they were asked to choose the correct referent, given three choices listed under the underlined "shortcut." Anaphoric cuing significantly increased students' understanding of the passage.

In the other set of exercises, CwA are taught to generate and respond to questions, using a story map framework. CwA increase the frequency of unprompted question generating and responding from the beginning to the end of the intervention. CwA require substantial prompting when generating and responding to inferential questions in comparison with stating facts from the story. This learning strategy relied on peer-tutoring or cooperative learning, giving CwA children an opportunity to develop their language skills in a social setting.

In teaching the oral language skills CwA should be taught to identify materials out of which common objects were made. Given common objects, such as a shirt, a paper napkin, or a leather shoe, the children need direct instruction that included modeling of correct responses, signals to cue students, choral student responses, and correction procedures for incorrect and non-responses. The caregiver can begin instruction using actual objects, then use representations (pictures), and finally move instruction to the abstract stage using words only. Ganz and Flores (2009) concluded that students increased their expressive language skills, based on an increasing number of correct responses to probes posed throughout instruction. The researchers also reported that some students spontaneously used language skills at home and at school, asking others to identify objects made of different materials. This study is significant in that it demonstrates that CwA can be guided to more abstract uses of language through direct instruction (Randi et al. 2010).

8.9 Evaluation of Training

In this section we describe our assessment of exercises in the short-term and long-term training settings.

8.9.1 Short-Term Evaluation

We present the results of the *short-term* evaluation in Table 8.3. The training exercises are categorized by the complexity of mental formulas for the entity to be taught. For each category, the reasoning skills were assessed before and after training (Fig. 8.31), with NL_MAMS assistance for one group (12 children) and without such assistance for the control group (10 children). Other than NL_MAMS-specific, the same set of exercises was offered to both groups. All children from both groups were registered with the same rehabilitation center.

Four task categories are shown: from first to fourth order (in accordance to how the complexity/intentionality of mental formulas has been specified,

Table 8.3 Evaluation of the short-term theory of mind training with and without NL_MAMS

Task category

Mental entity for the task	Autistic one-to-one training with NL_MAMS, 12 children, %		Autistic one-to-one training without NL_MAMS, eight children, %		Impact of NL_MAMS, % of improvement
	Before	After	Before	After	
First-order	22	69	21	62	6.2
Knowing an object and its attributes	25	67	25	75	
Not see – > not know	17	58	25	50	
Intention of others	25	83	13	62	
Second order	14	61	17	54	37.2
Informing	17	58	25	62	
False belief	8	58	13	50	
Questioning	17	67	13	50	
Third-order	8	33	7	22	31.2
Pretending	8	17	13	17	
Deceiving	0	17	0	17	
Offending	8	33	0	17	
Forgiving	8	50	13	33	
Reconciling	17	33	13	17	
Explaining	8	50	0	33	
Fourth-order	13	33	13	25	32
Resolving a conflict	8	33	17	17	
Negotiating	17	33	8	33	
Overall improvement of theory of mind skills due to using NL_MAMS, %					27.5

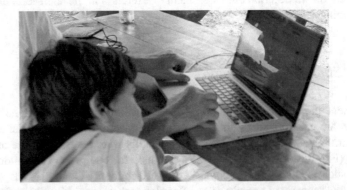

Fig. 8.31 Computers help to maintain trainee attention while doing reasoning skills assessment

Sects. 4.2 and 5.6). For each test exercise, a trainee is either assigned a pass or not, and the percentages of passed trainees are specified (shown in italic). Averaged percentages for groups are shown in normal font. The last (sixth) column indicates how the relative percentage of successful exercises is higher for the NL_MAMS-assisted training than for an unassisted training. It is calculated as

$$\frac{\%\ exper\ after}{\%\ exper\ before} : \frac{\%\ control\ after}{\%\ control\ before}$$

We select the experimental and control groups such that there is an insignificant deviation in initial ToM reasoning capabilities of the children from both groups (<4 % in spite of the different sizes of each group). We naturally observe that children's performances both before and after training are lower for the higher order of involved mental formulas (and respective task complexities) for both experimental and control groups. Unsurprisingly, theory of mind training is more fruitful for second-order than for the first order. However, the efficiency of training then drops for third and fourth orders. One can see that using NL_MAMS for first-order tasks is not as important as for higher-order tasks that require memorizing and operating with a larger amount of data. Overall, NL_MAMS improves the results of training by about a third in a short-term setting.

8.9.2 Long-Term Evaluation

The results of the *long-term* evaluation are shown in Table 8.4. The same evaluation exercises and result computation schema are used as in the short-term cases. We managed to conduct the long-term evaluation study with nine out of twelve children who were the subject of the short-term training (Fig. 8.32). The control group included ten children from another rehabilitation center.

We observe a similar natural phenomenon that handling of more complex mental expressions is harder. However, unlike the short-term evaluation where NL_MAMS has contributed almost equally to second-, third- and fourth-order mental formulas, in the long-term case one observes the following. Theory of mind training has improved the second-order performance by more than twice, and then the third- and fourth-order performance by more than eight times, compared with control group.

Overall performance in the long-term setting is improved by almost 40 % due to theory of mind training and by 280 % due to other forms of training and other reasons (judging on the control group, observed in the age range of 6–9, 7–10, ..., 10–13). 40 % may seem not as significant in respect to 280 % as a quantity, but it has a tremendous value as a portion of world knowledge, in terms of behavioral and emotional development of a child with autism. Moreover, we see that high-order mental formulas that are important for handling mental world indeed require NL_MAMS to be properly trained, as both long-term and short-term studies suggest.

Table 8.4 Evaluation of the long-term theory of mind training for the experimental and control groups

Task category

Mental entity for the task	Autistic one-to-one training with NL_MAMS, nine children, %		No theory of mind training, ten children		Impact of NL_MAMS-assisted theory of mind training, % of improvement
	Before	After 3 years	Before	After 3 years	
First-order	29	89	26	74	7.8
Knowing an object and its attributes	33	78	22	67	
Not see → not know	22	100	22	67	
Intention of others	33	89	33	89	
Second order	18	74	18	63	17.5
Informing	22	67	11	67	
False belief	11	78	22	56	
Questioning	22	78	22	67	
Third-order	11	48	13	35	62.0
Pretending	11	44	11	33	
Deceiving	0	33	11	22	
Offending	11	44	11	56	
Forgiving	11	67	22	33	
Reconciling	12	33	11	22	
Explaining	11	67	11	44	
Fourth-order	17	62	17	38	63.2
Resolving a conflict	11	56	22	33	
Negotiating	22	67	11	44	
Overall improvement of theory of mind skills due to using NL_MAMS-assisted and other forms of rehabilitation of mental reasoning, %					37.5

8.9.3   Evaluation of Intervention of Adjustment of Actions

To evaluate our methodology presented in this book, we observe the results of training triangulation structures of adjustment of actions (Sect. 6.4) to CwA. Triangulation structures are used to approach a proper application of default rules to handle properly the situations when it is important to adopt an action to an environment.

In the Table 8.4 we compare the trainees' performance completing the tasks they have been trained with, as well as new tasks of a similar complexity. Moreover,

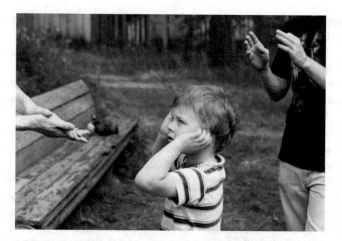

Fig. 8.32 Two trainers are interacting with a boy from different sides

we evaluate how the trainees perform applying learned reasoning patterns to real-world situations. The real time performance is evaluated before the training for each category of learners occurs.

This exercise does not validate whether the learners *understood* the decision making properly because it is expected to be easy just to memorize how to complete them.

1. *Performance completing the exercises which have been introduced earlier* verifies how learners can *reproduce* the decisions which have been shown to them earlier.
2. *Performance completing the exercises with similar rules in a new domain* demonstrates how learners are able to either *memorize* the patterns (rather than details of the offered contexts) of adapting an action to context or to apply them independently, having understood these patterns.
3. *Performance completing the exercises with new rules in a new domain* assesses learners' ability to form (invent) new rules on how to adopt an action to an environment.
4. Observing *correctness of decision-making in similar real-world situations* we can judge on how the learners can apply the skills developed in computer-assisted exercises on default reasoning to the real world environment. This step requires the learners to be capable of *transferring* acquired reasoning patterns from simulation to real world environment and their *application* to real-life objects. In this study we do not evaluate how the learners form new rules in the real world environment as this task is proved to be too hard for the audience of trainees.
5. As a baseline for our experiments, we assess the *Correctness of decision-making in a similar real-world situations without training.*

Our testing environment includes 20 exercises used for both training and evaluation (second column), 20 exercises using the same logic and structure in a distinct domain, 20 exercises for different domains and 20 imitations (or reproductions) of real world environments. A drop-down box-based exercise is considered as completed correctly if more than 80 % of choices are correct, when the exercise is run multiple times with different (randomly generated) initial conditions.

Naturally, each evaluation step is more complex than a previous one to complete: we observe the monotonic decrease of the rate of completion for all three categories of learners. For learners from both autistic and other mental disorder groups the performance is declining faster that that of controls.

For the autistic group of learners *similar rules in a new domain* is the hardest step, and for the group of other mental disorders *decision-making in similar real-world situations* is the hardest step; however it may not characterize these groups with respect to their overall skills of the real world abstraction.

On average autistic individuals perform about 5 % below individuals with other mental disorders for the first task, 2 % for the second task, 9 % for the third and fourth tasks but outperform the children with other mental disorders who did not do any training. This suggests that the case of autism indeed requires harder learning efforts.

The chart for the overall exercise completion is shown in Fig. 8.33. Four data points correspond to the columns 2,3,4 and 5 in Table 8.5. One can see that CwA and other mental diseases with comparable mental age complete exercise similarly compared to CC.

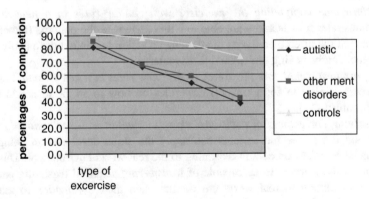

Completion of action adaptation exercise

Fig. 8.33 The chart for exercise performance for the tasks (2)–(3)

Table 8.5 The dynamics of trainee's development

		(1) Performance completing the exercises which have been introduced earlier	(2) Performance completing the exercises with similar rules in a new domain	(3) Performance completing the exercises with new rules in a new domain	(4) Correctness of decision-making in a similar real-world situations	Correctness of decision-making in a similar real-world situations without training
Autistic	A_Subject1	80	75	60	35	5
	A_Subject2	85	60	55	45	15
	A_Subject3	75	60	45	30	25
	A_Subject4	80	65	55	40	10
	A_Subject5	85	70	50	35	5
	A_Subject6	80	65	55	45	15
avg		80.8	65.8	53.3	38.3	12.5
Other mental problems (matched for	M_Subject1	95	60	55	45	15
	M_Subject2	85	55	55	55	20
	M_Subject3	80	65	60	35	5
	M_Subject4	80	70	55	40	15
	M_Subject5	85	75	65	35	10
	M_Subject6	85	70	60	45	5
	M_Subject7	85	75	60	40	10
avg		85.0	67.1	58.6	42.1	11.4
Controls	C_Subject1	90	85	75	75	60
	C_Subject2	95	90	80	70	65
	C_Subject3	95	85	85	65	65
	C_Subject4	90	85	90	80	70
	C_Subject5	85	90	85	75	70
	C_Subject6	95	90	80	75	65
avg		91.7	87.5	82.5	73.3	65.8

8.10 Discussion and Conclusions

There is no well-accepted medical treatment for autism, but it has become increasingly clear that early behavioral intervention is highly beneficial for autistic children (Green 1996; Jensen and Sinclair 2002; Galitsky 2005). Indeed, some experts argue that intensive behavioral intervention can even lead to normal behavior of autistic trainees (McEachin et al. 1993). So far, attempts to explain how a behavioral treatment can possibly eliminate autistic deficiencies were not very successful. It is still unclear why these treatments are successful in some cases but not in others (Lovaas 1987). Since a majority of experts consider behavioral intervention as the only approach to compensatory learning (see, e.g., Frith 2001; Howlin 1998), the claims of possible cures remain controversial.

We analyzed the results of assistance to individuals with autism in reasoning about mental world and other domains. This assistance is provided by a natural language multiagent simulator of mental states (NL_MAMS), introduced in Chap. 5. It assists in the tasks that are the hardest for autistic reasoning: operating with mental states and actions. Autistic patients are trained to perform a number of reasoning exercises.

We performed the simulator-assisted training and its evaluation at two levels: short-term and long-term. The short-term approach includes the theory of mind training with and without the simulator for two groups of autistic children of similar mental age and IQ. The evaluation is based on passing the set of tests including the seeing-leads-to-knowing (first-order) and Sally-Anne false belief (second-order) ones so that a uniform coverage of mental states and actions (up to the order three) is evaluated. In the short-term approach we perform a limited evaluation of the skills transfer from artificial situations to real life ones, but do not analyze how the training affects the socials skills of trainees. The short-term approach is utilized for the purpose of evaluation of theory of mind teaching efficiency, and the control group is subject to the simulator-assisted intervention after the evaluation.

The long-term approach has been applied for over a decade, where manual and simulator-assisted teaching of the ToM is combined with intervention strategies of various natures. The goal of our long-term approach is to teach theory of mind reasoning not just for the reasoning skills per se, but also for improvement of social behavior. Therefore, the evaluation criteria are based on tests of decision-making in the real world as well as tests of reasoning and choosing actions in artificial situations.

Educational approach we have developed here may sound too theoretical when compared with other approaches to learning (see e.g. Fry et al. 1999). Instead of teaching by explaining, showing examples, imitating or suggesting a hands-on experience, autistic trainees are taught formal entities, and automated reasoning software is used as a means to introduce these entities. As only the definitions of mental attitudes and links between them acquired by an autistic trainee, the further steps of applying the axioms to real-world situations are conducted in a conventional manner.

An educational strategy with a clear focus on mental states may seem as an exaggeration when it is applied to conventional students. However, there is a strong deviation in how people are capable of performing this task. Certain professions, including business and legal specialties, are quite demanding in this respect. Although average students do not require an intensive reasoning therapy concerning mental states as autistic trainees do, they may need some improvement. Building the educational strategy for autistic children where mental attitudes are crucial, the current study sheds a light on how this strategy may be applied to improvement of decision-making and negotiation skills in general higher education.

We have discovered that various kinds of emotions are built up at different speeds for the same trainees. As we learned from our intervention practice, training of each kind of emotion and mental reasoning should be conducted starting from the earlier ages, because for each mental task there is an age when this task becomes adequate to the current trainee's understanding of the mental world. Therefore, the training NL_MAMS-based toolkit is assumed to be suggested starting from the age when a trainee is able to read, till the full (possible) mental recovery in terms of interaction with other people.

In this chapter we evaluated how the learners transfer acquired default rules from artificial to real world situations, which is more feasible task for the target category of children with autism than forming new rules to match the real world environment. Therefore, having an artificial environments teaching children with autism and other mental illnesses how to adopt their actions in specific domains is beneficial. An alternative to this of postponing such training to the mental age when learners can be expected to form new rules in the real world would delay the overall development of learners and therefore seems unacceptable.

Using the literature domain for training to reason about the mental world takes advantages of the variety of plots, appealing and entertaining environment and rather complex mental states of literature characters. We believe such kind of training is essential for business, military, legal, psychological and other professional fields, which require rapid orientation and reaction in emergent situations with inconsistent goals and beliefs of opponents and customers. The system encourages the users (players, students) to demonstrate their knowledge of classical literature, from medieval to modern, asking questions about the mental states of the characters and compare the system results with your own imagination. The system stimulates the trainees to extract the mental entities, which can be formalized, from the totality of features of literature characters. After an answer is obtained, it takes some efforts to verify its relevancy to the question. It takes a little variation in the mental expression to switch from one work of literature to another.

We proceed to the comparison of other computer-assisted intervention technologies with the one based on default reasoning. Multiple technologies have been suggested for mental intervention, including a variety of virtual environments (Sik-Lnyi and Tilinger 2004), and the interactive tool for browsing and recognizing emotional expressions. These computer-based tools assist the development of a wide spectrum of behavioral and cognitive skills. However, this chapter is teaching default reasoning while choosing an action. The goal of this study is to build an intelligent reasoning-based intervention system that is at least capable of reasoning on its own, in contrast to the approaches mentioned above which are the infrastructures for providing access to various media. Dautenhahn and Werry (2004) discuss the potential of using interactive environments with a special focus on autonomous, mobile robots in autism therapy. Being a promising intervention strategy, it might be too expensive to help the majority of families with autistic children even in the Western Europe, US and Japan.

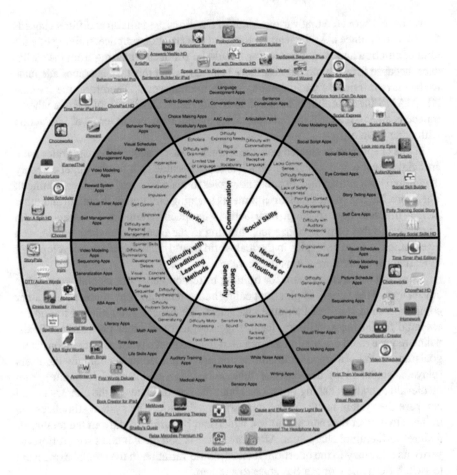

Fig. 8.34 A high-level chart depicting the classes of autistic difficulties, their instances and available training apps

There is a huge number of applications available to assist in autistic development, but none of them targets reasoning directly (Coppin 2012, Fig. 8.34).

The objective of CwA intervention is to make them adaptable. A trainer must accept CwA whoever he is, understand what are the weaknesses and what are the strengths. The trainer should then ground rehabilitation on the features of strength. Improving adaptation mechanisms, a member of intervention personnel should not fight with self-stimulation. Instead, the trainer should attempt to form activity and interaction mechanism with the external world more universal and stronger.

References

Boehner K, Vertesi J, Sengers P, Dourish P (2007) How HCI interprets the probes. In: Proceedings of the SIGCHI conference on human factors in computing systems. ACM Press, New York, pp 1077–1086

Cartwright KB (2006) Fostering flexibility and comprehension in elementary students. Read Teach 59:628–634

Cooley CH (1902) Human nature and the social order. Scribner's, New York. Conference pp. 183–184 for first use of the term "looking glass self".

Coppin M (2012). http://ausm.s3.amazonaws.com/docs/ASDAppWheel.pdf?javer=1303291138). Last downloaded July 15, 2016

Damasio A (2004) Descartes' error: emotion, reason, and the human brain. Avon Books, New York

Dautenhahn K, Werry J (2004) Towards interactive robots in autism therapy: background, motivation and challenges. Pragmat Cogn 12(1):1–35

Frith U (2001) Mind blindness and brain in autism. Neuron 32:969–979

Fry H, Ketteridge S, Marshall S (1999) A handbook for teaching & learning in higher education: enhancing academic practice. Routledge Falmer, London

Galitsky B (2000) Simulating autistic patients as agents with corrupted reasoning about mental states. AAAI FSS-2000 symposium on human simulation, Cape Cod, MA

Galitsky B (2001) Learning the axiomatic reasoning about mental states assists the emotional development of the autistic patients. AAAI FSS-2001 symposium on emotional and intelligent II, Cape Cod, MA

Galitsky B (2002) Extending the BDI model to accelerate the mental development of autistic patients. In: Second International Conference on Development & Learning. Cambridge, MA

Galitsky B (2003) Using mental simulator for emotional rehabilitation of autistic patients. FLAIRS conference 166–171

Galitsky B (2005) On a distance learning rehabilitation of autistic reasoning. In: Encyclopedia of online learning and technologies, vol 4. Idea Publishing Group

Galitsky B, Shpitsberg I (2015) Evaluating assistance to individuals with autism in reasoning about mental world. Artificial intelligence applied to assistive technologies and smart environments: Papers from the 2015 AAAI Workshop

Ganz JB, Flores MM (2009) The effectiveness of direct instruction for teaching language to children with autism spectrum disorders: identifying materials. J Autism Dev Disord 39(1):75–83

Green G (1996) Early behavioral interventions for autism: what does the research tell us? In: Maurice C (ed) Behavioral intervention for young children with autism. Pro-Ed, Austin

Greenspan SI (1997) Developmentally based psychotherapy. International Universities Press? New York

Greenspan SI, Wieder S (1998) The child with special needs: intellectual and emotional growth. Addison Wesley Longman, Reading

Hergott A (2016). http://heshergott.weebly.com/the-zones-of-regulation.html

Howlin P (1998) Children with autism and Asperger syndrome: a guide for practitioners and carers. Wiley, New York

Jain S, Asawa K (2015) EMIA: emotion model for intelligent agent. J Intell Syst 24(4): 449–465, ISSN (Online) 2191-026X, ISSN (Print) 0334-1860, doi:10.1515/jisys-2014-0071, January 2015. http://www.degruyter.com/view/j/jisys.2015.24.issue-4/jisys-2014-0071/jisys-2014-0071.xml?format=INT

Jensen VK, Sinclair LV (2002) Treatment of autism in young children: behavioral intervention and applied behavior analysis. Infants Young Child 14(4):42–52

Lewis M, Haviland-Jones JM, Barrett LF (2010) Handbook of emotions. The Guilford Press, New York

Lovaas OI (1987) Behavioral treatment and normal educational and intellectual functioning in young autistic children. J Clin Consult Psychol 55:3–9

Massumi B (2002) Parables for the virtual. Duke U. Press, Durham

McEachin J, Smith T, Lovaas O (1993) Long-term outcome for children with autism who received early intensive behavioral treatment. Am J Ment Retard 97:359–372

McNamara DS (ed) (2009) Reading comprehension strategies: theories, interventions, and technologies. Erlbaum, Mahwah

Minsky M (2007) The emotion machine: commonsense thinking, artificial intelligence, and the future of the human mind. Simon & Shuster, New York

Oatley K, Johnson-Laird PN (1987) Towards a cognitive theory of emotions. Cognit Emot 1:29–50

Picard RW (1997) Affective computing. MIT Press, Cambridge, MA

Quek FKH (1995) Eyes in the interface. Image and Vision Computing 13, August

Randi J, Tina N, Grigorenko EL (2010) Teaching children with autism to read for meaning: challenges and possibilities. J Autism Dev Disord 40(7):890–902

Rosenschein J, Zlotkin G (1994) Rules of encounter: designing conventions for automated negotiation among computers. MIT Press, Cambridge, MA

Shouse E (2005) Feeling, Emotion, Affect. M/C Journal 8(6). http://journal.media-culture.org.au/0512/03-shouse.php

Sik-Lnyi C, Tilinger A (2004) Multimedia and virtual reality in the rehabilitation of autistic children. ICCHP: 22–28

Swettenham J, Baron-Cohen S, Gomez J-C, Walsh S (1996) What is inside someone's head?Ó. Conceiving of the mind as a camera helps children with autism acquire an alternative to a theory of mindÓ. Cogn Meuropsychiatry 1:73–88

Uras C, Verri A (1995) Hand gesture recognition from edge maps. In: Proceedings of IWAFGR'95, (Zurich), pp 116–121, June 1995

Viterbi AJ (1967) Error bounds for convolutional codes and an asymptotically optimum decoding algorithm. IEEE Trans Inf Theory 13(2):260–269

Werbos PJ (1994) The roots of backpropagation. From ordered derivatives to neural networks and political forecasting. Wiley, New York

Chapter 9
From Reasoning to Behavior in the Real World

This is the final chapter of the book. We now know a lot about how reasoning and cognition works in control children and perfect engineering systems. We have also explored the mechanism of corruption for reasoning and learning, and how it affects the behavior. Based on our findings and hypotheses of this mechanism, we outlined the reasoning rehabilitation strategy. And in this chapter we are making a last stop of this journey: what kind of behavior we can expect as a result of our remediation, and what we have observed in the children who have completed the training presented in the previous chapter.

9.1 Origination of Autism

While the specific causes of autism are not known, an etiological framework, shown in Fig. 9.1, has been traced out that leads from genetic and possibly environmental factors, through neurobiological development and cognitive functioning, and finally to behavioral manifestations (adapted from Minshew and Goldstein 1998).

Some scientists believe that much of the upsurge is the result of increased awareness of ASDs or changes in diagnostic criteria, which would suggest that the true prevalence of the disorders has been stable over time. If the number of cases is truly on the rise, then it would seem likely that some change in the environment is driving up the total. This observation has divided scientists into opposing camps with focus on the relative importance of genetic and environmental factors in the disorders' etiology. A few cases of ASD have been clearly linked to environmental insults. These include prenatal exposure to chemical agents such as thalidomide and valproic acid, as well as to infectious agents such as the rubella and influenza viruses. The correlation here is not 100 %, therefore a genetic predisposition is necessary for chemical and microbial factors to act as triggers.

© Springer International Publishing Switzerland 2016
B. Galitsky, *Computational Autism*, Human–Computer Interaction Series,
DOI 10.1007/978-3-319-39972-0_9

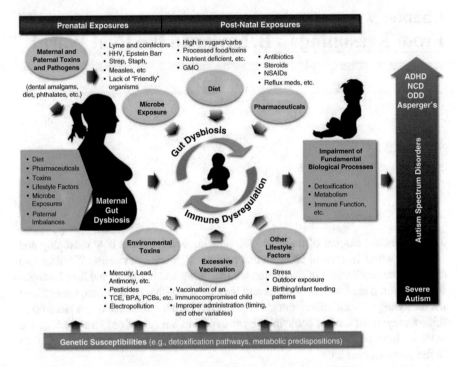

Fig. 9.1 Origination of autism (Adapted from Minshew and Goldstein 1998)

As to the other conditions and syndromes (comorbidities) related to or commonly occurring alongside autism, they are as follows (Fig. 9.2):

- Attention deficit/hyperactive disorder (ADHD) describes children who have overactive behavior (hyperactivity), impulsive behavior, and difficulty in paying attention.
- Epilepsy, a brain disorder involving recurrent seizures. Seizures are sudden changes in behavior due to an excessive electrical activity in the brain.
- Learning Disability (mental retardation) and intellectual disability, which are the permanent conditions, arising during childhood or adolescence, characterized by a state of incomplete development of mind that includes significant impairments of intelligence and social functioning.
- Non-verbal learning disorder (NVLD), which covers people with the social behavior pattern of Asperger syndrome, who also have problems with the non-verbal skills of arithmetic and some visuo-spatial skills.
- Semantic-pragmatic disorder is characterized by good grammatical language but lack of ability to use language in a socially appropriate manner.
- Tourette's syndrome is characterized by multiple tics characteristically involving the face and head (twitches, blinking, nodding) as well as vocal tics.

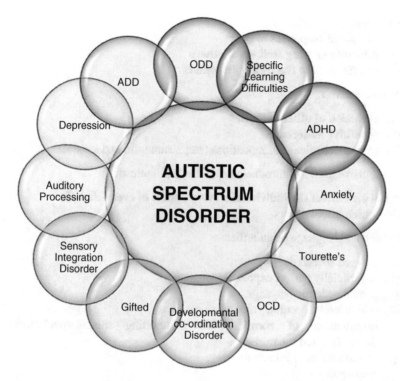

Fig. 9.2 Co-occurrence of ASD and other mental disorders (From WordPress 2015)

9.2 Diagnosing Autism

We enumerate the diagnostic criteria for Asperger syndrome (Gillberg and Gillberg 1989; Szatmari et al. 1989) and highlight the ones which are the target of intervention methods associated with "Computational" issues of autism:

1. Social impairment

    (a) difficulties interacting with peers
    (b) **indifference to peer contacts**
    (c) **difficulties interpreting social cues**
    (d) **socially and emotionally inappropriate behavior**
    (e) **approaches others only to have own needs met**
    (f) extreme egocentricity

2. Social isolation

    (a) no close friends
    (b) **avoids others**
    (c) **no interest in making friends**

(d) a loner

(e) **one-sided responses to peers**

(f) **difficulty sensing feelings of others**

(g) **indifference to the feelings of others**

3. Narrow interest:

(a) **exclusion of other activities**

(b) **repetitive adherence**

(c) more mechanical and repetitious than meaningful and sensible

4. Compulsive need for introducing routines and interests:

(a) **which affect the individual's every aspect of every-day life**

(b) **which affect others**

5. Speech and language peculiarities:

(a) delayed speech development

(b) superficially perfect expressive language

(c) formal pedantic language

(d) odd prosody, peculiar voice characteristics

(e) **impairment of comprehension including misinterpretations of literal/implied meanings**

(f) abnormalities of inflection

(g) over-talkative

(h) **non-communicative**

(i) **lack of cohesion to conversation**

(j) idiosyncratic use of words

(k) repetitive patterns of speech

6. Non-verbal communication problems:

(a) limited use of gestures or large and clumsy gestures

(b) clumsy and gauche body language

(c) limited facial expression

(d) inappropriate facial expression

(e) peculiar, stiff gaze

(f) avoids looking at others

(g) **does not use hands to aid expression**

(h) **impossible to read emotions through facial expression of the child**

7. Motor clumsiness

(a) poor performance in neuro-developmental test

Now we enumerate the characteristics of autistic behavior (highlighting affected by reasoning and cognition):

- Obsessions with objects, ideas or desires.
- Ritualistic or compulsive behavior patterns (sniffing, licking, watching objects fall, flapping arms, spinning, rocking, humming, tapping, sucking, rubbing clothes).
- **Fascination with rotation. autistics can have unusual attachments**
- **Play is often repetitive.**
- Many and varied collections.
- Unusual attachment to objects.
- Quotes movies or video games.
- **Difficulty transferring skills from one area to another.**
- **Perfectionism in certain areas.**
- Frustration is expressed in unusual ways.
- **Feels the need to fix or rearrange things.**
- Transitioning from one activity to another is difficult.
- Difficulty attending to some tasks.
- Gross motor skills are developmentally behind peers (riding a bike, skating, running).
- Fine motor skills are developmentally behind peers (hand writing, tying shoes, scissors).
- Inability to perceive potentially dangerous situations.
- Extreme fear (phobia) for no apparent reason.
- Verbal outbursts.
- Unexpected movements (running out into the street).
- **Difficulty sensing time** (Knowing how long 10 min is or 3 days or a week).
- **Difficulty waiting for their turn** (such as in a line).
- Causes injury to self (biting, banging head).

9.3 Autistic Spectrum

Autism is a developmental disorder characterized by deficits in social interactions and communication (including language) skills, along with limited imagination and a tendency toward a repetitive pattern of behavior (American Psychiatric Association 1994). AS is characterized by these same impairments but without language delay. Researchers have found that individuals with AS demonstrate better imaginative abilities and demonstrate more circumscribed interests than those with high functioning autism (HFA) at the age of 13, but that their early histories show more pronounced differences in language and communication development, with individuals with HFA showing more delays than those with AS (Ozonoff et al. 2000). Individuals with AS and HFA have similar cognitive and behavioral profiles but differ in degree of impairment; those with AS have a better chance of successful rehabilitation than those with HFA. AS is different from autism based on different neurological profiles. AS is at the far end of the ASD continuum, being a "bridge" between autism and typical development (Baron-Cohen et al. 2001).

9.4 Applied Behavior Analysis and Rehabilitation of Reasoning

Obviously, the main target of autistic intervention activity is behavior. There is a number of approach to cure behavior directly, and Applied Behavior Analysis (ABA) is one of them. Behavior analysis focuses on the principles that explain how learning takes place. Positive reinforcement is one such principle. When a positive, productive behavior is followed by some sort of reward, this behavior is more likely to be repeated. Instead of explaining CwA a rule *why* he should behave in a certain way to achieve something, ABA rewards him without explanation, without providing a rationale behind the decision.

Behavior analysts began working with young CwA in the 1960s. Early techniques often involved adults directing most of the instruction. Some allowed the child to take the lead. Since that time, a wide variety of ABA techniques have been developed for building useful skills in learners with autism of various ages. ABA can be used in a formal educational environment such as a classroom as well as in everyday situations at home. ABA therapy sessions involve one-on-one interaction between the behavior analyst and the participant or group instruction. ABA can be complementary to the reasoning rehabilitation technique presented here. In this work we distance ourselves from ABA for verbal CwA since we believe reasoning is a proper foundation of behavior control in humans and not controlling the behavior directly. For non-verbal CwA ABA can be the only available remediation strategy.

Pivotal Response Treatment is derived from ABA and aims at the development of communication, language and positive social behaviors and relief from disruptive self-stimulatory behaviors, and the "pivotal" areas of a child's development. These include motivation, response to multiple cues, self-management and the initiation of social interactions. By targeting these critical areas, this treatment is believed to produce substantial improvements in sociability, communication, behavior and academic skills. A targeted technique meant to improve social engagement among children with autism spectrum disorders, PRT forgoes the focus on specific skills, like block-building, to concentrate instead on so-called "pivotal areas," such as motivation, in hopes of inducing a cascading effect with similar impact across multiple areas.

Voos et al. (2013) used fMRI as the tool for measuring the impact of Pivotal Response Treatment on both lower- and higher-functioning children with autism receiving this treatment for the first time. fMRI allows researchers to see what areas of the brain are active while processing certain stimuli, in this case human motion. Comparing pre- and post-therapy data from the fMRI scans of their 5-year-old subjects, the researchers observed noticeable changes in how the children were processing the stimuli. After 4 months of treatment, CwA starting to use brain regions that typically-developing kids are using to process social stimuli.

If one looks at this approach from the software standpoint, it would look like updating a training set for a faulty machine learning system. But all software engineers understand that the most straightforward way to improve an algorithm is to update its source code, and altering the training set can only take the system so far in its development.

9.5 Dealing with Challenging Behavior

Disordered receptive communication leads to confusion and anxiety when CwA are unable to understand what other people are talking about. When they are unable to understand what is happening around them or what is about to happen, the confusion and anxiety may cause a challenging behavior.

Behavioral problems are easier to be solved when they are formulated as logical and predictable responses to particular situations. Once the meaning behind a behavior is understood, solutions or modifications to the environment can be applied.

Understanding of behavior relied on the knowledge that behavior is a communication means as a logical response to a given situation (Janzen 1996). Challenging behavior is an attempt to regulate encountered conditions that deviate from CwA needs. Behavior is a logical response to the environment where this behavior was first learned. Over time this behavior is generalized to other situations that are not appropriate and the purpose behind original behavior may be abandoned. Also, behavior is an attempt by a person to keep the brain in active mode and in a kind of equilibrium (examples here are self-stimulation and repetitive behavior). Furthermore, behavior is an outward expression of an inward mental state of an individual. Fears and phobias, disease, anxiety and fatigue all have a significant effect on a person's tolerance and control in different situations.

A promising approach in behavioral remediation is Popular Behavior Approach. It emphasizes the observation and most challenging behaviors are learned rather than inherited. It is unacceptable to justify a certain behavior by saying that "a person has always been like that". A challenging behavior is also communicative as it serves as a means to send clear message to others. The cause of problematic behavior is associated with either receptive language difficulties or difficulties with expression. Once communicative skills are improved (through the use of visual strategies), the behavior improvement is expected to follow (Dodd 2003). Positive behavior approach teaches the skills that are required to function in the general community and decrease stress and anxiety level (Fig. 9.3). The approach's focus is developing communicative strategies that are pitched at each CwA level of understanding.

A *multi-element approach* to behavior remediation looks beyond the behavior itself to understand the background of the problem and identify skill deficit. A

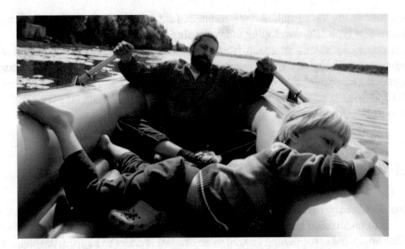

Fig. 9.3 Group exercise in attention focus

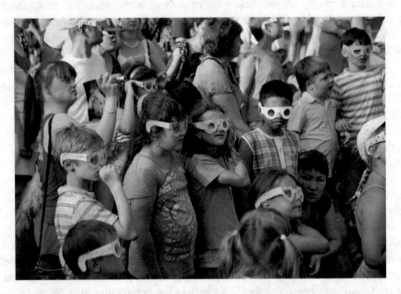

Fig. 9.4 An attempt to put a CwA into a new, interesting, non-stressful environment encouraging exploration

multi-element approach provides an environmental support taking into account the necessary physical, social and program changes to prevent anxiety, develop independence and competence, teaching alternative, more functional ways of communicating needs and wants. This approach provides a positive reinforcement to encourage desired behaviors and established the crisis management plan (Fig. 9.4).

9.6 Rehabilitation Case Studies

We present the case studies of NL_MAMS-assisted treatment of reasoning that has been developed in 1997–2001, evaluated in 1999–2002 and used on a regular basis since 2002. Usually, each child is suggested the developed series of exercises during three half an hour session; success in each exercise is recorded. If some progress is detected in a particular component of mental reasoning, it is subject to further development during consecutive sessions. If the exercises are performed easily, ones with more complex mental states are suggested. In case of a complete failure, the same exercises are planned to be attempted in a few month time, when a trainee gets may acquire some background knowledge and skills that are essential to perform these exercises.

Such strategy fits well into the methodology of rehabilitation center "Our Sunny World" (Moscow, Russia), where the objective is to stimulate all phases of child development process assuming some of them failed in comparison with control children (Fig. 9.3). Not all children are worth applying the totality of developed exercises. Some kinds of exercises like "show a person in a certain mental state" are applicable to non-verbal children with rich internal world; questions about "attributes of an object held by a person with specified mental state" are well-suited for the trainees with least developed world knowledge. We believe, however that all trainees should be encouraged to complete the totality of developed exercises on mental reasoning as a long-term goal. NL_MAMS helps to assure a totality of mental states of given complexity has been covered; frequently intervention of a member of rehabilitation personnel is not required.

We present two case studies for two pairs of children with high-functioning autism (Table 9.1). Their mental and emotion capabilities are believed to have been developed by the suggested approach in addition to the traditional combination of treatments. This pair was chosen from the group of 12 children mentioned in Sect. 8.9 (from 6 to 10 years old, diagnosed with one of the autism syndromes) because the training seemed to better fit their mental age. Alexandra (F) and Leon (M), 10 years old, have attended "Sunny World" on a regular basis, participating in common games with other children, speech therapy, animal-assisted therapy, general training for reading, writing, mathematics and other skills. We track the progress of their mental capabilities from the winter of 2001/2002 to the autumn of 2002 (Table 9.2). One can see that both children have dramatically improved their overall skills of behavior in the mental world. As we can judge given the data for two children, each has his/her own problems that were the direct or implicit targets of the training. However, certain capabilities have been developed insignificantly; they may be weakly affected by the suggested methodology. The reader might notice that a lot of additional training has to be performed so that the mental and emotional development proceeded towards the normal skills for their age (Figs. 9.5 and 9.6).

Table 9.1 The progress of mental development for two trainees

Ability to understand or to perform a mental action or state	Child	Alexandra		Leon	
Testing year		2001	2002	2001	2002
Good will deception		Unable	Deception on a wide spectrum of topics	Deception on limited number of topics	Deception on an arbitrary topic
Pretending		Unable	Pretending concerning a subject, concerning own mental state	Pretending on limited number of topics	Pretending on a wider, but still limited number of topics
Being surprised		On rare occasions	Systematically with proper timing, playing with the teacher	Randomly	Systematically with proper timing, playing with the teacher
Feeling sorry for another person		Non-systematically	Almost always when appropriate	Never	Sometimes, when logically deduced
Feeling happiness for another person		Randomly	Frequently when appropriate	Sometimes, when appropriate and inappropriate	Frequently when appropriate, seldom when inappropriate
Understanding jokes		Unable	Irregular understanding of some kinds of jokes	Randomly	Randomly, but with clear reaction
Cooperating with others when performing a collaborative task		Willing to cooperate without understanding the common goal	Cooperation on different matters with responsiveness and understanding intentions of others	Avoiding any cooperation	Cooperation on demand from the teacher
Analysis of own behavior		Incapable	Can characterize separate fragments of own mental actions without analysis of motivations. Happy to follow intentions of others	Believes that everyone has opposite (and the same) intention and behavior to his own	Can speak about re-adjustment of his behavior to match the intentions of others

Analysis of other's behavior	Easily described physical (but not mental) states of others	Can reveal the sequence of mental states/actions without clear explanation of motivations	Easily describes physical (but not mental) states of others	Can reveal the sequence of mental states/actions without clear explanation of motivations
Understanding of intention of others	Understanding of only own intentions	Can understand others' intentions of limited complexity	Can understand intentions of others, but ignores them	Able to analyze both own and other's intentions
Understanding of knowledge and beliefs of others	Strongly distorted	Can understand knowledge and beliefs of others in practical situations; still confused with own and others' knowledge	Fully understands knowledge and belief of others up to solving the "muddy children" problem Fagin et al. (1996). The mental age with respect to understanding knowing is therefore approaching 20 years old!	
Understanding derived mental states	No recognition of pretending	Understands pretending if it affects her wishes	Understands pretending if it affects her wishes	Understands pretending if it affects his wishes
Good will deception	Unable	Limited deception on a wide spectrum of topics	Deception on a limited number of topics after it was explained for these topics	Deception on an limited but broad range of topics
Pretending	Mostly-unable	Pretending concerning a subject, concerning own mental state	Pretending on some number of topics after being shown them	Still limited number of topics to pretend about
Being surprised	On rare occasions	Systematically with proper timing, playing with the teacher	Randomly	Systematically with proper timing, playing with the teacher
Feeling sorry for another person	Non-systematically	Almost always when appropriate	Never	Sometimes, when logically deduced
Feeling happiness for another person	Randomly	Frequently when appropriate	Sometimes, when appropriate and inappropriate	Frequently when appropriate, seldom when inappropriate

(continued)

Table 9.1 (continued)

Ability to understand or to perform a mental action or state	Child	Michael		Andrew	
Testing year		2012	2013	2012	2013
Understanding jokes		Unable	Understanding of some kinds of jokes on selected relevant topics	Unable	Mostly unable
Cooperating with others when performing a collaborative task		Declined to cooperate	Cooperation performing some tasks; understanding intentions of others in some cases	Avoiding any cooperation	Cooperation on demand from the teacher
Analysis of the behaviour of your own		Believes that all peers have the same intentions, and they all behave the same way as himself	Can characterize separate fragments of own mental actions, but no without analysis of motivations.	Believes that everyone has opposite intention and behavior to his own	Can speak about re-adjustment of his behavior to match the intentions of others. Follows intentions of others
Analysis of the behaviour of others		Rudimentary descriptions of mental states of others	Capable of detection of some sequences of mental states and actions. Although without clear explanation of motivations	Easily describes physical (but not mental) states of others	Can follow a sequence of mental states/actions but lacking explanations of them
Understanding intention of others		Understanding of only own intentions	Can understand others' intentions of order one	Can understand intentions of others, but ignores them	Able to analyze both own and other's intentions
Understanding of knowledge and beliefs of others		Very rudimentary	Can understand intentions of others in practical situations; still confused with own and others' knowledge	Understands knowledge and belief of others well in most cases	
Understanding derived mental states		No recognition of pretending	Understands pretending if correlated with his intentions	Understands pretending if it affects his wishes	

Table 9.2   A sample log for a training session

Name	Key success features	Problems unsolved so far
Eugenia O	Fast understanding of interactions (memorizes information that has been explained and then answers repetitive questions in a much more complete manner)	Lack of understanding for motivations, causal links, mental expressions with complexity above one
Daniel O.	Good understanding of characters participating/not participating in a given activity	Lack of understanding/prediction of an intention of characters participating/not participating in a given activity. Misunderstanding of negations in cases with no direct effect
		Lack of complete explanations of characters' behavior, motivations and causal links
Alexey Y.	Capability of supporting a conversation; understanding the modes of sharing/gaining information	Avoiding mental terms in conversation
Ivan B.	Acquiring the definitions of *cheating/pretending* and *offending/forgiving*	Failure of revealing motivations and predicting scene characters' behavior for scene characters
Victor N.	Partial detecting hide-and-seek scenario from the scene and transferring it to realistic hide-and-seek behavior	Lack of understanding characters participating/not participating in a given activity
Andrew G.	Acquiring the definitions of *cheating/pretending* and *offending/forgiving*	Improper conduct of the dialog, distorted understanding of discourse
	Demonstration of its applicability to real-world situations	

As to the other trainees in this group, each of them improved certain emotional skills and capabilities of reasoning about mental states to a various degree. Ten other trainees of "Sunny World" have participated in the emotional rehabilitation training using NL_MAMS. (Table 9.2 shows only six autistic trainees among them, summer 2003). Observations of a sample training session are outlined, including the strong and weak points for each trainee. Given a definition of a mental entity (for example, via the form with multiple choices for agents and entities, Section 5.6), the trainees are suggested to describe a scene to reveal the learned forms of behavior from the scenes.

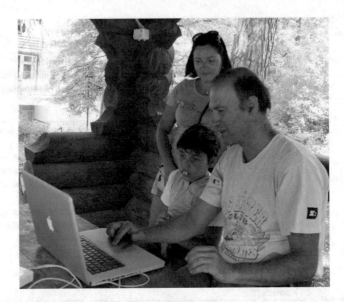

Fig. 9.5 Computer-assisting training involves a parent and a trainer

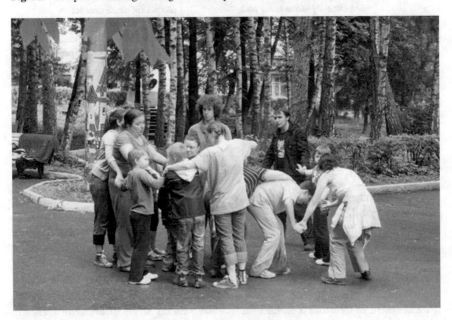

Fig. 9.6 Development of basic communication/interaction skills

9.7 Relying on Hyper-Systematizing Skills

There is a strong evidence for hypersystemizing in autism, which should be relied upon while choosing remediation strategies. PwA have an increased rate of savant skills in systems such as calendars, calculation, or train timetables (Hermelin 2002). Ideally, CwA should form calendars, calculations and timetables for something related to mental states. The PwA score high on tests of attention to detail (O'Riordan et al. 2001) and can achieve high levels in domains such as mathematics, physics, or computer science. Also, they may have an "exact mind" when it comes to art (Myers et al. 2004).

A number of studies confirm our approach to teaching emphasizing via systemizing. According to (Golan et al. 2006), the efforts to teach CwA to mind read succeed only when taking the fairly artificial approach of presenting mental states (such as emotional expressions) as if they are lawful and can be systemized, even if they are not. Such an approach tailors the information to the learning style of the learner so that at least they can begin to process it.

On the picture-sequencing task, CwA perform above average on sequences that contain temporal or physical-causal (i.e., systematic) information (Baron-Cohen et al. 1986). Their obsessions cluster in the domain of systems, such as watching electric fans go round (Baron-Cohen and Wheelwright 1999). Given a set of colored counters, they show extreme "pattern imposition" (Frith 1970)—they hypersystemize. The evidence for systemizing being part of the "broader autism phenotype" includes the finding that fathers—and even grandfathers—of children with ASC are twice as likely to work in the occupation of engineering (a clear example of a systemizing occupation) (Baron-Cohen et al. 1997). Students in the natural sciences (engineering, mathematics, physics) also have a higher number of relatives with autism (Baron-Cohen et al. 1998). Mathematicians have a higher rate of autistic spectrum, and so do their siblings (Baron-Cohen et al. 2007). Both mothers and fathers of children with AS have been found to be strong in systemizing on the Embedded Figures Test (Baron-Cohen and Hammer 1997). Finally, there is some evidence that above average systemizers have more autistic traits. There is the strongest correlation of AS and math skills (Baron-Cohen et al. 2001). These findings suggest a link between systemizing talent and autistic traits, the link being likely to be genetic.

9.8 Estimating Real-World Performance

The critical point of suggested methodology is the estimate of the real-world performance we have approached in Chap. 8. One needs to see how well the trainees can transfer the acquired skills from the class exercise with hypothetical characters to the human agents of real world. We conducted the case study with Andrew G. (age 11, Table 9.2). After training session, when Andrew was suggested the *cheating* exercise, the author encouraged Andrew's participation in the following scenario, when it became clear that Andrew can properly handle *cheat* in the training scenarios.

Passing by the children playing soccer, Andrew was encouraged to bring the attention of a goalkeeper by telling his something loudly right before the goal attempt, when the goalkeeper was expected to focus on the ball. Assumed to be motivated to distract the goalkeeper from catching the ball, Andrew shouted "there is a cat passing by" in the right time. Andrew was capable of analyzing the goalkeeper's actions that were caused by Andrew's cheating attempt: "the goalkeeper looked around trying to locate a cat and missed the ball".

It is quite hard to precisely evaluate the impact of NL_MAMS-assisted rehabilitation of reasoning on the resultant capabilities of the trainees in real world. We outline two following levels at which the resultant trainees' skills are evaluated:

1st level: answering questions and behaving during the evaluation session;
2nd level: interacting with other people in real world.

Accurate estimate of the set of acquired axioms is currently performed by the parents, reporting how their children associate patterns of *cheating* and *pretending*, being *jealous*, *offending* and *forgiving*, etc. As to the 2nd level, we have a rough estimate of 60 % of the entities that have been introduced in a training scenarios have been adequately identified while interacting with other people.

The high-level view of how a remediation strategy should be chosen is shown in Fig. 9.7.

9.9 Assisting in Autistic Cognition

CwA does not believe that learning from experience leads to a good result, because of a long history of failures in solving real world problems. The belief is that everything is permanent, and let it be that way. CwA believe that they never succeeded in anything.

The purpose of training is to make CwA believe that it is not the case and they can successfully learn how to recognize new stuff and apply new cognitive skills in the real life. Training autistic cognition, a caregiver is expected to give a child the feelings that can potentially be used to learn and succeed. We need to demonstrate that with recognized information CwA can do something, apply it to the problems of the real world, and take her to a state she would enjoy (Fig. 9.8).

Stimulation of learning is also done in ABA by making CwA do something good, like acquiring some skills, but it is hard to explain *what is good* within ABA framework. So a teacher gives something tasty once CwA performs a particular good thing, and CwA forms association "good-tasty" which is neither reasoning or cognitive advantageous step but nevertheless a step towards normal behavior. A usual ABA approach is unable to change adaptation mechanism. ABA does not

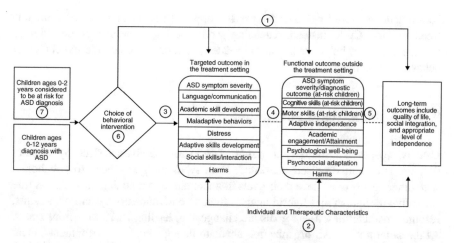

Fig. 9.7 Decision-making chart for chosing remediation strategy

Fig. 9.8 Evaluating the performance in the orienteering exercise

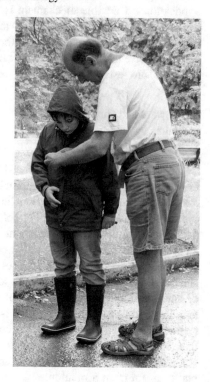

motivate the successful recognition. Instead, it strengthen motivation to receive positive feeling directly, skipping the cognition loop.

Another source of critics for ABA is that every individual has a freedom of choice and ABA limits it. By training certain behavior forms directly, without

building the required reasoning layer to support these behaviors, we limit this
freedom for a CwA. Instead, reasoning should be taught before the behavior so
that the choice of behavior becomes broader and more rational, and the choice of
behavior is voluntary.

9.10   Autistic Team Formation

Usually, agents of a multiagent system (MAS) can be characterized by whether
they are cooperative or self-interested. Both types of agents need to collaborate
with other agents to achieve their goals in uncertain, dynamic domains. This is true
for software, human and hybrid agents. In such environments system constraints,
resource availabilities, agent goals are changeable, leading MAS to various states.
At the same time, MAS organization needs to be adjusted for environments, there
is no single best organization for all possible states. In a broad range of MAS
applications, a flexible mechanism is required to facilitate automated forming of
teams and autonomous adaptation to the environment (Bai and Zhang 2005a). Both
software and human agents develop their team forming skills in the due course, as a
result of active learning with reward (Lopes and Oudeyer 2010).

There are established research areas of team formation in the following
settings:

- software and hardware agents;
- human agents;
- hybrid/mixed teams.

A vast body of literature addressed team formation scenarios in the above cases,
in a broad range of application domains (Bai and Zhang 2005b). These scenarios
are usually complex and very domain-specific, so it is hard to judge how general
the conclusions can be drawn. For software and hardware agents, a lot of technical
details need to be taken into account. In the case of human agents, psychological
analysis makes considerations rather complex and possibly ambiguous.

In this study we focus on the case of *autistic team formation*, which is expected to
shed the light on the fundamental properties of the team formation process. Behavior
of small children with autism is not as complex as that of controls of the same
age. Furthermore, autistic behavior is simpler than that of software agents, since
engineering details do not need to be taken into account. Hence we hypothesize
that a team of small children with autism is a much more "pure" environment for
studying the phenomenon of team formation compared to conventional investigation
platforms for team formation.

9.10.1   How Trust Develops in a Baby

Trust is baby's inner certainty that the mother is going to help when it is needed
(Erikson 1968; Serhan 2011). This certainty is derived from predictability and

consistency of the mother's actions. If mistrust (a model of danger) emerges during the first half year, then the baby is at disadvantage and this is a path to autistic adaptation. Developing trust in first half year is necessary to acquire a control over one's affairs. This is also true when a baby grows into a toddler, is expected to succeed in toilet training, feeding independently, bathing and interacting with known people.

Mistrust in child's surrounding combined with the impression that the world is unpredictable is another feature of autistic adaptation and keeps the child from expanding his world and exploring her opportunities. For a CC, if the mother is inconsistent in her availability and her care for the baby then there is a risk that this baby develops into a mistrusting and will be withdrawn from the world. Success in this stage will lead to the virtue of hope. By developing a sense of trust, the infant can have hope that as new crises arise, there is a real possibility that other people will be there are a source of support. Failing to acquire the virtue of hope will lead to the development of fear.

For example, if the care has been harsh or inconsistent, unpredictable and unreliable, then the infant will develop a sense of mistrust and will not have confidence in the world around them or in their abilities to influence events. This infant will carry the basic sense of mistrust with them to other relationships. It may result in anxiety, heightened insecurities, and an over feeling of mistrust in the world around them.

The repetitiveness and sameness of actions (Sect. 7.3.4), behavior and facial expressions carried out by the mother at the initial step of development eventually create a set of symbols in the baby's mind. This is how baby's trust is developing. These symbols come to represent safety in interaction and having a calming effect. Then when these symbols of familiarity and predictability come up later in toddler life they will be associated with social comfort. Trust development vary in how much time it takes to be accomplished. A mother can recognize if her baby develops trust in her constant presence is through the following. When the mother leaves the room and observes the baby reaction, one of two can be seen:

1. The baby reacts with anxiety, frowning, erratic movements, crying spell.
2. The baby does not react and continues without changing.

The former means that the trust has not been established yet. Once the trust has been established (2) the mother can be more flexible with delegation of caregiving. When the baby acquired, tension in the baby significantly decreases and he will ask for attention less frequently; separation between self and environment proceeds along with baby's feeling of independence.

9.10.2 Assessing Mental Reasoning Capability to Form Teams

We explore how children with autism form teams to perform simple tasks. The focus of our experiment is to find a correlation between how children do reasoning about mental world, and how they perform team formation tasks. The underlying model for our correlation is a belief-desire-intention (BDI, Rao and Georgeff 1995) model for a multiagent system (Chap. 4).

To assess reasoning capabilities of children, we ask them questions about mental states of characters, and evaluate the correctness of their answers (Galitsky et al. 2011). We hypothesize that while team formation, they have to initiate the same or similar questions before they perform speech acts with their proponents and possibly opponents. The questions involve first order mental states (*do you know ... ?, does she want ... ?*), second order (*do you want him to believe ... ?*), third order (*he believes she wanted him to know that she wanted ...*), and fourth-order (*he know she wanted him to know that she does not want ...*).

We used the following team formation tasks. These are the tasks CwA of the age 6–10 usually experience difficulties with, being fairly easy for the CC. These tasks rely on various physical actions, but the commonality between them is the necessity to reason about beliefs and intentions of other team members:

- hide-and-seek game, where children need to agree who is hiding and who is searching (Sect. 8.7);
- "hiding an object in a bag" game;
- making one participant do something with the second participant what the third participant wants;
- form a team of buyers to shop for the items of mutual interested;
- form small soccer, football or basketball teams, two vs two;
- form chess playing team taking turns in moves, two vs two.

Each task required 3–4 participants. Sixteen children of the age 6–10 participated in all team-building tasks and completed all reasoning exercises.

We split CwA into four groups with respect to their capabilities in team formation:

1. Active team builder who can initiate a new team;
2. Active team builder which can maintain the team performing tasks and encourage others to do so;
3. Passive team members who can be maintained to be a part of the team being encouraged by other members. They cannot initiate team formation themselves, but they can resume the team activity after it stopped;
4. Passive team members who can be maintained to be a part of the team. They can neither initiate team formation themselves, nor resume the team activity (Fig. 9.9).

For each child, we assign him to a group if he is capable of performing the required team formation function in more than a half of scenarios. Notice that some team building scenarios require verbal communication, and some rely on non-verbal one.

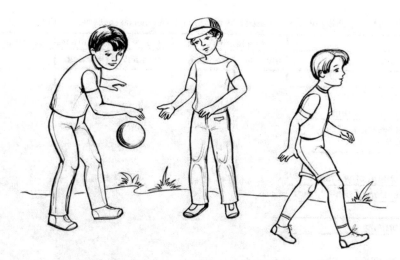

Fig. 9.9 An illustration for basketball team formation

The joint results of the reasoning assessment and team formation assessment are shown in Table 9.3. Rows indicate the percentages of successfully completed reasoning tasks for each group of team formers (averaged through 4 individuals). Rows are grouped from top to bottom according to the order of formulas required to answer the respective question. Dark grey area shows good performance of reasoning tasks (>70 %) and light-grey show lower performance (60–70 %). The white area shows the level of reasoning complexity this group of team formers cannot reliably achieve. Mental states and actions of reasoning exercise are ordered in the way of increasing complexity (averaged performance). Columns are formed according to four groups of children above.

We observe a direct correlation between the reasoning order and team forming capabilities. If children cannot perform even the first-order reasoning tasks, they are neither capable of team forming nor understanding of team forming by others. To be capable of team forming, second-order reasoning needs to be satisfactory.

The third-order mental states are the ones the trainees experience most difficulties with. Various skills at these tasks differentiate children with autism into two groups:

- those who can initiate new teams, and
- those who can maintain team activities and resume team operations.

For the former group, substantial third-order reasoning is required, and for the latter, just rudimentary third-order skills suffice.

Finally, fourth order mental states are difficult for both children with autism and controls of comparable age (see the rightmost column for evaluation of team formation by the control group).

Table 9.3 Capability of team formation vs reasoning about mental states capabilities

Roles	Active team builder		Passive team members		Controls
	Initiate	Maintain	Maintain	Resume	
Knowing an object and its attributes	95	91	82	72	95
Not seeing-> not knowing	90	93	78	80	90
Intention of yourself	88	90	80	76	95
Intention of others	92	87	71	70	95
Informing	87	84	78	73	90
Information request	91	89	72	71	85
Asking to do an action	78	83	80	75	90
Asking to help	85	80	70	75	90
Questioning	81	83	68	70	85
Explaining	72	70	61	64	85
Agreeing	76	73	64	60	90
Pretending	81	76	65	62	90
Deceiving	70	64	62	54	80
Offending	73	68	58	50	85
Forgiving	72	62	61	46	80
Reconciling	65	64	50	39	85
Disagreeing	72	69	42	40	75
Inviting to help	62	59	39	46	70
Asking to leave	64	57	40	51	85
Interfere	70	50	38	32	70
Disagreeing	62	46	32	28	65
Resolving a conflict	42	37	17	12	65
Negotiating	48	24	12	7	60

9.10.3   *Autistic Cooperation in the Real World*

We observed the team formation behavior in the real world as a part of the intervention program conducted by the Center for children with special needs "Our Sunny World" (www.solnechnymir.ru). The children in the summer camp were forming teams with the help of intervention personnel and parents, performing

Fig. 9.10 A team of children at work (Sunny World 2014)

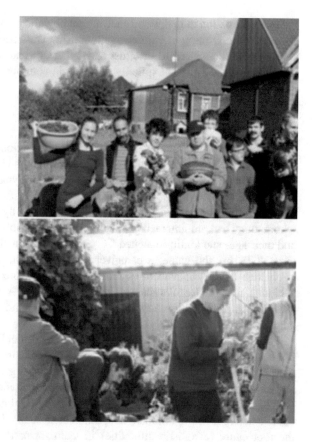

various farming tasks. These tasks include harvesting and packaging vegetables into boxes. Children had to agree on who is doing what, how to store and pass vegetables between each other and in what order, and how to handle varying harvesting conditions (Fig. 9.10). The difficulty level for this task is of the order two and three in most cases.

The children who participated in our evaluation study and successfully formed teams in artificial scenarios were also capable of forming teams for the farming tasks. On the contrary, those who could not adequately participate in our assessment had significant difficulties in performing the tasks requiring interaction with other team members.

It was hard to do a performance assessment in farming teams because of lack of repetition and systematic framework in the farming tasks. Unlike the team formation exercises, which also included conflict scenarios, farming ones involved cooperation only, avoiding any kinds of conflicts. However, the overall impression of the personnel and the parents was that doing abstract team formation helped some children to understand mental states sufficiently to form cooperative teams.

Team formation in real world shed a light how the notion of *trust* is perceived by the reduced reasoning of children with autism. Trust becomes a mental state with certain rules, compared to the trust states that are learned by control human and software agents. Trust is explicitly defined via communicative actions of *promise* and *believe:*

$$trust(Who, Whom) :- \forall Subject promise(Whom, Who, Subject), believe(Who, Subject).$$

and serves as an additional constraint for team formation rule: engage with trusted partners. In this respect the notion of trust is simpler than in general case of adequate reasoners, who need to acquire trust in the course of dynamic process.

Yi et al. (2013) investigated whether children with ASD had an indiscriminate trust bias, believe in any information provided by an unfamiliar adult with whom they had no interactive history. Young school-aged children with ASD and their age- and ability-matched CC participated in a simple hide-and-seek game (Sect. 8.7). In the game, a caregiver with whom the children had no previous interactive history pointed to or left a marker on a box to indicate a location of a hidden reward. Results showed that although CwA did not blindly trust any information provided by the unfamiliar adult, they tend to be more trusting in the adult informant than CC.

For an abstract reasoning system, experiencing difficulties in forming teams does not necessarily mean that deficiencies are in the domain of reasoning about mental world. It could be general incapability to adjust to a given environment (Galitsky and Peterson 2005), general problems in non-monotonic reasoning (Galitsky and Goldberg 2003; Galitsky 2007), autistic planning (Galitsky and Jarrold 2011) and autistic active learning (Galitsky and Shpitsberg 2014). However, it turned out that the root cause of autistic difficulties in team formation are due to reasoning in the mental domain, as demonstrated by its direct correlation with the real world performance.

We explored team formation at the following level:

1. Abstract reasoning in mental world related to team formation
2. Team formation in controlled, assessment tasks

We found a strong correlation between (1) and (2), and a weak qualitative correlation between (2) and (3). We used the computational tool capable of solving similar problems (reasoning about mental states, Galitsky 2013) to what were given to children to simulate the peculiarities of autistic reasoning on one hand and support intervention exercises on the other hand. We used the following hybrid teams of agents: autistic + autistic, autistic + control and autistic + software (educational, assessment).

We found that the main determining feature of autistic team formation is their reasoning capabilities. This observation can be extended to the case of software agents, where behavioral algorithms can be affected by a broad range of circumstances. For software agents, the bottleneck of reasoning about mental states can be less noticeable, but we expect it to be as almost as strong as for the case of autistic reasoning.

Our study has certain implications for how the autonomy features of abstract agents can be modeled via aspects of human behavior. Our finding confirms the theory of social interdependence in its simple form, applied to naïve autistic reasoners: once agents become capable of operating in mental world, they are able to form teams: no special, additional skills are required. Once children form teams, their mental reasoning capabilities improve, but they don't need to learn anything besides mental states and actions to learn forming simple teams. In this respect, our findings back up the traditional individual methodological perspectives (e.g., cognitive architectures).

9.11 Preparing Autistic Children for School

When a parent is getting his child ready to start school, planning ahead is a good idea. And as a general rule, slow and steady works best. There are also some simple strategies that can help make the transition successful. Parents should building familiarity with school, practice it, organize their CwA for school and make transition plans.

Once the parent chosen her child's school, it can be very helpful to slowly introduce the things that she'll need for the school day. This way she can get familiar with them before she starts school. It can also help reduce anxiety about having too much change in one go. You could have your child's new school bag, books, lunch box or clothes lying out in the open so he can get used to seeing it around.

Helping CwA get used to the school itself can be done gradually. A parent could start with just walking or driving past when you're on normal trips to other places. This will help your child see the school as part of her everyday routine. Visiting the school with CwA after hours could be the next step. If possible, the parent should try to do this several times so that her child gets to know the school environment.

The parent could also encourage CwA to train with a school attendance scenario about starting school or a visual storybook with photos of the school. This can help CwA understand what to expect as well as to anticipate what other people will expect him to do. Having a practice at home before CwA starts school can help CwA feel familiar with the new routines and activities. It can also help the parent to spot any potential problems and resolve them before the child actually starts.

Being organized and ready for when your child starts school will ease the stress and help it go well. It's a good idea to make sure the child has everything she needs well in advance. Schools usually give the parent a comprehensive list of what the child will need.

When a parent has decided on a school for her autistic child, whether a specialist school or a mainstream school, she should go in and meet the teachers. Although the teachers will receive medical notes about each child, it is best for both the teacher and the child to meet in person. Usually, prior to the start of term, the teachers arrange transition visits for every child and their family. The teachers need to be able to understand each individual's needs before term starts as every CwA is different, but they can also provide plenty of advice for parents.

The parents should take a camera on their school visit, and take pictures of all the new classrooms, canteen, sports halls and toilets your child may use. With these images the parent can create your own picture book, to help your child become familiar with the environment. Planning is key when it comes to helping CwA to have an easy transition into school life. The parents need to be prepared to face any situations that may arise, even if your child's been fine in the past. Sometimes CwA may just not feel well, but the parents should stay calm and work things through together.

9.12   Preparing Autistic Adults for Work

We share our experience on how to apply reasoning intervention methodology to a child to be included in a regular education process. Also, reasoning and math exercises for teenagers and young adults are included. We discuss vocational training adjusted to the strength and weaknesses of adults with various forms of autism.

One of the key barrier for an AwA to engage in a work activity is *avoidant personality* (Fig. 9.11). A person with *avoidant personality* experiences a long-standing feeling of inadequacy due to the lack of social skills that result from mind-blindness. This influences the AwA to be socially inhibited. Because of these

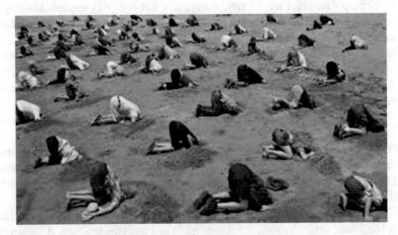

Fig. 9.11 Exaggerated representation of a group of people with avoidant personality (From http://www.emotionalaffair.org 2016)

feelings of inadequacy and inhibition, these individuals will often seek to avoid work, school, or any activities that involve socializing or interacting with others (e.g., many young PwA with avoidant personality are still living with their parents and playing video games rather than working, going to college, getting married, etc.).

The treatment of choice is psychotherapy. While individual therapy is usually the preferred modality, group therapy can be useful if the AwA can agree to attend enough sessions. Because of the basic components of this condition, though, it is often difficult to have the individual attend group therapy early on in the therapeutic process. It is a modality to consider as the AwA approaches termination of individual treatment, if additional therapy seems necessary and beneficial to her. We suggest the following strategies for such adults:

1. Actively seek out and join supportive social environments.
2. Challenge negative, unhelpful thoughts that trigger and fuel social anxiety, replacing them with more balanced views.
3. Challenge social anxiety one step at a time. While it may seem impossible to overcome a feared social situation, you can do it by taking it one small step at a time. The key is to start with a situation that you can handle and gradually work your way up to more challenging situations, building your confidence and coping skills as you move up the "anxiety ladder" (e.g., if socializing with strangers makes you anxious, you might start by accompanying an outgoing friend to a party, and once you're comfortable with that step, you might try introducing yourself to one new person, and so on).
4. Group therapy for social anxiety is a good idea. It uses acting, videotaping and observing, mock interviews, and other exercises to work on situations that make you anxious in the real world. As you practice and prepare for situations you're afraid of, you will become more and more comfortable and confident in your social abilities, and your anxiety will lessen.
5. Know that avoidance leads to more problems. While avoiding social situations may help you feel better in the short term, it prevents you from becoming more comfortable in social situations and learning how to cope. In fact, the more you avoid certain social situations, the easier it is to become even more unsociable. Avoidance may also prevent you from doing things you'd like to do or reaching certain goals.
6. Learn how to control the physical symptoms of anxiety through relaxation techniques and breathing exercises.
7. Take a social skills class or an assertiveness training class. These classes are often offered at local adult education centers or community colleges.
8. Use cognitive-behavioral techniques for social anxiety, including role-playing and social skills training.
9. Volunteer doing something you enjoy, such as walking dogs in a shelter, or stuffing envelopes for a campaign — anything that will give you an activity to focus on while you are also engaging with a small number of like-minded people.

10. Work on your communication skills. Good relationships depend on clear, emotionally-intelligent communication. If you find that you have trouble connecting to others, learning the basic skills of emotional intelligence can help.

A number of skills such as self-regulation, independence, social relationships, and self-advocacy are important for getting and keeping a job. Being able to get and hold a job is an essential result of all the life skills acquired at autism intervention facilities. For someone to be accepted by a company, they must be able to control themselves emotionally and also in their sensory space. Substantial independence is required to perform job responsibilities. Understanding that an employee should speak to his boss differently than he would to a colleague is important to know in most work situations. Self-advocacy skills are necessary in order to request what you need to get the job done.

Life skills in general should be broken down into step-by-step sets and translated into the intermediate training goals and objectives. Obviously, the skill level reached at each of these steps is different depending on the person, but every CwA student is expected to learn a minimum in order to live and work in the community.

Employers usually look for the following characteristics: honesty, integrity, a strong work ethic, analytical skills, computer skills, teamwork, time management, organizational skills, communication skills (oral and written), flexibility, interpersonal skills, motivation and initiative. Most AwA are not the employee who will be caught stealing or cheating. A strong work ethic applies to most of AwA: they the ones who do not like a change in routine and are going to be there rain or shine. They will be very devoted to the workplace (Baron-Cohen and Wheelwright 1999) and will not be calling in sick because of some personal circumstances, or leave early because they have an event to attend.

Analytical skills are really 'obsessive attention to detail,' and many of CwA have that. The child who likes to line up blocks and trains probably has good organizational skills. Teamwork and flexibility are difficult areas for many CwA and a lot of attention should be paid to these skills (Sect. 9.10). Teachers should be teaching flexibility at schools, such as exercises from Chap. 8. The teamwork can be handled by ensuring the AwA has one person on the team that he is in contact with for all needed information.

Recently, technical recruiters started recommending employees with AS as preferred (Romano 2016). They are described as living on open-source forums, having no social skills as their advantage for a company, "generally marry the first girl they date", making no eye contact, having their resume poorly written and education background as a mess. However their main advantage for their employers is that they work like machines, don't engage in politics, don't develop attitudes and never switch jobs.

For some professions, AwA have strong advantages due to their analytical skills and hypersensitivity. Military analytics is one of such professions. Many autistic soldiers who would otherwise be exempt from military service have found a place in a selective intelligence squad in Israel where they can leverage their advanced perceptual skills. For a full day, AwA sits in front of multiple computer screens, scanning high-resolution satellite images for suspicious objects or movements. As a

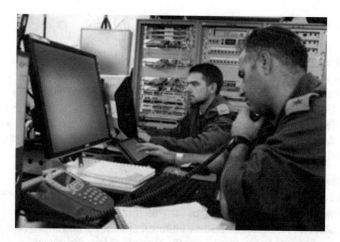

Fig. 9.12 Intelligence unit using soldiers with autism produces stellar results (algemeiner.com 2014)

decoder of complex and heavily civilian battlefield, AwA is critical in preventing the loss of life of soldiers on the ground in several different situations. For CC, looking through each millimeter of the same location from various angles would be tedious work—but AwA describes his job as relaxing and hobby-like (Fig. 9.12).

Israel Defense Force's "Visual Intelligence Division," employs a hundred of Israelis on the autism spectrum among its members. The relationship between this unit and AwA is a mutually beneficial one, being a chance for these young people to have an active, satisfactory lifestyle that might otherwise be closed to them. And for the military, it is an opportunity to take advantage of the unique cognitive capabilities for visual thinking and attention to detail. Both these skills are critical for the highly specialized task of aerial analysis.

There is a socially innovative company "Specialisterne" (Danish as "The Specialists") where many employees have an ASD diagnosis. AwA work as business consultants on tasks such as software development, quality assurance and data-entry. The company takes advantages of the special characteristics and talents of PwA and use them as a competitive advantage, and as a means to help people with autism secure meaningful employment. Specialisterne has operations in numerous locations around the Europe and US.

There is individual who has autism and a cum laude degree from Yale. He got a job as a telemarketer and lasted a day and a half. He is now a research assistant testing computer code. His co-workers are all work study undergraduate students. He comments, "So, rather than just looking at the rumpled suit and diffident eye contact, employers might be well advised to give candidates with autism a second look. After all, what good is it to hire a normal guy who dresses well and gives you a presentation worthy of a drum major if he or she is going to move on in six months? Besides someone like that will probably be making personal phone calls all day, whereas people with autism would seldom or ever do so. If these people are really looking for diligent, loyal employees, they just might find that people with autism fit the bill."

9.13   Cross-Cultural Differences and Autism

Cross-cultural psychology research and ethnographic methods in cognitive anthropology have shed some light on which of these two perspectives, constructivism or nativism, best characterizes our abilities to reason about the minds of others. (Lillard 1998) reviews the evidence for and against differences between the standard European/American commonsense psychological model and that of non-European/American cultures, and argues that meaningful variations can be found in the following areas:

- Not all cultures appear to view the mind as equal to the self, as internal to and distinct from the body, or as an important topic of conversation and attention.
- There are variations in the degree to which other cultures view behavior as a result of mental processes. In some cultures, situational and social factors prevail in driving behavior stronger than in the European/American view.
- Whereas the primary way of affecting the mind in the European/American view is through perception of the world, several cultures hold beliefs that the mind is also affected by ritual acts or by transgressions of people in their past.
- The characterizations of specific mental processes, particularly perception, emotion, and thinking, can vary widely across cultures, and can include the beliefs that hearing applies to non-acoustic phenomenon, that the cause of sadness is an illness, and that thinking about something is only a superficial means of understanding something.

In summarizing the evidenced cultural differences in common-sense psychological theories, Lillard recommends caution: systematic cross-cultural studies of adult theories of the mind have yet to be completed. Moreover, (Lillard 1998) points out that cultural differences should not be seen as proof of cultural relativism in commonsense psychology; underlying the differences seen between cultures is a substantial amount of similarity, with many common beliefs that might be candidates for human universals.

As with many findings of cross-cultural studies, the universality of any psychological trait is likely to be a matter of degree. On one hand, Avis and Harris (1991) demonstrated the universality of the human ability to reason about the beliefs and desires of others in their experiments with children of the Baka, a group of pygmies living in the rain forests of southern Cameroon. On the other hand, (Wu and Keysar 2007) studied people's ability to take the perspective of another in a visual perception task, and demonstrated significant differences between Chinese and American-raised adults attending the same university on the south side of Chicago. While significant differences such as these suggest a role for enculturation in the development of commonsense psychology, the current cross-cultural evidence does not strongly favor either the constructivist or nativist perspective.

People in collectivistic cultures such as India are believed to have interdependent self-perception, and people in individualistic Western European cultures such as the US are believed to have independent selves. To assess the role of culture,

(Wu and Keysar 2007) observed Chinese and American individuals playing a communication game that is a perspective-taking based. The measures of Eye-gaze showed that the interdependent self-perception participants were more tuned into their partner's perspective than were the independent selves participants. Moreover, independent selves often completely failed to take the perspective of their partner, whereas interdependent self-perception almost never did. Cultural patterns of interdependence focus attention on the other, causing Chinese to be better perspective takers than Americans. Although members of both cultures are able to distinguish between their own perspective and that of another persons, cultural patterns give Chinese a chance to effectively use this ability to quickly decode other people's actions and intents.

9.14 Discussion and Conclusions

We observed how the account of autism *reasoning engine → behavior* presented in this book yielded the intervention strategy that helps children with autism to develop skills for everyday life. Reasoning skills are the main target of training to achieve adequate behavior among peers, and the more advanced these skills are, the more complete and satisfactory is the feeling of CwA at school, at a social event and at home.

To tackle the mental world, CwA needs to acquire its axioms and apply them as strict rules. Since living in the mental world is the hardest thing for CwA, the more axioms about it are learned and being followed literally, the better. For the physical world, where CwA is already more comfortable, she is expected to not just follow its rules but to be capable of adjusting them to the context, handling exceptions properly. We conducted the evaluation for how using the training strategy according to *reasoning engine → behavior* account helps in better living in both these worlds.

PwA have preference for systems that change in highly lawful or predictable ways (such as mathematics, repetition, objects that spin, routine, music, machines, collections) and why they become disabled when faced with systems characterized by less lawful change (such as social behavior, conversation, people's emotions, or pure fiction), since these cannot be easily systemized and are not oriented towards discovering "truth" (defined as lawfulness). PwA have a "need for sameness" or "resistance to change" (Kanner 1943) in such "random" contexts as the social world. Although CwA are not native inhabitants of the social world, their hypersystemizing can bring their talent in problem domains that can be represented in a systematic way. The majority of PwA have their hypersystemizing skills focused on a massive collection of facts and observations (lists of schedules and cycles of home appliances) or on massive repetition of behavior of physical systems. However PwA who go beyond a life at home, become data scientists and propose a law or a pattern of the data can substantially contribute to human knowledge.

Autistic genes for increased systemizing have strongly affected human history (Fitzgerald 2002). The "Assortative Mating" theory of (Baron-Cohen 2006) proposes that the cause of ASC is the genetic combination of having two strong systemizers as parents. This theory may help explain why the genes that can cause social disability have also been maintained by natural selection in the gene pool. These genes comprise all the advantages that strong systemizing can bring on the first-degree relatives of PwA.

This Chapter summarizes the results of the proposed intervention strategy. Having read this Chapter, the reader is expected to be fluent with the main concepts related to autistic reasoning and behavior, be prepared to complete a broad spectrum of proposed exercises and also be ready to assess how her child is progressing. A parent should now be prepared to deal with challenging behavior, involve her child into a team work, and have the child ready for school and the adult ready for work.

We want to conclude this Chapter from the standpoint of theoretical foundations of educational approaches. The cognitive domain has been the principal focus for developing educational goals and objectives while the affective and psychomotor domains have received less attention. (Bloom 1956) taxonomy has been used by generations of curriculum planners in both traditional and special needs education areas (Magnusen 2005). Bloom's taxonomy of Educational Objectives identified the following levels of cognitive learning that we apply here to the mental world:

- Knowledge – The remembering of learned mental states and actions; this involves the recall of a basic and derived mental entities
- Comprehension – The ability to grasp the meaning of previously-learned mental entities; this may be demonstrated by translating material from one form to another, interpreting material (explaining or summarizing), or by predicting consequences or effects of communicative actions.
- Application – The ability to use learned material about the mental world in new and concrete situations; this may include the application of rules for individual communicative actions and mental states to concrete situations of interaction between people.
- Analysis – The ability to break down the events in the mental world into its component parts so that its organizational structure may be understood; this may include the identification of the parts of this event of interaction between people, analysis of the relationships between these parts, and recognition of the structural principles on what drives the communication between people.
- Synthesis – The ability to put parts together to form a new whole scenario of interaction between people. This may involve the production of a scenario of an encounter between people, or a plan of operations to resolve a conflict between people, or a set of abstract relations in the mental world.

References

American Psychiatric Association (1994) Diagnostic and statistical manual of mental disorders, 4th edn. American Psychiatric Association, Washington, DC

Avis J, Harris P (1991) Belief-desire reasoning among Baka children: evidence for a universal conception of mind. Child Dev 62:460–467

Bai Q, Zhang M (2005a) Dynamic team forming in self-interested multi-agent systems. AI2005, Sydney, Australia, LNAI Vol 3809, Lect Notes Artif Intell, Springer, Berlin Heidelberg, pp 674–683

Bai Q, Zhang M (2005b) Flexible agent team forming in open environments. In: Proceedings of the fifth international conference on intelligent technology, Phuket, Thailand, pp 402–407

Baron-Cohen S (2006) The hyper-systemizing, assortative mating theory of autism. Prog NeuroPsychopharmacol Biol Psychiatry 30:865–872

Baron-Cohen S, Hammer J (1997) Parents of children with Asperger syndrome: what is the cognitive phenotype? J Cogn Neurosci 9:548–554

Baron-Cohen S, Wheelwright S (1999) Obsessions in children with autism or Asperger syndrome: a content analysis in terms of core domains of cognition. Br J Psychiatry 175:484–490

Baron-Cohen S, Leslie AM, Frith U (1986) Mechanical, behavioural and intentional understanding of picture stories in autistic children. Br J Dev Psychol 4:113–125

Baron-Cohen S, Wheelwright S, Stott C, Bolton P, Goodyer I (1997) Is there a link between engineering and autism? Autism Int J Res Prac 1:153–163

Baron-Cohen S, Bolton P, Wheelwright S, Short L, Mead G, Smith A et al (1998) Does autism occurs more often in families of physicists, engineers, and mathematicians? Autism 2:296–301

Baron-Cohen S, Ring H, Wheelwright S, Bullmore ET, Brammer MJ, Simmons A et al (1999) Social intelligence in the normal and autistic brain: an fMRI study. Eur J Neurosci 11:1891–1898

Baron-Cohen S, Wheelwright S, Skinner R, Martin J, Clubley E (2001) The autism-spectrum quotient (AQ): evidence from Asperger syndrome/high-functioning autism, males and females, scientists and mathematicians. J Autism Dev Disord 31(1):5–17

Baron-Cohen S, Wheelwright S, Burtenshaw A, Hobson E (2007) Mathematical talent is genetically linked to autism. Hum Nat 18(2):125–131

Dodd SM (2003) Understanding autism. Elsevier, Australia

Engelhart MD, Furst EJ, Hill WH, Krathwohl DR (1956) Taxonomy of educational objectives. In: Bloom BS (ed) Handbook I: the cognitive domain. David McKay Co Inc, New York

Erikson EH (1968) Identity: youth and crisis. Norton, New York

Fagin R, Halpern JY, Moses Y, Vardi MY (1996) Reasoning about knowledge. MIT Press, Cambridge, MA/London

Fitzgerald M (2002) Asperger's disorder and mathematicians of genius. J Autism Dev Disord 32:59–60

Frith U (1970) Studies in pattern detection in normal and autistic children: II. Reproduction and production of color sequences. J Exp Child Psychol 10:120–135

Galitsky B (2007) Handling representation changes by autistic reasoning. AAAI fall symposium – technical report FS-07-03, pp 9–16

Galitsky B (2013) A computational simulation tool for training autistic reasoning about mental attitudes. Knowl-Based Syst 50:25–43

Galitsky B, Goldberg S (2003) On the non-classical reasoning of autistic patients. In: International conference on neural and cognitive systems Boston University, MA

Galitsky B, Jarrold W (2011) Discovering patterns of autistic planning. AAAI workshop – technical report WS-11-16, pp 2–9

Galitsky B, Peterson D (2005) On the peculiarities of default reasoning of children with autism FLAIRS-05

Galitsky B, Shpitsberg I (2014) Finding faults in autistic and software active inductive learning. AAAI spring symposium – technical report

Galitsky B, de la Rosa J-L, Kovalerchuk B (2011) Discovering common outcomes of agents' communicative actions in various domains. Knowl-Based Syst 24(2):210–229

Gillberg IC, Gillberg C (1989) Asperger syndromeÑsome epidemiological considerations: a research note. J Child Psychol Psychiatry 30(4):631–638. doi:10.1111/j.1469-7610.1989.tb00275.x

Golan O, Baron-Cohen S, Wheelwright S, Hill JJ (2006) Systemising empathy: teaching adults with Asperger syndrome to recognise complex emotions using interactive multi-media. Dev Psychopathol 18:589–615

Hermelin B (2002) Bright splinters of the mind: a per- sonal story of research with autistic savants. Jessica Kingsley, London

Janzen JE (1996) Assess and plan interventions for severe behavior problems. In: Janzen JE (ed) Understanding the nature of autism: a practical guide. Therapy Skill Builders, Texas

Kanner L (1943) Autistic disturbances of affective contact. Nerv Child 2:217–250

Lillard A (1998) Ethnopsychologies: cultural variations in theories of mind. Psychol Bull 123(1):3

Lopes M, Oudeyer P-Y (2010) Active learning and intrinsically motivated exploration in robots: advances and challenges (guest editorial). IEEE Trans Auton Ment Dev 2(2):65–69

Magnusen C (2005) Teaching children with autism and related spectrum disorders. Jessica Kingsley publishing, London/Philadelphia

Minshew NJ, Goldstein G (1998) Autism as a disorder of complex information processing. Ment Retard Dev Disabil Res Rev 4:129–136

Myers P, Baron-Cohen S, Wheelwright S (2004) An exact mind. Jessica Kingsley, London

O'Riordan M, Plaisted K, Driver J, BaronCohen S (2001) Superior visual search in autism. J Exp Psychol Hum Percept Perform 27:719–730

Ozonoff S, South M, Miller J (2000) DSM-IV defined Asperger syndrome: cognitive, behavioral, and early history differentiation from high-functioning autism. Autism 4:29–46

Rao M, Georgeff P (1995). BDI-agents: from theory to practice. In: Proceedings of the first International Conference on Multiagent Systems (ICMAS' 1995)

Romano A (2016) Everything wrong with Silicon Valley culture in one gross presentation. http://www.vox.com/2016/4/19/11451092/alex-st-john-tech-recruiting-millennials-women

Serhan R (2011) Psyche-smart autism ePub

Sunny World (2014) http://solnechnymir.ru/. Last downloaded June 23, 2014

Szatmari P, Bremner R, Nagy J (1989) Asperger's syndrome: a review of clinical features. Can J Psychiatry 34(6):554–560

Voos Avery C, Pelphrey KA, Tirrell J, Bolling DZ, Wyk BV, Kaiser MD, McPartland JC, Volkmar FR, Ventola P (2013) Neural mechanisms of improvements in social motivation after pivotal response treatment: two case studies. J Autism Dev Disord 43(1):1–10

WordPress (2015) https://the7flowers.wordpress.com/tag/mood-disorder/2015

Wu S, Keysar B (2007) Cultural effects on perspective taking. Psychol Sci 18:600–606

Yi L, Pan J, Fan Y, Zou X, Wang X, Lee K (2013) Children with autism spectrum disorder are more trusting than typically developing children. J Exp Child Psychol 116:755–761

Chapter 10
Conclusions

It has been discovered two decade ago that autistic people cannot properly understand and reproduce mental states and emotions. The proposed account of autism, *reasoning engine → behavior*, is based on the observation that people with autism suffer from difficulties in learning social rules from examples but nevertheless can memorize and apply rules independently. Many remediation strategies have not taken this into account. Therefore an appropriate intervention strategy is to teach not simply via examples but to teach the rule along with it. In this book we suggested a reasoning intervention strategy, based in particular on playing with a computer based mental simulator that is capable of modeling mental and emotional states of the real world. A model of the mental world has been presented in twenty-three steps. We described our implementation of the natural language multiagent system NL_MAMS that implements this model. In addition, we described the system's user interface for autistic intervention. This system was subject to short-term and long-term evaluation of rehabilitation of autistic reasoning. Case studies with children who used it extensively are presented. Implications specifically in terms of autistic rehabilitation as well as generally in terms of reasoning about mental states are discussed.

The main contribution of this book is the model of reasoning about mental world and the simulation means for children with autism to learn this model. The following steps were accomplished in the path from the former to the latter:

1. The theory of mind is subject to a formal treatment from the standpoint of logical artificial intelligence;
2. The possibilities of the theory of mind teaching are re-evaluated, taking into account the developed formal framework for reasoning about the mental world;
3. Appropriateness of formal reasoning as an educational means and associated cognitive issues are assessed;
4. The model of mental world is constructed to serve as a basis for education means;

© Springer International Publishing Switzerland 2016
B. Galitsky, *Computational Autism*, Human–Computer Interaction Series,
DOI 10.1007/978-3-319-39972-0_10

5. The simulation-based hybrid algorithm of deriving consecutive mental states and its software implementation is designed and evaluated;
6. Theory of mind teaching using this software is evaluated on a short-term and long-term basis;
7. Implications for the practical intervention strategies are analyzed;

Results of short-term and long-terms rehabilitation of autistic reasoning have been presented, and we demonstrated the benefits of using the tool in autism intervention centers. We showed that children with NL_MAMS-based training perform better than those without theory of mind training, both in testing environment and interacting with other children in real world. Hence we recommend using the developed tool, NL_MAMS, in autism rehabilitation facilities in various languages across the world, having tested it in "Our Sunny World" center and other organizations. A number of intervention tools and exercises are available at relevance-based-on-parse-trees.googlecode.com/files/autistic_rehabilitation.zip.

A computational approach to studying the phenomena of autism has been introduced. We critiqued modern accounts of autism, proposed a computationally-centered one and explained how a reasoning-based account can assist in understanding the nature of autism as well as in curing it. We also explained how autistic reasoning due to its purity can help computer scientists evaluate their reasoning models. It has been demonstrated that knowledge in a formalized form is more suitable to reproduce the peculiarities of autistic reasoning on one hand and to directly teach reasoning and domain-specific rules to children with autism on the other hand. We outlined the common features of teaching autistic children and computers various forms of reasoning and machine learning. We also discussed how our experience accumulated while teaching children with autism in the above domains can be applied to the design of intelligent software systems.

We showed that CwA are not alone in their problems with reasoning. The real world multiagent systems such as groups of people performing the common goals, partnerships and corporations, as well as engineering AI systems, frequently experience similar difficulties to CwA. In this book we attempted to find a common cure for human and engineering reasoning systems to overcome these difficulties, and demonstrated the remediation results for the former case. Additional material is available at http://extras.springer.com.

Printed in the United States
By Bookmasters